Effects of A-Bomb Radiation
on the Human Body

Effects of A-Bomb Radiation on the Human Body

edited by

Hiroshima International Council for Medical Care of the Radiation-Exposed

Itsuzo Shigematsu
Radiation Effects Research Foundation
Hiroshima

Chikako Ito
Hiroshima Atomic Bomb Casualty Council
Hiroshima

Nanao Kamada
Hiroshima University
Hiroshima

Mitoshi Akiyama
Radiation Effects Research Foundation
Hiroshima

and

Hideo Sasaki
Radiation Effects Research Foundation
Hiroshima

translated by

Brian Harrison
Chuo University
Tokyo

harwood academic publishers
Australia • Austria • Belguim • China • France • Germany • India •
Japan • Malaysia • Netherlands • Russia • Singapore • Switzerland •
Thailand • United Kingdom • United States

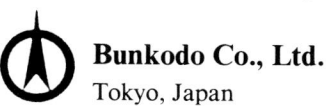

Bunkodo Co., Ltd.
Tokyo, Japan

Harwood Academic Publishers
Poststrasse 22
7000 Chur, Switzerland

Edited by

Hiroshima International Council for Medical Care of the Radiation-exposed
c/o Atomic Bomb Victim's Affairs Department
Health and Environmental Affairs Department
Hiroshima Prefectural Government
10-25 Motomachi, Naka-ku, Hiroshima-shi 730 Japan

British Library Cataloging in Publication Data

Effects of A-Bomb Radiation on the Human Body
  I. Shigematsu, Itsuzo II. Harrison, Brian
  616.9897

ISBN 3-7186-5418-0

CONTENTS

FOREWORD

Ever since the unprecedented human toll wrought by the atomic bombs, research has continued into the health effects on the survivors of Hiroshima and Nagasaki. The first and foremost objective of the studies on late atomic bomb effects was to obtain knowledge that could be applied to the care and medical treatment of atomic bomb survivors. However, it is also clear that the knowledge relating to the effects of radiation on the human body has benefited the entire human race.

For example, the International Commission for Radiation Protection (ICRP), the most authoritative organization in the field of radiation protection, has long placed great emphasis on data obtained from Hiroshima and Nagasaki when establishing dose limits (i.e. the standards for the maximum exposures deemed acceptable for both ordinary people and the occupationally exposed).

Recent years have witnessed people being exposed to radiation in various parts of the world, e.g. those exposed in the nuclear accident at Chernobyl. In order to help with the medical care of such people, Hiroshima and Nagasaki have been asked to publish and disseminate the information and knowledge which they have accumulated. The International Council for the Medical Care of the Radiation-exposed was established to facilitate this. Functions performed include both educational activities such as the acceptance of medical personnel from abroad for training, the dispatch of specialists overseas and the presentation of lectures, as well as the compilation of documents relating to the medical care of the atomic bomb survivors.

Genbaku Hoshasen no Jintai Eikyou (Effects of A-Bomb Radiation on the Human Body) is one such document. Based on the data obtained to date, and focusing particularly on the health effects on the human body, it is an attempt to explain radiation effects with respect to different diseases in a manner that is easy to comprehend. The authors are mainly people in Hiroshima who are at the forefront of medical care, health management and research concerning the atomic bomb survivors. Consequently, the book can be considered a reference manual incorporating the latest and most relevant information for the medical care of atomic bomb survivors.

We hope that this book will foster widespread understanding of the health effects of atomic bomb radiation and will prove useful in the medical care of radiation-exposed people throughout the world.

Itsuzo Shigematsu
President
International Council for the Medical Care of the Radiation-exposed

FOREWORD TO THE ENGLISH EDITION

The detonation of the atomic bombs in 1945 devastated the cities of Hiroshima and Nagasaki, with great loss of life. Approximately half a century has passed since then, and from their ashes new and modern cities have arisen, with the disappearance of virtually all the remains symbolizing that tragic time.

Nagasaki was the last city to suffer an atomic bombing. But in recent years fresh damage due to radiation exposure has become evident in various parts of the world as the result of nuclear testing and accidents at nuclear power plants, etc.

In order to help the victims of such events, the Hiroshima prefectural and municipal governments, with the co-operation of various local organizations, established the International Council for the Medical Care of the Radiation-exposed in April 1991. During a discussion at the predecessor of this organization (a committee founded in November 1990), the need was expressed for publication of a book detailing the medical care of radiation-exposed individuals. A compilation of data pertaining to the medical effects of atomic bomb radiation on the human body was published in 1979 and covered knowledge acquired until approximately 1976. Since then, however, rapid advances have been made in studies on the late effects of atomic bomb radiation, which have been presented in individual research papers but not brought together in a single volume. It was felt that all current knowledge should be summarized in one book, which could then be employed as a text for medical personnel coming to Hiroshima from overseas to undergo training. This book has been compiled to meet that objective.

The authors are involved with the treatment of atomic bomb survivors in Hiroshima and are active at the forefront of research and medical care concerning people who have been exposed to radiation. Despite the severe restrictions imposed by tight scheduling, and the need to write within limited space in such a manner that both specialist and non-specialist would understand, while presenting the material in standardized format, the authors readily incorporated suggestions from the editors and enabled the project to be completed on schedule; the editors are extremely grateful to the authors for their co-operation and effort.

It is difficult to convey the considerable and unremitting efforts of the 39 authors and their colleagues who have made this first English edition possible. Through their dedicated and unselfish contributions it will be possible to publish updated editions more easily in the future and thus increase our understanding of atomic radiation, which is vital for the future of humanity.

Chikako Ito
Deputy Director
Hiroshima Atomic Bomb Casualty Council
Health Management Center

LIST OF CONTRIBUTORS

AKIBA, Suminori
Kagoshima University School of
Medicine

AKIYAMA, Mitoshi
Radiation Effects Research Foundation

AWA, Akio
Radiation Effects Research Foundation

CHOSHI, Kanji
Hiroshima University School of
Medicine

DOHI, Kiyohiko
Hiroshima University School of
Medicine

DOHY, Hiroo
Hiroshima Red Cross Hospital and
Atomic Bomb Survivors Hospital

EZAKI, Haruo
Tsuchiya General Hospital

FUJIMURA, Kingo
Research Institute for Nuclear Medicine
and Biology
Hiroshima University

FUJITA, Shoichiro
Radiation Effects Research Foundation

FUJIWARA, Saeko
Radiation Effects Research Foundation

HASAI, Hiromi
Hiroshima University School of
Engineering

HAYAKAWA, Norihiko
Research Institute for Nuclear Medicine
and Biology
Hiroshima University

HOSHI, Masaharu
Research Institute for
Nuclear Medicine and Biology
Hiroshima University

ITO, Chikako
Hiroshima Atomic Bomb Casualty
Council

KAMADA, Nanao
Research Institute for Nuclear Medicine
and Biology
Hiroshima University

KATO, Hiroo
The National Institute for Minamata
Disease

KODAMA, Kazunori
Radiation Effects Research Foundation

KUSUMI, Shizuyo
Radiation Effects Research Foundation

KUSUNOKI, Youichiro
Radiation Effects Research Foundation

MABUCHI, Kiyohiko
Radiation Effects Research Foundation

NAKAMURA, Nori
Radiation Effects Research Foundation

NOMA, Kouji
National Kure Hospital

OGAWA, Junichiro
Hiroshima Atomic Bomb Casualty
Council

OGUMA, Nobuo
Research Institute for Nuclear Medicine
and Biology
Hiroshima University

OKUSAKI, Ken
Hiroshima University School of
Medicine

OTAKE, Masanori
Radiation Effects Research Foundation

SASAKI, Hideo
Hiroshima Atomic Bomb Casualty
Council

SASAKI, Hideo
National Kure Hospital

SATOW, Yukio
Research Institute for Nuclear Medicine
and Biology
Hiroshima University

SATOH, Chiyoko
Radiation Effects Research Foundation

SHIGEMATSU, Itsuzo
Radiation Effects Research Foundation

SHIMIZU, Yukiko
Radiation Effects Research Foundation

SHIZUMA, Kiyoshi
Hiroshima University School of
Engineering

TAKEICHI, Nobuo
Hiroshima University School of
Medicine

TATSUMI-MIYAJIMA, Junko
Kyoto University School of
Medicine

TOKUNAGA, Masayoshi
Kagoshima City Hospital

YAMADA, Michiko
Radiation Effects Research
Foundation

YAMAKIDO, Michio
Hiroshima University School of
Medicine

YOSHIMOTO, Yasuhiko
Radiation Effects Research
Foundation

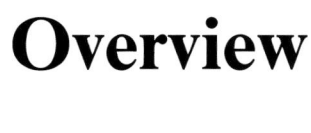

Overview

OVERVIEW

INTRODUCTION

Atomic bombs were dropped on Hiroshima and Nagasaki in August 1945. Within a few months the bomb blast, heat and radiation emitted by the atomic explosions had led to approximately 114,000 fatalities in Hiroshima and about 70,000 deaths in Nagasaki. The radiation in particular continued to exert an effect on the human body over a long period of time, resulting in the development of tumors and functional abnormalities in various organs. This overview will briefly touch on the physical destruction wrought at the time of the explosion, and then outline the acute and late damage inflicted on the human body.

1. PHYSICAL DESTRUCTION CAUSED BY THE ATOMIC BOMB[1]

The Hiroshima bomb was detonated at 8.15 am on August 6th 1945 at a height of 580 meters above the Shima Hospital, near the A-bomb dome (the site of the former Hiroshima Prefectural Industrial Promotion Hall).

The Hiroshima atomic bomb, known as "Little Boy," employed ^{235}U (uranium-235) and packed the equivalent of 15 kilotons of TNT. The atomic bomb differed from conventional explosions in that besides the bomb blast it was accompanied by intense heat and radiation, with the dissipation of energy believed to have been in the ratio of bomb blast (50%), heat (35%), and radiation (15%) (Fig. 1).

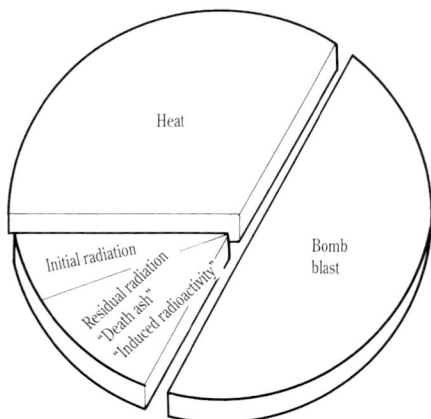

Figure 1   Distribution of energy released by the atomic bomb

A. Bomb Blast

The explosion created an extremely high pressure at the point of detonation equal to several hundred thousand atmospheres; the surrounding air expanded greatly to form the bomb blast, which is believed to have attained a velocity of 280 m/sec around the hypocenter and a velocity of 28 m/sec at a point 3.2 km away. The leading edge of the bomb blast advanced as a shock wave, which had traveled a distance of approximately 3.7 km after about 10 seconds, and covered a distance of about 11 km after 30 seconds. The shock wave spread outwards; at the instant that the wind had abated, a weaker blast blew inwards from the outside (due to the reduced pressure at the hypocenter) and participated in the formation of a mushroom cloud.

B. Heat

A fireball was created in mid-air at the same time as the explosion. At the instant of detonation the temperature reached a maximum of approximately one million degrees Centigrade, with the temperature on the surface of the fireball registering approximately 7,000°C after 0.3 seconds; the heat content was calculated to be 99.6 cal/cm^2 in the vicinity of the ground below the point of detonation, and 1.8 cal/cm^2 at a point 3.5 km away. Within 3 seconds of the explosion, 99% of the thermal radiation emitted by the fireball had affected the surface of the ground. The heat caused the scorching of wood etc. for a distance of approximately 3 km from the hypocenter, and for a distance of 3.5 km caused the burning of any human flesh that was not covered with clothing. The burns resulting from exposure to the thermal radiation proved fatal to any unprotected people within about 1.2 km of the blast; estimates attributed 20–30% of the total deaths to these burns. Figure 2 shows those areas within the vicinity of the hypocenter of the Hiroshima bomb which were completely gutted as a result of the thermal radiation (indicated by solid squares) and also the areas in which buildings were destroyed by the bomb blast (indicated by diagonal lines)[2].

C. Radiation

It is possible to classify the radiation released by the mid-air atomic explosion into two categories: the initial radiation, which was emitted from mid-air within one minute of the explosion and which accounted for approximately 5% of the total energy, and the residual radiation, which was released later at ground level over a long period of time and which accounted for approximately 10% of the total energy.

i) *Initial Radiation*

The initial radiation was composed primarily of gamma rays and neutrons. Several estimates have in the past been advanced for the initial dose of radiation. The tentative T65D dose estimates (established in 1965) were revised in July 1987 by the US-Japan Committee for Reassessment of Atomic Bomb Radiation Dosimetry in Hiroshima and Nagasaki, and the new DS86 dosimetry system was adopted[1] (Table 1).

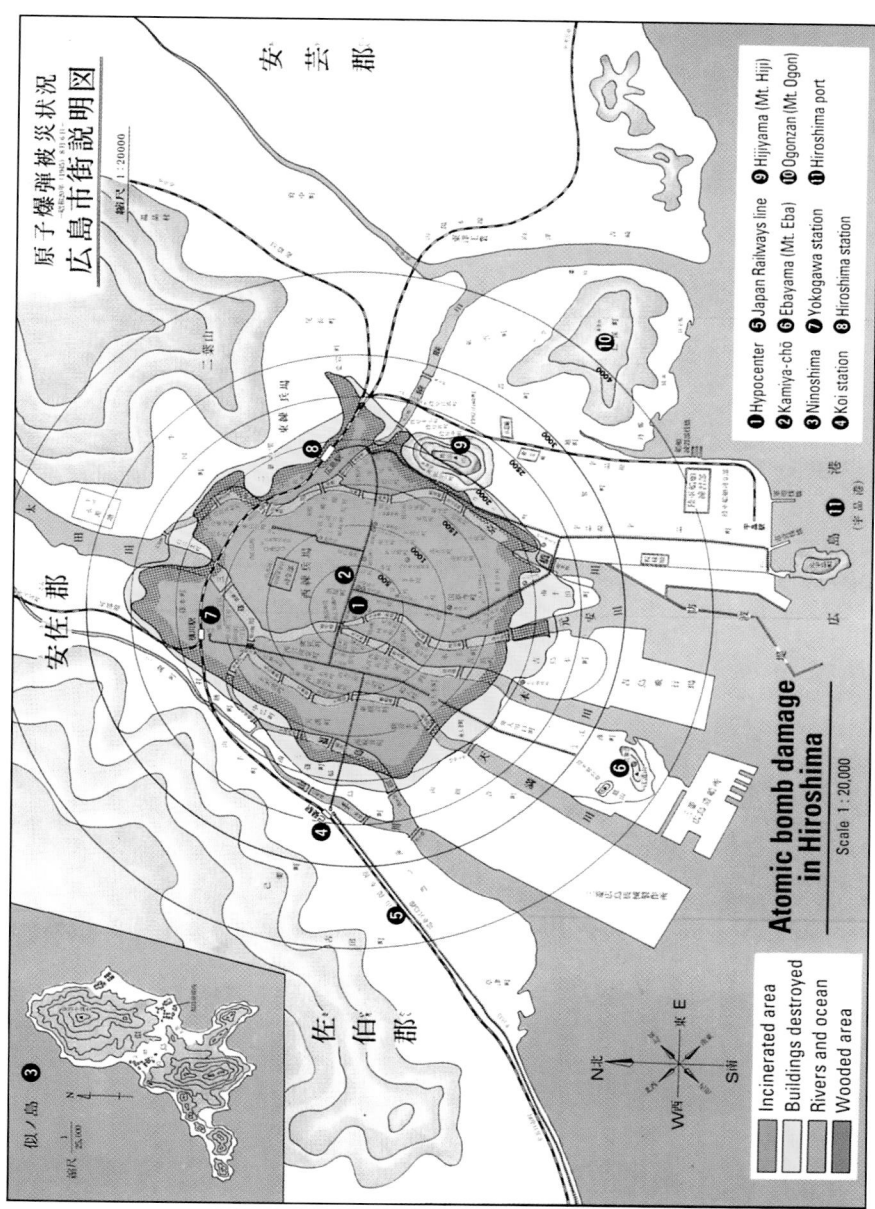

Figure 2 Atomic bomb damage in Hiroshima[2]

Table 1   Initial radiation doses (DS86)[1]

Distance from epicenter (m)		Distance from hypocenter (m)	Gamma-ray dose (Gy)	Neutron dose (Gy)
0	Hiroshima	580	—	—
	Nagasaki	503	—	—
500	Hiroshima	766	35.0	6.04
	Nagasaki	709	78.5	3.31
1,000	Hiroshima	1,156	3.93	0.227
	Nagasaki	1,119	7.83	0.143
1,500	Hiroshima	1,608	0.487	0.008
	Nagaski	1,582	0.893	0.006
2,000	Hiroshima	2,082	0.071	0.0
	Nagasaki	2,062	0.127	0.0
2,500	Hiroshima	2,566	0.012	0.0
	Nagasaki	2,550	0.021	0.0

N. B. Since the above values are the mid-air doses, they can be deemed appropriate as values of the radiation dose absorbed by surface human skin in unshielded victims. For the effect on internal parts such as the bone marrow, it is necessary to convert the dose measured in grays into sieverts because of weakening of the dose by any shielding. Consequently, the simple addition of gamma-ray and neutron doses in the table is not strictly correct, but is perhaps acceptable in the first stage of the debate. Studies are still in progress with respect to distances greater than 2,000 m from the hypocenter.

ii) *Residual Radiation*

The residual radiation is classified into two types. First, the products of nuclear fission and the uranium 235 that had not undergone nuclear fission dispersed in mid-air; after one minute of the explosion these had been converted into a radiation source consisting of gamma rays, beta rays and alpha rays, which were termed "death ash." Second, the initial radiation that bombarded the ground (neutrons) collided with the nuclei of atoms in the ground and in building materials and provoked nuclear reactions which led to induced radioactivity. It is extremely difficult to find a general expression to describe the extent of injury suffered as a result of residual radiation since this was governed by the circumstances surrounding each individual's activities, but it is possible to summarize the general trends in the following way.

It has been estimated that those people who entered the hypocenter area on the day following the blast and who worked there for 10 to 20 hours a day for one week were exposed to approximately 0.10 Grays (Gy) of induced radioactive gamma rays. For anybody present at the hypocenter from immediately after detonation of the bomb, the maximum received dose is estimated at approximately 0.80 Gy in Hiroshima, and approximately 0.30–0.40 Gy in Nagasaki. However, fires raged at the hypocenter for over 6 hours, probably making it impossible to enter the area immediately after the explosion.

Immediately following detonation of the bomb, the so-called "black rain" fell from the northern to western districts of Hiroshima, and in the eastern parts of Nagasaki, thus spreading the residual radioactivity to distant places. In particular, it is believed that external irradiation with gamma rays occurred due to radioactivity produced as a result of nuclear fission. However, the maximum level of this residual radioactivity is believed to have been only 0.01–0.03 Gy in Hiroshima and 0.20–0.40 Gy in Nagasaki. The effect of the residual radioactivity was different from that of direct exposure to the bomb, and was characterized by long-term exposure to low doses of radiation.

Besides the effects of external gamma ray radiation described above, there is also the question of the radioactivity which was absorbed into the body, causing direct irradiation of various internal organs. In this case beta rays and alpha rays acted in addition to the gamma rays. The people who absorbed large quantities of dust when they entered the city in later days in order to dispose of the corpses and deal with the debris from the buildings, and particularly those people who were exposed to the great cloud of dust that was present immediately after the explosion, may have been exposed to a level of radioactivity greater than the maximum permitted dose recommended by the International Commission on Radiological Protection for workers facing occupational exposure to radiation.

Figure 3 shows the physical effects resulting from the detonation of the atomic bomb in Hiroshima. Figure 3a shows the situations pertaining to the thermal radiation immediately after the explosion, the fireball and bomb blast, and the initial radioactivity[3–5]. Figure 3b shows the altitude and state of the cloud at 1 minute, 2–3 minutes, and 20–30 minutes after the explosion.

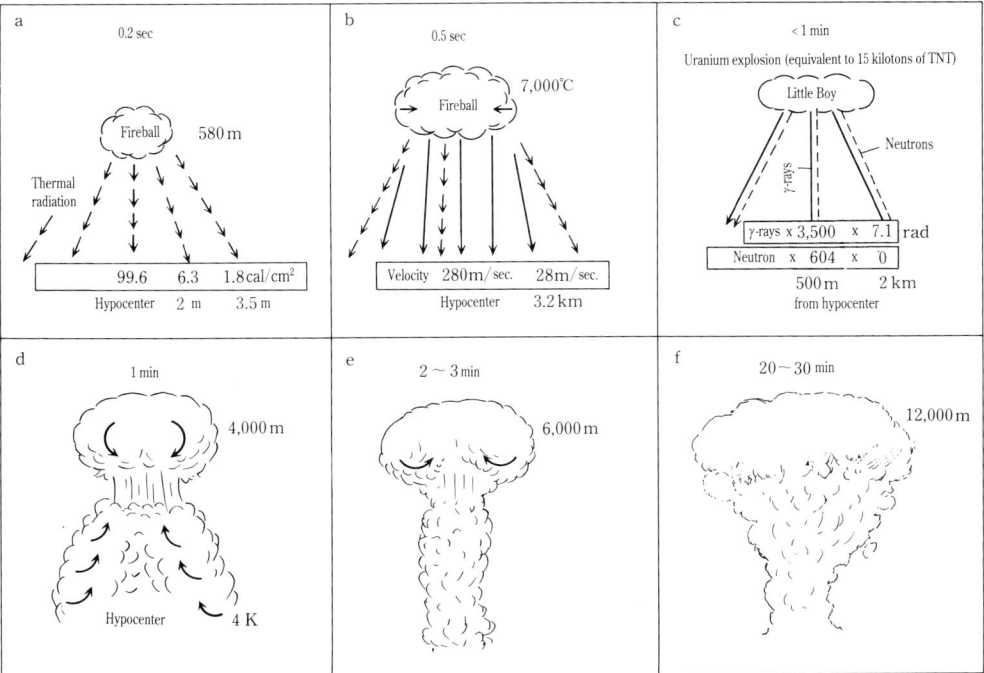

Figure 3 Physical effects of the Hiroshima atomic bomb[3–5]

2. EFFECTS ON THE HUMAN BODY

A. Number of Fatalities (by December 1945)

In a book entitled "Hiroshima Genbaku Sensaishi" (Record of the Hiroshima A-bomb War Disaster)[6] (published in 1971) the Information Department of Hiroshima City Office presented the number of casualties in Hiroshima based on the documents already collected by around 1947 (Table 2). This refers to the number of dead and injured on August 10th 1946, but since the number of fatalities occurring between January and August 1946 is estimated as approximately 3,915, the number of casualties up until December 1945 (the so-called short-term casualties) amounted to approximately 114,000. The figures in Table 2 do not include the 20,000 killed, who were among approximately 40,000 military personnel or Koreans working in Hiroshima. In either case the records are scarce, and the actual situation is extremely unclear.

Various figures have so far been put forward regarding the number of deaths caused by the atomic bomb[7-9], but there is good agreement between the number given by the early official survey of atomic bomb victims (Table 2) and the estimated numbers determined by other methods, and thus it would seem that this figure is reliable.

LD_{50}: When humans are exposed to radiation, those doses which lead to the deaths of 50% of the people within either less than 30 days or less than 60 days are respectively referred to as the $LD_{50/30}$ and $LD_{50/60}$ doses. A contoured map indicating the average mortality rates was constructed from data obtained in a survey of 6,000 households in December 1945 (Fig. 4)[10]. The general trends were for the contours representing equal mortality rates to be slightly distended towards the south and south south-west, but for the arc to be slightly drawn in towards the east and south-east. Based on this curve, it is believed that the point at which a 50% mortality rate occurred lies at a distance of 1 km in an easterly direction and at a distance of around 1.5 km in a southerly direction. The data obtained from the Atomic Bomb

Table 2   Relationship between number of casualties and distance from the hypocenter in Hiroshima (Aug. 10th 1946, excluding military personnel)[6]

Distance from hypocenter (km)	Deaths	Seriously injured	Slightly injured	Missing	Uninjured	Total
< 0.5	19,329	478	338	593	924	21,662
0.5 ~ 2.0	42,271	3,046	1,919	1,366	4,434	53,036
1.0 ~ 1.5	37,689	7,732	9,522	1,188	9,140	65,271
1.5 ~ 2.0	13,422	7,627	11,516	227	11,698	44,490
2.0 ~ 2.5	4,513	7,830	14,149	98	26,096	52,686
2.5 ~ 3.0	1,139	3,046	2,923	32	19,907	30,796
3.0 ~ 3.5	117	474	1,934	2	10,250	12,777
3.5 ~ 4.0	100	295	1,768	3	13,513	15,679
4.0 ~ 4.5	8	64	373		4,260	4,705
4.5 ~ 5.0	31	36	156	1	6,593	6,817
> 5.0	42	19	136	167	11,798	12,162
Total	118,661	30,524	48,606	3,677	118,613	320,081

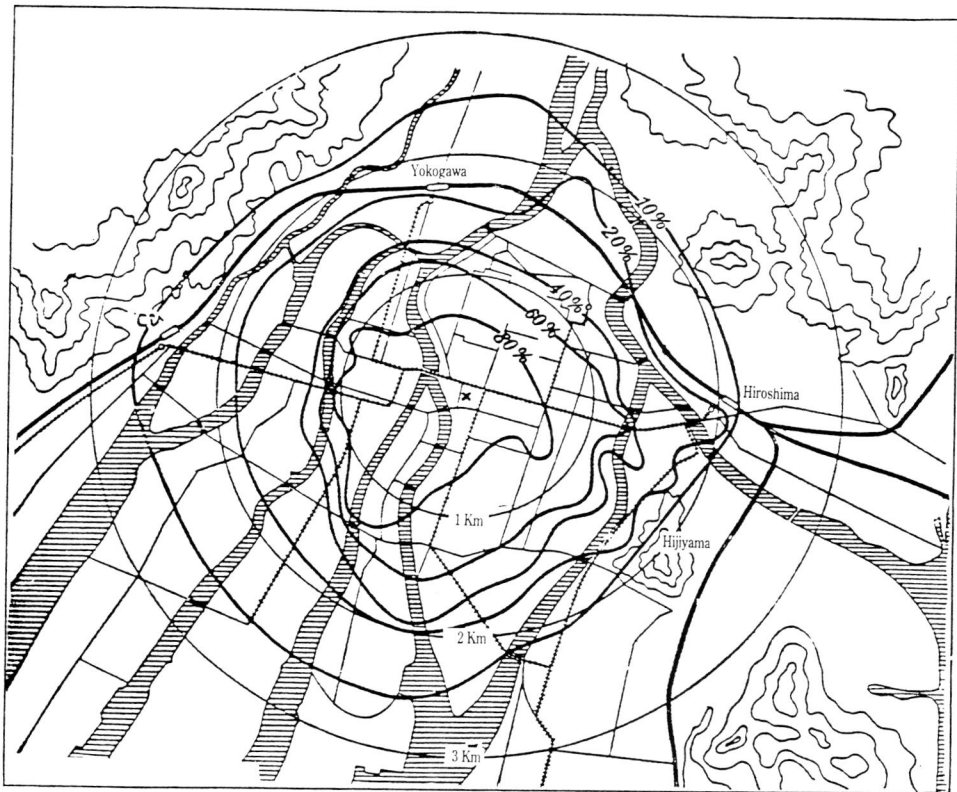

Figure 4   Mortality rate contours in the Hiroshima area

Disaster Overall Picture Survey conducted between 1969 and 1975 showed that the LD_{50} among atomic bomb victims who were inside wooden buildings occurred at a point 1,002 meters from the hypocenter[11]. Also, a separate study on 2,500 people who were inside Japanese-style buildings within 1,600 meters of the hypocenter estimated that the LD_{50} radiation dose was equivalent to a bone marrow dose of 2.3–2.6 Gy[12]. In addition, a survey on 90 of the members of a volunteer corps from the Shintoku Girls' High School who were exposed to radiation at the Hiroshima Central Telephone and Telegraph Office (situated at a distance of 530–580 meters from the hypocenter), together with a study of the frequency of chromosome aberrations in the survivors, was used to estimate the LD_{50} dose; employing T65D air kerma estimates, the estimated value was 6 Gy (approximately 4 Gy if adopting DS86 dosimetry)[13]. This latter rather high figure for the LD_{50} was for 15 year old girls, who can be regarded as having been less affected by the bomb. In the Hiroshima atomic bomb approximately half of the victims at a point 1 km from the bomb died, which suggests that the bone marrow dose received at that time was approximately 3 Gy.

Timing and Primary Cause of Deaths: If the total number of deaths occurring among victims within 2 km of the hypocenter is taken as 100%, then an analysis of the changes in mortality rate with respect to time up to the end of December reveals that 88.7% of the fatalities occurred within the first two weeks, and that 11.3% died between the 3rd and 8th weeks. With regard to the cause of death, 20% of the total number of dead lost their lives due to trauma caused entirely by the bomb blast which struck them when they were within 1.2 km of the hypocenter; a further 20% died due to radiation-caused effects; and the remaining 60% died because of burns produced as a result of thermal radiation and secondary fires.

B. Acute Effects[10]

Various acute effects were observed since variations in the effects of the bomb blast, heat and radiation from the atomic bomb produced variations in the extent of the damage inflicted on the human body, the principal organs suffering injury, and the degree to which different types of injury are inter-related. Differences also occurred in the symptoms exhibited. Table 3 shows the general extent of injury suffered as a function of distance from the hypocenter and exposure status[10]. It can be seen that moderate radiation damage were evident within 1.5 km of the hypocenter even by those who were inside buildings, and that a moderate level of trauma was experienced by those inside wooden buildings up to a distance of 4 km.

The acute symptoms are defined as those appearing between the time of bombing in August 1945 and the end of the following December, and can be divided into three phases (Table 4). During the first phase, which covered the period from immediately after exposure to the end of the second week (August 19th), various acute symptoms were observed and are described below. The second phase covered the period between the third week and the end of the eighth week (early October); during the first half of this period subacute symptoms were observed, with complications appearing in the latter half. During the third phase, up to the end of December 1945, various signs of recovery were observed.

1. *Acute Symptoms*

The causes of death for most victims who were killed instantaneously included being crushed to death by collapsing buildings, receiving external injuries over their entire body, being burnt to death after it proved impossible to escape from collapsed buildings, or suffering burns over the whole body surface. Although escaping instantaneous death, those victims who suffered severe burns over more than 20% of their body surface and those who suffered severe trauma complained of fever, thirst and vomiting within several hours of the bombing, and then lapsed into shock, with most dying by the end of the first week.

Even when the burns and trauma were slight, many of the victims who were exposed to intense radiation immediately exhibited weakness and feelings of exhaustion, nausea and vomiting etc., and within a few days experienced fever, diarrhea,

Table 3   General relationship between atomic bomb radiation effects and distance from the hypocenter[10]

Distance from hypocenter (km)		0	1	2	3	4	5	6
Outdoors (exposed)	Trauma	Severe	Slight					
	Burns	Severe	Moderate	Slight				
	Radiation effects	Severe	Moderate	Slight				
Outdoors (shielded)	Trauma	Slight						
	Burns	Slight						
	Radiation effects	Moderate		Slight				
Inside wooden buildings	Trauma	Severe			Moderate		Slight	
	Burns	Slight						
	Radiation effects	Moderate		Slight				
Inside concrete structures	Trauma	Slight						
	Burns	Slight						
	Radiation effects	Moderate	Slight					

Mortality rates
Severe symptoms 50 ~ 100%
Moderate symptoms 10 ~ 50%
Slight symptoms 0 ~ 10%

Table 4   Appearance of acute effects with respect to time

Phase 1:	From immediately after atomic explosion to end of the 2nd week — acute symptoms
Phase 2:	From 3rd week to end of the 8th week (6 weeks) 1st half (3rd week to 5th week) — subacute symptoms 2nd half (6th week to 8th week) — complications
Phase 3:	From 3rd month to end of December 1945 (11 weeks) — signs of recovery

hemoptysis, hematemesis, bloody stool, and hematuria. The whole body became debilitated and death occurred within about ten days of exposure.

Pathological observations on those who died at this time revealed that the radiation had caused destruction of hematopoietic tissue such as the bone marrow, lymph nodes and spleen etc., and swellings and degeneration in the epithelial cells of the intestines, in the reproductive organs, and in endocrine gland cells. In addition, various other characteristics were observed which are believed to have had their origin in burns and trauma, such as dilation of the right ventricle, acute liver congestion, pulmonary emphysema, and pulmonary hydrops etc.

2. *Subacute Symptoms*

The main subacute symptoms included nausea, vomiting, diarrhea, epilation, weakness, fatigue, hematemesis, bloody stool, hematuria, nose bleeds, gum bleeding, genital hemorrhage, subcutaneous hemorrhage, fever, sore throat, stomatitis, leukopenia, erythropenia, aspermatism, and emmeniopathy etc.

Pathologically the most significant change was the radiogenic destruction of tissue such as the bone marrow, lymph nodes and spleen etc., which led to a decrease in hematocytes, especially granulocytes and platelets. This resulted in a decreased resistance to infection, and hemorrhaging. Many of the deaths in this period were due to sepsis. Although not directly related to the causes of death, atrophic damage due to radiation was observed in endocrine glands such as the pituitary gland, thyroid, and adrenal gland.

The main acute effects of radiation exposure were epilation, hemorrhaging (including purpura), pathological changes in the oropharynx, and leukopenia. The frequencies of epilation, hemorrhaging and pharyngeal lesions became more marked with an increase in the radiation dose; the relationship was virtually linear from a figure of 5–10% for a total dose of 0.50 Gy to a level of 50–80% for a dose of 3 Gy, but at greater doses the rate gradually leveled off.

Epilation was conspicuous up to 8 weeks after exposure, and at the latest by the 10th week, but any epilation that occurred after that time can not be termed an acute radiation effect. Also, from the 3rd to 5th weeks there was a distinct correlation between the severity of leukopenia and the mortality rate. In particular, the number of leukocytes in the 3rd week is the strongest indicator of a correlation with acute radiation.

3. *Complications*

Comparatively mild symptoms that began to disappear and which represented the start of recovery were cessation of fever, ending of inflammation, and the disappearance of a bleeding tendency. However, in some patients symptoms of pneumonia, empyema and severe colitis appeared, in which case it was then common for patients who had once improved to again exhibit a worsened condition. The appearance of these complications can be considered due to a radiation-caused decrease in resistance.

4. *Signs of Recovery*

During the third phase, a trend towards recovery was seen in the trauma, burns, and radiation-caused functional damage of blood and various internal organs, with most having been cured by the end of this period. Hair began to grow in cases of mild epilation, leukocyte counts returned to normal, and there was increased proliferation of granulocytic and erythroblastic cells in the bone marrow, etc. On the other hand, the effects of radiation on the reproductive organs continued, with male sperm counts down and women displaying menstrual disorders. Also in this period various types of damage became evident, such as the appearance of cicatrical contraction and keloid formation.

3. *Late Effects*

Late effects are considered to be those effects on the human body that were caused by radiation and which began to appear from 1946. As far as observations were able to determine, the symptoms displayed were not unique to radiation but exactly the same as in diseases due to other causes, and it is impossible to discern whether or not they were caused by radiation. However, since examination of the exposed population reveals a high frequency of the diseases, there is a strong likelihood that such diseases can be ascribed to radiation. The existence of late radiation effects are thus characteristically clarified by advanced statistical analyses. Consequently, before discussing the long-term effects on the human body, it is necessary to touch briefly on the survey program and subjects covered in the human effects study in Hiroshima, and it is also necessary to refer to the radiation dose used in order to correctly evaluate the long-term effects.

A. Studies and Subjects

The institutions in Hiroshima and related professional organizations directly involved in research into the long-term effects of the atomic bomb are shown in Table 5 in order of establishment. These are at the present time the main institutions, but prior to their establishment the Hiroshima Atomic Bomb Survivors' Treatment Council (which was organized through the efforts of the Hiroshima prefectural and city medical societies) was formed in 1953 and dealt with surveys and treatment concerning the atomic bomb victims. Details of the main study

Table 5   Main institutions and organizations connected to Hiroshima and directly concerned with studies on the late effects of atomic bomb radiation (listed in chronological order of foundation)

Institutions	• Atomic Bomb Casualty Commission (ABCC, 1947), renamed Radiation Effects Research Foundation (RERF, 1980) • Hiroshima Red Cross and Atomic Bomb Hospital • National Institute of Radiological Sciences • Research Institute for Nuclear Medicine and Biology, Hiroshima University (1953) • Hiroshima Atomic Bomb Casualty Council Health Management and Promotion Center (1953)
Organizations	• Meeting on Late Effects of the Atomic Bomb • Japan Radiation Research Society • Research Team for Investigation of the Late Effects of the Atomic Bomb

Table 6   Main research projects

Name of institution	Study	No. of subjects	Year of commencement of study
Radiation Effects Research Foundation	• Atomic bomb survivors		
	Life span study	120,000	1958
	Pathology study	70,000	1961
	Adult health study	20,000	1958
	In utero study	2,800	1956
	• Children of A-bomb survivors		
	Mortality study	77,000	1960
	Biochemical genetic study	45,000	1975
	Cytogenetics study	33,000	1967
Research Institute for Nuclear Medicine and Biology, Hiroshima University	Study on the mortality of atomic bomb survivors	269,000	1968
	Study on the families of atomic bomb survivors	350,000 (87,000 families)	1976
	Study on proximally exposed atomic bomb survivors	600	1973
	Medical and sociological study on A-bombed twins	460 pairs	1980
	Study on the children of atomic bomb survivors	12,000	1986
	Serum cohort study	9,700	1990
Hiroshima Atomic Bomb Casualty Council Health Management Center			
	Study on atomic bomb survivors who received health examinations	150,000	1968
	Study on atomic bomb survivors who did not receive health examinations	14,000	1971
	Study on contents of health examinations	2,000	1973
	Epidemiological study on diabetes mellitus	110,000	1963
	Study on gastric cancer incidence	110,000	1964
	Study on lung cancer incidence	110,000	1976

programs of existing institutions and the number of subjects involved are shown in Table 6. From a supplementary survey accompanying the national censuses of October 1950 and November 1955, the Atomic Bomb Casualty Commission (ABCC) established a cohort of approximately 120,000 based on atomic bomb survivors; of these 82,000 (including 20,000 who were not exposed to the bomb) were in Hiroshima, and 38,000 in Nagasaki (including 6,000 non-exposed). This marked the beginning of studies on the predicted late effects due to radiation, i.e. studies on atomic bomb survivors with respect to leukemia, cataracts, growth and development of young children exposed to the bomb, and the effects on prenatally exposed survivors and their offspring.

The Research Institute for Nuclear Medicine and Biology, Hiroshima University, collected and registered atomic bomb survivors and their families scattered throughout Japan, and then classified the family records. As a special project, medical and sociological studies were begun on proximally exposed survivors and also on twins who had been exposed to atomic bomb radiation. Also, in every field theoretical studies have been performed in order to investigate the medical and biological effects of atomic bomb radiation (and particularly the late effects), and at the same time treatment has been provided to those survivors suffering from internal disorders and external injuries.

The Hiroshima Atomic Bomb Casualty Council Health Management and Promotion Center has continued to carry out medical examinations on all atomic bomb survivors twice every year, and for those survivors for whom detailed examinations are deemed necessary referrals are given to special institutions, and consultations and tests conducted by specialists. In addition, based on these data, consideration has been given to the question of how to conduct studies on those who did not participate in initial examinations and to measures to improve health surveys. On the other hand, based on the data from the detailed examinations, studies are performed on the incidence of malignant tumors (gastric cancer, lung cancer, uterine cancer, breast cancer, and multiple myeloma) among the exposed population.

B. Radiation Dose Estimates

For evaluation of the late effects of atomic bomb radiation on the human body, besides understanding the effects from the health point of view, it is at the same time important to estimate as accurately as possible the radiation dose received by each atomic bomb survivor, which will permit more appropriate investigations into the dose-response relationship. The effort to accurately estimate received doses has been continued by Japanese and American specialists since immediately after the atomic bomb was detonated (Table 7). In the beginning estimates of the received dose for each individual were calculated based on the distance from the hypocenter and the

Table 7   Advances in estimates of atomic bomb radiation doses

1956	Relationship between distance from the hypocenter and acute symptoms (epilation, oral erosion, subcutaneous hemorrhaging)
1957	Establishment of tentative 1957 dosimetry system (T57D doses)
1965	Establishment of tentative 1965 dosimetry system (T65D doses)
1976	Errors perceived in T65D system by US investigators
1981–1985	Joint Japanese-American project
1986	Creation of 1986 dosimetry system (DS86 doses)

appearance of acute radiation symptoms. In 1957, based on the results of the Ichiban project that had been performed the previous year, the United States for the first time presented figures for the air kerma dose (T57D) according to distance from the hypocenter. However, these T57D doses were revised in 1965 to the T65D dose, and until very recently analyses of the dose-response relationship were performed exclusively on the basis of T65D doses. However, since it became apparent that the T65D dose contained errors in such points as the estimate of the neutron dose, Japanese and American specialists worked on a joint project from 1981 to 1985 and, in the spring of 1986, completed a new system for determining the radiation dose which was termed DS86 dosimetry. Compared to T65D dosimetry, the new system used more detailed information concerning the situation of each individual at the time of bombing, and eventually the DS86 dose was calculated for 87,000 (92%) of the approximately 90,000 subjects in the Radiation Effects Research Foundation (RERF) Life Span Study sample for whom a T65D dose had been estimated. Dose estimates have also been conducted at other research institutions, but it is only for the approximately 87,000 atomic bomb survivors in the RERF study that the received dose has been calculated for each individual person.

C. Late Effects of Atomic Bomb Radiation on the Human Body

Table 8 shows the findings of ABCC-RERF studies, and also includes observations made at other institutions. The late effects produced by atomic bomb radiation can generally be classified into three categories. The first category consists of "confirmed increases," in which a statistically significant difference in the frequency of the disorders exists between the atomic bomb survivors and non-exposed individuals, and where a dose-response relationship is found when the data are examined with

Table 8   Late effects of atomic bomb radiation

Confirmed increase	Increase indicated but not confirmed	No increase

• Malignant tumors
  Leukemia
  Thyroid cancer
  Breast cancer
  Lung cancer
  Gastric cancer
  Colon cancer
  Multiple myeloma
• Cataracts
• Chromosome aberrations
  (lymphocytes and bone marrow cells)
• Somatic cell mutations
• Mental retardation (microcephaly) in
  survivors exposed to radiation as fetuses
• Growth and development retardation
  in survivors exposed at a very early age
• Functional abnormalities in organs
  (thyroid gland; parathroid gland)
	• Malignant tumors
	  Esophageal cancer
	  Salivary gland cancer
	  Urinary tract cancer
	  Ovarian cancer
	  Malignant lymphoma
	  Skin cancer
	• Mortality rates due to causes
	  other than malignant tumors
	• Changes in specific humoral
	  immunocompetence and cellular-
	  mediated immunocompetence
		• Malignant tumors
		  Chronic lymphocytic leukemia
		  Osteosarcoma
		• Increased incidence with aging,
		  including cardiovascular disease
		• Sterility
		• Congenital abnormalities,
		  increases in mortality rate,
		  chromosomal aberrations and
		  protein abnormalities etc. in
		  children of atomic bomb survivors

respect to received dose. With regard to the same relationships, the "increase suggested" and "no increase" categories respectively include types of damage that are suggested but not confirmed, and those for which no increase is observed. However, even if a certain disorder is placed in the "no increase" category, it does not necessarily mean that no relationship exists, since the possibility remains that significant differences will become apparent as a result of continued observations, an increase in the number of subjects for study, or the development of more sensitive techniques, etc.

One of the most important late effects appearing in the human body as a result of exposure to atomic bomb radiation is the development of malignant tumors. The RERF surveys over the 35-year period from 1950 to 1985 show a clear correlation with radiation dose for leukemia, breast cancer, thyroid cancer, lung cancer, gastric cancer, colon cancer, and multiple myeloma etc. For each type of malignant tumor, Fig. 5 shows the period during which an increased incidence was observed (indicated by a dashed line) and also the period for which a large increase was noted (indicated by a solid line). Significant increases were observed in leukemia from approximately 1950; in thyroid cancer from approximately 1955; in breast and lung cancer from about 1965; and in gastric cancer, colon cancer, and myeloma from around 1975[14]. The incidence of many malignant tumors began to increase as the age of the atomic bomb survivors increased.

1. *Disorders for which an Increase has been Confirmed*

i) *Malignant Tumors*

1) Leukemia

A high leukemia incidence was observed among atomic bomb survivors who had been exposed to a large single dose of radiation. The leukemia contracted by the atomic bomb survivors has four characteristics: (a) the leukemia believed attributable to atomic bomb radiation peaked in approximately the period 1950–53 (Fig. 6);

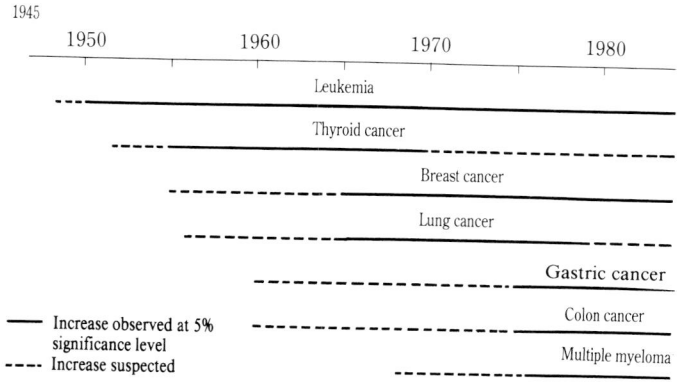

Figure 5 Year of development of malignant tumors[11]

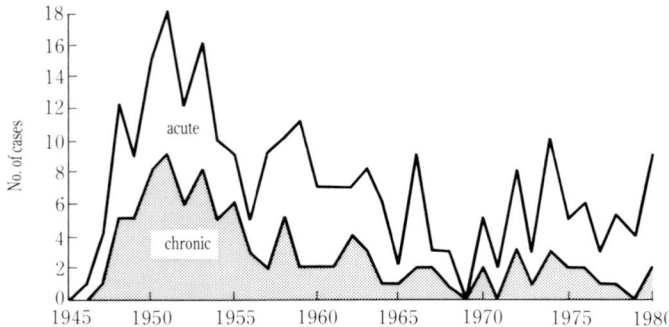

Figure 6   Number of leukemia cases among Hiroshima atomic bomb survivors by year of onset (exposed within 2,000 m)

(b) the leukemia incidence increased with dose in an approximately linear fashion (Fig. 7); (c) even within a population that received the same dose, the leukemia incidence increased with a decrease in age at the time of bombing (ATB); (d) classification according to cell type showed that the ratio of acute leukemia to chronic myelocytic leukemia was 1.5 : 1, compared to a national average in Japan of 4.5 : 1, thus indicating an extremely high incidence of chronic myelocytic leukemia among Hiroshima survivors[15,16].

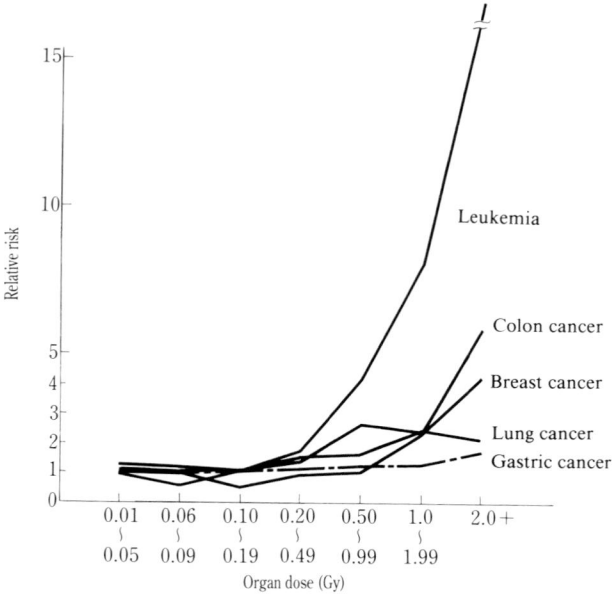

Figure 7   Estimated relative risks for various malignant tumors observed in atomic bomb survivors[15] (in comparison with the non-exposed (0 Gy) population)

2) Thyroid Cancer

Thyroid cancer began to increase approximately 10 years after exposure, with an increased incidence continuing until about 1970. Many of these cases were survivors aged under 20 ATB, and included many who had been exposed to over 0.5 Gy[17–19]. No special characteristics with respect to histologic type were detected in radiation-induced thyroid cancer.

3) Breast Cancer

Breast cancer began to increase approximately 10 years after exposure, and showed a significant increase 20 years after the bombing, with a linear correlation observed with the dose received by the breast tissue (Fig. 7). An excess incidence of radiation-related breast cancer was observed among women aged under 10 years ATB, with the breast cancer risk tending to increase with a decrease in age ATB. With regard to the histologic type of breast cancer, no special characteristics in radiation-induced breast cancer were observed with respect to age at the time of bombing, or to radiation dose, etc.

4) Gastric Cancer

Gastric cancer began to exhibit a significant increase from around 1975 (Fig. 5), with the incidence significant among the heavily exposed (Fig. 7) and individuals aged under 30 ATB. Classification by histologic type reveals a high incidence of well-differentiated adenocarcinoma among the low-dose population, and conversely a high incidence of poorly-differentiated adenocarcinoma among the heavily exposed[20]. Furthermore, recent research has shown that the gastric cancer risk is particularly high among those survivors with low serum ferritin levels.

5) Lung Cancer

Lung cancer began to increase from around 1955, with a significantly high increase being observed after 1965 (Fig. 5). The lung cancer risk rises with an increase in smoking, and it is believed that radiation acts with the effect of smoking in an additive manner; the lung cancer risk also rises with increased exposure to radiation (Fig. 7). In the same manner as leukemia and gastric cancer, the lung cancer risk tends to rise with a decrease in age ATB, but for those who were young at the time (aged ≤ 10 years) a final conclusion cannot be made since those survivors are still only in their fifties. With regard to histologic type, there is a strong tendency for the development of adenocarcinoma rather than squamous cell carcinoma, but this is not yet conclusive.

6) Multiple Myeloma

Along with the aging of the exposed population, multiple myeloma began to increase from around 1975, and in the second half of the 1970's the relative risk among the > 1 Gy population was 5.3 times greater than among those exposed to 0 Gy. With regard to the type of multiple myeloma, cases have been detected among the exposed group which have a form intermediate between benign paraproteinemia and malignant paraproteinemia (multiple myeloma), and are referred to as premyeloma and intermediate-type multiple myeloma.

ii) *Cataracts*

Cataracts are a direct effect of radiation and are greatly affected by the type and dose of radiation. A perfect correlation exists between the dose and lenticular opacity. Also, since the Hiroshima bomb contained a much higher neutron dose than the Nagasaki bomb, for an identical dose the proportion of Hiroshima survivors exhibiting opacities is higher. Cataracts caused by atomic bomb radiation are characterized by their location in the central region of the posterior pole of the lens. Recent medical examinations show that atomic bomb survivors, who have now entered old age, also exhibit age-related cataracts (characterized by opacities spreading from the peripheral regions) so that opacity spreads from both the central and peripheral regions, resulting in a variety of forms.

iii) *Chromosomal Aberrations and Somatic Cell Mutation*

With regard to chromosome aberrations in atomic bomb survivors, reports have appeared on T- and B-lymphocytes in the peripheral blood, and on bone marrow cells and skin fibroblasts, all of which demonstrate a positive correlation with radiation dose. Atomic bomb survivors exposed to > 2 Gy often exhibited chromosomal aberrations in over 30% of lymphocytes and bone marrow cells, including cells carrying identical chromosome aberrations, termed "clones." More important is the evidence that chromosomal aberrations exist in the bone marrow stem cells, which form the basis of hematopoietic processes, and this is believed to be the reason for the increase in the leukemia incidence, and also for the persistence of chromosomal aberrations even forty years after exposure to the atomic bomb. Somatic cell mutations can be determined from the differences in the proteins expressed in the lymphocytes and/or erythrocytes, and have demonstrated a positive correlation with radiation dose.

iv) *Mental Retardation and Microcephaly in Prenatally Exposed Survivors*

The incidence of mental retardation among prenatally exposed survivors varies according to the gestational age at exposure and the dose received. Fetuses in the 8th to 15th week of life are the most vulnerable, with the severity of mental retardation being directly proportional to the dose received. Unlike other disorders, the threshold value appears to be approximately 0.2 Gy.

v) *Functional Abnormalities*

Functional abnormalities have recently become clarified in certain organs, with suggestions that these abnormalities are related to radiation dose.

It is possible to detect hyperparathyroidism as continued elevated hypercalcemia and high serum parathyroid gland hormone levels. As can be seen from Fig. 8, the

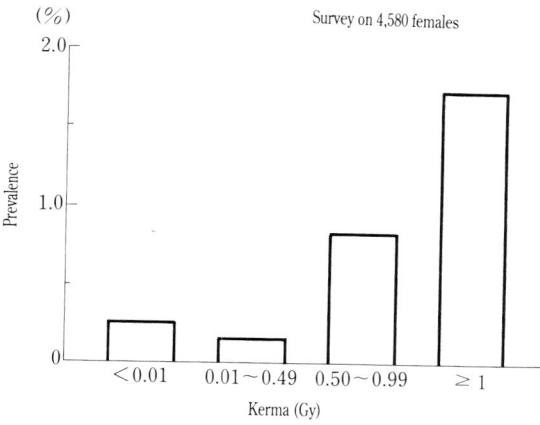

Figure 8   Relationship between radiation dose and hyperparathyrodism[22]

rate increases significantly with doses in excess of 0.5 Gy. Also, this tendency increases with a decrease in age ATB[22]. Surgical evidence has shown that some of the hyperparathyroidism cases are due to adenoma or hyperplasia. Hypothyroidism is also believed to be related to radiation dose.

2. Disorders for which an Increase has been Suggested

Some malignant tumors are included in the "increase suggested" category as a definitive increase has not yet been determined e.g. esophageal cancer, cancer of the salivary glands, cancer of the urinary tract, ovarian cancer, and malignant lymphoma etc. Research on skin cancer has been performed since around 1987[23], and it has been reported that skin cancer in atomic bomb survivors is increasing, although the relationship with radiation dose is not yet known. With regard to histologic type, there is a high incidence of basal cell carcinoma, which is different from the general population. A change is also indicated in specific humoral immunocompetence and cellular-mediated immunity tests, but this is not conclusive since many factors are involved, including age.

Recent reports concerning the mortality rate from causes other than malignant tumors (approximately half of which are due to cardiovascular disease) show that the mortality rate is rising among survivors aged < 40 ATB who were exposed to > 1.5 Gy (Fig. 9)[24].

3. Disorders for which no Increase has been Observed

No statistically significant relationship with exposure to atomic bomb radiation has yet been observed in malignant tumors such as chronic lymphatic leukemia and osteo-sarcoma etc. Infertility rates have not increased. In addition, despite the vigorous research that has continued over many years, no results have directly implicated radiation exposure in disorders such as congenital abnormalities, mortality rates,

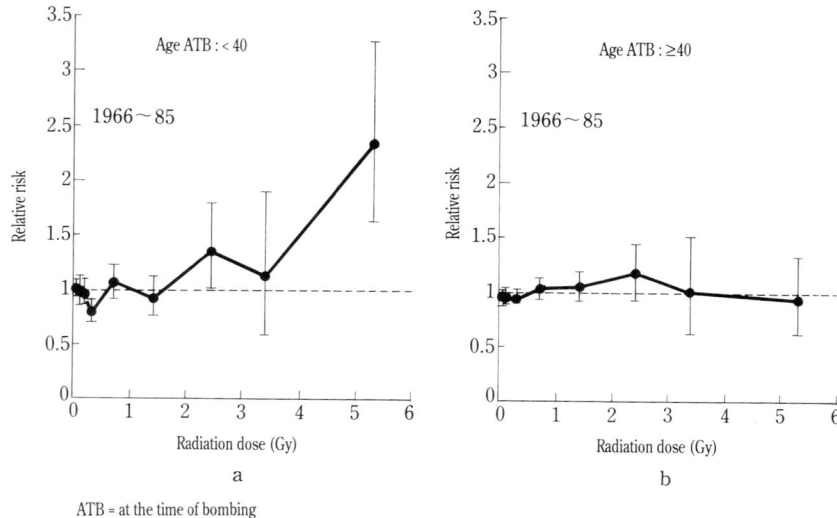

ATB = at the time of bombing

Figure 9   Relative mortality risk by dose for all diseases except cancer and hematologic diseases[21]

chromosomal aberrations, and blood protein mutations etc. in the children of atomic bomb survivors.

CONCLUSION

Great advances have been made in the last decade in studies of the effects of atomic bomb radiation on the human body. Firstly, in 1986 a dosimetry system was completed that enabled received doses to be estimated for each human organ, and which provided accurate dose-response relationships. Secondly, diseases appeared with the aging of atomic bomb survivors. The many years of research have clarified a large number of questions relating to the late effects of atomic bomb radiation, but numerous problems still remain. The clarification of disorders which result from radiation exposure is related to treatment and is an important problem yet to be resolved. Thirdly, now that the survivors who were exposed to the atomic bomb at an early age are about to reach the age at which various types of cancer frequently develop, it is possible that a higher incidence will occur than has yet been observed, thus making it even more imperative in the future to perform thorough medical observations of the atomic bomb survivors. In addition, there is an obvious necessity to carry out long-term follow-up studies on the genetic effects.

(Itsuzo Shigematsu, Chikako Ito, Nanao Kamada)

REFERENCES

1. Roesch WC. US-Japan reassessment of atomic bomb radiation dosimetry in Hiroshima and Nagasaki. Vol. 1. Hiroshima, RERF, 1987.

2. Summary of A-bomb Survivors Measures Projects (1990). Hiroshima: Hiroshima Prefecture, 1990: 1–31.

3. Hiroshima District Meteorological Observatory. Report on the investigation of the Hiroshima atomic bomb casualties (meteorological conditions related). Hiroshima District Meteorological Observatory, 1947.

4. Hiroshima Prefectural Office. History of Hiroshima prefecture war disaster. Hiroshima, 1988.

5. Hirschfelder JO, Parker DB, Kramish A, *et al.* The effects of atomic weapons. Washington: U.S. Government Printing Office, 1950.

6. Hiroshima City Office. Record of the Hiroshima A-bomb war disaster, vol. 1. Hiroshima, 1971.

7. Committee of Experts appointed by the Japan Council against Atomic and Hydrogen Bombs. White paper on damages by atomic and hydrogen bombs. Tokyo: 1975.

8. Shohno N, Iijima S. Nuclear radiation and atomic bomb disease. Tokyo: Japan Broadcasting Publishing, 1975.

9. Oughterson AW, Warren S. Medical effects of the atomic bomb in Japan. New York: McGraw-Hill, 1956.

10. Special Committee for the Investigation of the Effects of the Atomic Bomb. Medical report on atomic bomb effects. National Research Council of Japan, Japan Society for the Promotion of Science, Tokyo, 1953.

11. Hayakawa N, Munaka M, Kurihara M, *et al.* Analysis of early mortality rates of survivors exposed within Japanese wooden houses in Hiroshima by exposed distance. *J Hiroshima Med Ass* 1986; **39**: 126–9.

12. Fujita S, Kato H, Schull WJ. The LD$_{50}$ associated with exposure to the atomic bombing of Hiroshima. *J Radiat Res* 1989; **30**: 359–81.

13. Kamada N, Shigeta C, Kuramoto A, *et al.* Acute and late effects of A-bomb radiation studied in a group of young girls with a defined condition at the time of bombing. *J Radiat Res* 1989; **30**: 218–25.

14. Shimizu Y, Kato H, Schull WJ. Life Span Study report 11. Part 2: cancer mortality in the years 1950–1985 based on the recently revised doses (DS 86). RERF TR 5-88, 1988.

15. Ichimaru M, Ishimaru T, Belsky JL. Incidence of leukemia in atomic bomb survivors belonging to a fixed cohort in Hiroshima and Nagasaki, 1950–71. Radiation dose, years after exposure, age at exposure and type of leukemia. *J Radiat Res* 1978; **19**: 262.

16. Ichimaru M, Tomonaga M, Amenomori T, *et al.* Atomic bomb and leukemia. *J Radiat Res* 1991; **32** (Suppl): 162–7.

17. Ezaki H, Shigemitsu T. Studies on thyroid cancer induced by A-bomb exposure. *Proceedings of the 7th Meeting of the Research Society for Late Effects of Atomic Bomb*; 1965 Oct 16–17; Hiroshima. Hiroshima: Research Society for Late Effects of Atomic Bomb. 1965; 336–47.

18. Parker LN, Belsky JL, Yamamoto T, *et al.* Thyroid carcinoma after exposure to atomic radiation. *Ann Intern Med* 1974; **80**: 600–4.

19. Ezaki A, Takeichi N, Yoshimoto Y. Thyroid cancer: epidemiological study of thyroid cancer in A-bomb survivors from extended Life Span Study cohort in Hiroshima. *J Radiat Res* 1991; **32** (Suppl): 193–200.

20. Ito C, Kato M, Yamamoto T, *et al.* Study of stomach cancer in atomic bomb survivors. Report 1. Histological findings and prognosis. *J Radiat Res* 1989; **30**: 164–75.

21. Akiba S, Neriishi K, Blot W, *et al.* Serum ferritin and stomach cancer risk among A-bomb survivors. RERF TR 14-89, 1989.

22. Fujiwara S, Ezaki H, Sposto R, *et al.* Hyperparathyroidism among atomic bomb survivors in Hiroshima, 1986–1988. RERF TR8-90, 1990.

23. Sadamori N, Honda T, Mine M, *et al.* The incidence of skin cancer in Nagasaki atomic bomb survivors, 1955–1984. *Proceedings of the 28th Meeting of the Research Society for Late Effects of Atomic Bomb*; 1978 June 7; Hiroshima. Hiroshima: Research Society for Late Effects of Atomic Bomb. 1987, 86–94.

24. Shimizu Y, Kato H, Schull WJ, *et al.* Life Span Study report 11, Part III. Non-cancer mortality, 1950–1985, based on the revised doses (DS 86). Tech Rep RERF TR 2-91, 1991.

1

Malignant Tumors

1.1 CANCER MORTALITY RATES IN ATOMIC BOMB SURVIVORS

INTRODUCTION

It is estimated that when the atomic bombs were dropped on Hiroshima and Nagasaki in August 1945, the populations of those cities were 330,000 and 250,000 respectively. It is further estimated that of these the number of people who perished within four months of the atomic bombing due to the effects of the bomb blast and the heat and radiation released by the explosion amounted to 110,000 in Hiroshima (33% of the population), and 70,000 in Nagasaki (28%)[1]. Amongst the atomic bomb survivors who escaped such short-term fatalities, the effects of the bomb were seen later in the increased mortality rates due to cancers such as leukemia and lung cancer. This chapter summarizes the cancer mortality rates observed amongst atomic bomb survivors, focusing on the results of a recent analysis of a mortality study covering the 35-year period from 1950 to 1985, which was carried out on the Life Span Study sample by the Radiation Effects Research Foundation (RERF)[2,3].

1. SUBJECTS AND METHOD OF INVESTIGATION

Due to the post-war confusion the first national survey on atomic bomb survivors in Japan was not carried out until the 1950 census, five years after the atomic bombs were dropped. The survey revealed that there were 280,000 atomic bomb survivors in Japan, of whom approximately 180,000 were living in Hiroshima and Nagasaki. Staff from RERF visited the 180,000 survivors and examined in detail both the sites where they were at the time of bombing and also the shielding conditions.

Based on the results, the Life Span Study was conducted on a total of 120,000 subjects (Table 1). The 34,000 survivors exposed within 2,000 meters of the hypocenter (the so-called proximally exposed survivors) were considered to have received a significant dose of radiation; the control population was a random sample comprised of equal numbers of people from two groups: those who were exposed at a distance greater than 2,500 meters from the hypocenter (the distally exposed survivors), and people who were not exposed to the bombing. The fact that this study was carried out on a fixed population (or cohort) obtained from a sound population base was extremely beneficial from the point of view of follow-up studies. In addition, autopsies were performed on a high percentage of the deceased members of this population.

Deaths were ascertained by periodic examinations of family registers; causes of death were obtained from the death columns in the lists of population changes kept by public health centers throughout the country, which had been transferred from the death certificates. However, a problem existed concerning the accuracy of these listed causes of death since they were based on clinical diagnoses performed by clinical physicians. When the cause of death based on the death certificate for those

Table 1 Original Life Span Study sample (1950) and subjects for whom DS86 doses were estimated[3]

a) Original sample

	Estimated population at time of bombing (August, 1945)	Number and percentage of short-term deaths (within 4 months of bombing)	Number of atomic bomb survivors in 1950 census (All Japan)	Number of subjects in Life Span Study (1950)		
				A-bomb survivors	Non-exposed	Total
Hiroshima	330,000	110,000 (33%)	159,000	62,000	20,000	82,000
Nagasaki	250,000	70,000 (28%)	125,000	32,000	6,000	38,000
Total	580,000	180,000 (31%)	284,000	94,000	26,000	120,000

b) Number of subjects by DS86 dose

	DS86 dose (Gy)										
	0	0.01–0.05	0.06–0.09	0.10–0.19	0.20–0.49	0.50–0.99	1.0–1.99	2.0–2.99	3.0–3.99	4.0 +	Total
Hiroshima	20,346	12,745	3,376	4,360	5,407	2,911	1,422	483	167	173	51,390
Nagasaki	13,926	6,447	753	812	1,151	705	524	154	44	85	24,601
Total	34,272	19,192	4,129	5,172	6,558	3,616	1,946	637	211	258	75,991

cases in which an autopsy was performed is compared with that stated in the autopsy report, and the accuracy of the cause of death expressed in terms of a diagnostic accuracy rate[4], then there is a high degree of accuracy for leukemia, breast cancer and gastric cancer (85–95%), whereas for lung and rectal cancer a rather low diagnostic accuracy rate of 60–70% is obtained. For cancers at sites for which the diagnostic accuracy rate is low, or where the mortality rate is low (such as with thyroid and breast cancer), it is inappropriate to perform risk estimates based solely on mortality studies; it is then necessary to also utilize data from tumor tissue registries.

Although the deaths occurring in the Life Span Study sample are periodically ascertained and the results of analyses regularly published, the discussion here is based on recent reports covering the period 1950–1985[2,3]. In addition, the present analysis considers the revised DS86 dose estimates[2] instead of the T65 doses which have hitherto been used. Table 1 shows the number of subjects considered by DS86 dose for both Hiroshima and Nagasaki.

2. RESULTS

A. Cancer Mortality Rates by Site

Figure 1 shows, for various organs, how many times greater is the risk of dying (i.e. the relative risk) from cancer in the group exposed to 1 Gy (shielded kerma) in comparison with the mortality rates observed in the control population (0 Gy). The errors in the computation of relative risk were statistically estimated within the 90% confidence limit and are indicated in the diagram by the length of the horizontal line.

Although there was a distinct increase in the frequency of leukemia amongst atomic bomb survivors, an increase could also be observed in other forms of cancer;

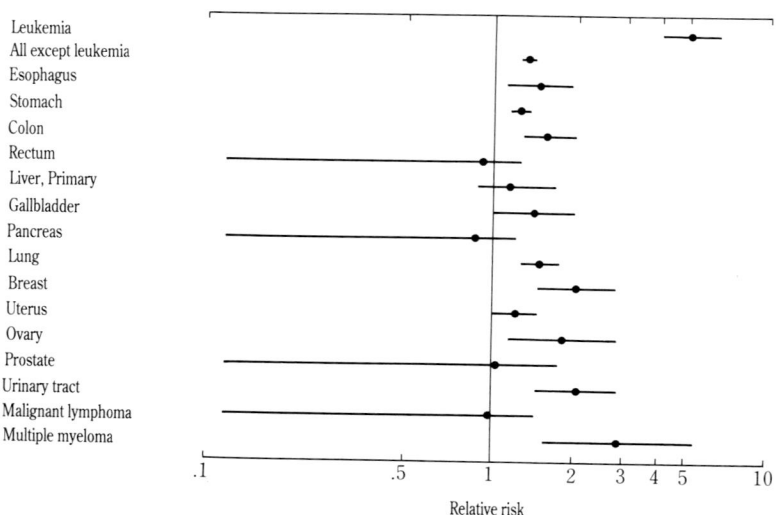

Figure 1   Relative risk at 1 Gy (shielded kerma) and 90% confidence limit, 1950–85[3]

however, this tendency was not seen at all sites. Even within the leukemia population, no increase was observed in chronic lymphatic leukemia[5]. With regard to the digestive tract, radiation increased the risk of cancer of the esophagus, stomach and colon, whereas no relationship to radiation was found with cancer of the rectum, liver, gall bladder and pancreas. With respect to cancers in organs other than the digestive organs, a significantly increased risk was observed in cancers of the lung, breast, ovaries, urinary tract, and in multiple myeloma. However, no such tendency was found in uterine cancer, prostate cancer or in malignant lymphomas. In incidence studies, an increased risk due to radiation was also observed in thyroid cancer[6]. These results indicate that radiosensitivity and induction of cancer vary with the organ concerned.

B. Latency Periods for Radiation-Induced Cancers

Instead of appearing immediately after exposure, the effects of radiation are manifested after a certain interval of time. When a human being is exposed to radiation, changes occur in the irradiated cells, which proliferate and result in the appearance of clinical symptoms (the onset of cancer) and, if no treatment is successful, result in death. The period of time between exposure and the onset of cancer (or death when date of onset cannot be determined) is referred to as the latency period.

In the case of chronic irradiation, such as occurs in occupational exposure to radiation or in medical treatment, it is difficult to determine the period of irradiation. With atomic bomb survivors, however, the date and time of exposure is known exactly, and moreover the radiation dose measurements and follow-up studies were carried out almost perfectly, with the result that these data are virtually the only data for detailed study of the modifying factors such as radiation dose and age at the time of exposure that cover the whole of the latency period from exposure to onset of cancer.

A significant difference was observed in the post-exposure temporal development of radiation-induced cancer between leukemia and solid cancers such as lung cancer and breast cancer (Fig. 2). Radiation-induced leukemia appeared after a minimum

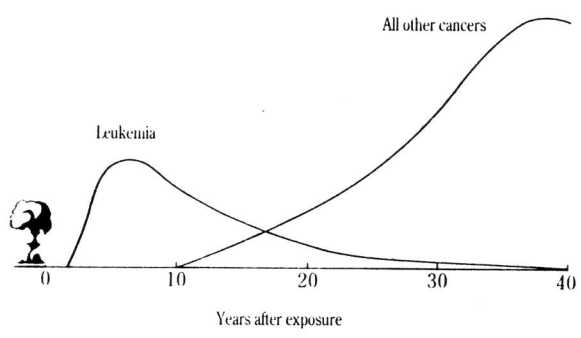

Figure 2   Incidence of radiation-induced cancer after atomic bombing

latency period of 2–3 years, reached a maximum after 6–7 years, and then decreased with time. No significant increase in mortality rate has been observed in Nagasaki since 1970; in Hiroshima, however, although the number of deaths recorded in the recent study (1981–1985) was extremely small (4 people in the $\geq$ 1 Gy population), the mortality rate is significantly higher than in the control population. The latency period for radiation-induced leukemia is thus between 3 and 40 years. In addition, illness tends to develop earlier with heavy exposure, i.e. the latency period decreases dose-dependently.

However, the situation is different for solid tumors such as lung cancer. As shown in Fig. 2, radiation-induced solid cancers appear after a long minimum latency period of ten or more years, and then increase with time. Lung cancer was selected as an example of a solid cancer, and the time at which the effect of the radiation appeared was examined by age at the time of bombing (ATB) (Fig. 3). The cumula-

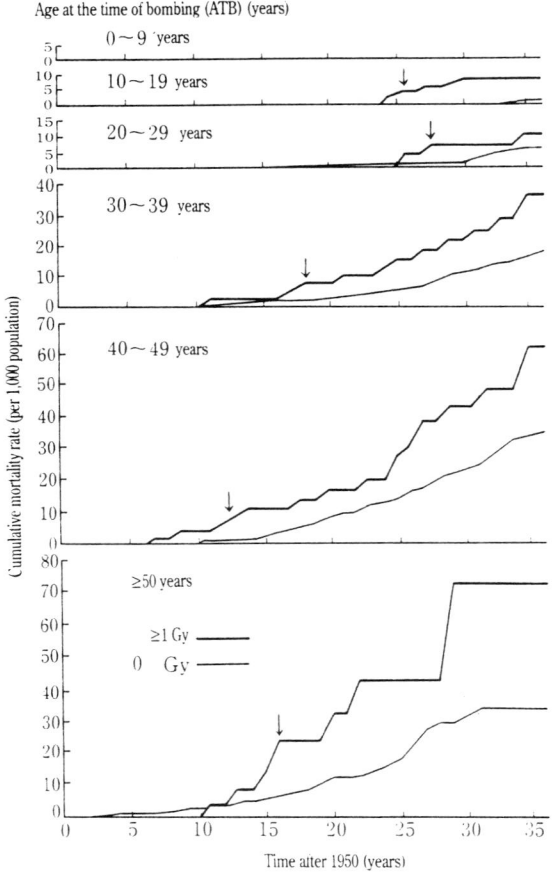

Figure 3   Cumulative lung cancer mortality rates for the heavily exposed ($\geq$ 1 Gy) and control population (0 Gy) between 1950 and 1985 by age at the time of bombing[3]

tive death rates since 1950 for the high-dose population ($\geqslant 1$ Gy) and control population (0 Gy) were compared according to age ATB. The arrows in the diagram indicate the time at which the difference in mortality rates between the two populations first became statistically significant (the time at which the radiation-induced cancers clearly appeared for the first time). For the population aged 40–49 years ATB, an excess number of radiation-related deaths was first observed after 15–20 years (around 1960–1965), after which it continued to increase. Amongst the young atomic bomb survivors, the mortality rate in the heavily exposed population tended to increase at a much later date. For example, the increase in the 10–19 year old ATB population was discerned after an interval of 30 years. In short, unlike leukemia, in lung cancer the effect of radiation appears clearly at the age at which the cancer frequently occurs, with no reduction in latency period observed in the heavily exposed population. Recently the multi-step theory concerning the onset of cancer has been widely accepted. This is based on *in vitro* and animal experiments, including molecular biology techniques. The theory holds that it is necessary for an initiator, a promoter, and also a proliferation factor to act in sequential stages, and it can be considered that the radiation is involved in all these three stages.

When malignant solid tumors such as lung cancer and breast cancer etc. occur in the young ATB populations, the radiation can be considered to have acted as an initiator (for example, by activation of oncogenes) resulting in cell transformation. When a factor other than radiation acts as a promoter, the second stage occurs (the process up to this time probably being reversible), and in the third stage a proliferation factor acts, irreversible proliferation occurs, and clinical symptoms of cancer may also appear. If this hypothesis is correct, then there is no relationship between the radiation dose that initiates the carcinogenic process, and the time at which the promoter and proliferation factors act in the second and third stages of the process; consequently, the latency period is unrelated to the dose. For any particular cancer site, radiation-induced cancer is believed to develop at the age at which cancer frequently develops at that site; i.e. cancer develops at the age at which the promoter and proliferation factors frequently act. At the time of bombing, the older populations had already reached an age at which cancer frequently occurs. Since another carcinogen (for example, a female hormone such as prolactin etc.) can be assumed to have already promoted the first stage, the radiation probably acted as the promoter in the second stage or as the proliferation factor in the third stage (for example, by inactivation of the cancer-suppressing genes); therefore, clinical symptoms of cancer appeared after the minimum latency period. Various animal experiments have been performed with the aim of directly verifying this hypothesis[7–9], with all the experimental results supporting the previously mentioned findings concerning the onset of cancer for solid tumors (lung cancer and breast cancer etc.) in atomic bomb survivors. Since radiosensitivity in the case of leukemia is extremely high, the changes occurring in the first, second and third stages are produced by the radiation either at the same time or else at extremely short intervals thereafter. Consequently, the appearance of leukemia can be viewed as virtually unrelated to the age at the time of bombing, with tumor development occurring more rapidly with increasing doses. Although possibly an over-simplification of the mechanism by which radiation causes cancer, this hypothesis is effective in explaining the discrepancies in observations relating to the latency period.

C. The Relationship Between the Onset of Radiation-Induced Cancer and Time (The Additive Risk and Multiplicative Risk Models)

As previously mentioned, the incidence of radiation-induced solid cancer increases with age. Two models which can be considered when examining the manner of this increase are described in reports by the United Nations[10] and the Committee on the Biological Effects of Ionizing Radiation (BEIR-III)[11] (Fig. 4). The first is known as the additive model (previously referred to as the absolute risk model), which postulates that the number of excess cancer deaths due to radiation is constant and bears no relationship to the age at the time of death. The other is the multiplicative model (previously referred to as the relative risk model), which postulates that the risk relative to the rate of natural occurrence is constant and unrelated to the age at the time of death, and that in this case the number of excess cancer deaths naturally increases with an increase in age at death. The risk of developing radiation-related cancer is usually expressed as the number of radiation-induced cancer cases occurring during the lifetime of the population that is exposed to a certain amount of radiation ("lifetime risk of radiation-induced cancer"), and the above models adopted when such an estimation is performed. However, when the multiplicative model is used, the estimated value is 3–4 times greater than that obtained with the additive model, as is clearly shown by Fig. 4. Thus the choice of model profoundly affects the estimated lifetime risk.

Table 2 shows the relative risk of all cancers except leukemia following exposure to a dose of 1 Gy, by both age at death and also by age at exposure (ATB). For the

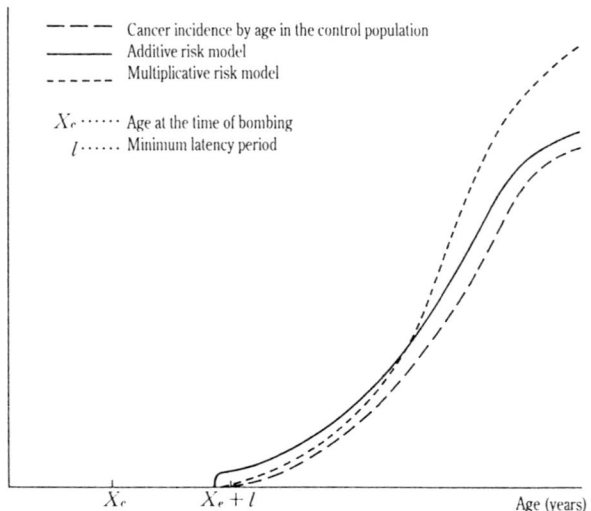

Figure 4 The additive and multiplicative risk models for estimation of risk of radiation-induced cancer

Table 2   Relative risk and number of excess by age at the time of bombing (ATB) and age at death[3]. (All cancers except leukemia, shielded kerma)

Age ATB (yrs)	Age at death (years)					
	< 30	30–39	40–49	50–59	60–69	70 +
Relative risk (at 1 Gy)						
< 10	7.49	1.96	1.86			
10–19	(1.37)	1.66	1.59	1.68		
20–29		(1.38)	2.09	1.74	1.37	
30–39		(0.84)	(1.12)	1.11	1.23	1.48
40–49			(1.25)	1.11	1.13	1.33
50 +				(2.58)	(0.95)	1.15
Excess deaths per 10,000 person years (per Gy)						
< 10	0.88	2.85	5.16			
10–19	(1.37)	2.00	5.84	13.91		
20–29		(1.39)	9.40	15.71	14.33	
30–39		(−1.32)	(1.33)	3.16	11.00	41.01
40–49			(2.48)	(3.37)	7.31	37.30
50 +				(35.29)	(−2.88)	17.21

Parentheses indicate estimates based on the assumption that the minimum latency period is less than 10 years

population aged ⩾ 10 years ATB, the relative risk is approximately constant and unrelated to the age at the time of death, i.e. the data supports the multiplicative model and not the additive model. A recent British follow-up study on ankylosing spondylitis[12] indicated that even for solid cancers the relative risk has recently been decreasing. In the 1990 American BEIR-V report, the lifetime risk was estimated using the multiplicative model based on the British data, in which the risk decreases with age. However, in the case of the atomic bomb survivors even a recent mortality study (1950–1985) shows that, with the exception of leukemia, the relative risk at all cancer sites was constant and did not decrease with age (Table 2).

Moreover, a chronological examination of the data for individual sites reveals no significant change in relative risk with time, even for cancers of the lung, stomach and breast.

D. Modifying Factors

The cancer risk due to radiation varies with sex and age (both age ATB and the age at death), and is modified by carcinogens such as tobacco and hormones.

1. Age at the Time of Bombing

The mortality rates for all solid cancers for the same age at death show that both the relative and absolute risks increase with decreasing age ATB (Table 2). For example, for those who died aged 20-29, the absolute risk for the population aged ⩾ 10 years

ATB was 2.85, which was 2.1 times greater than that for the population aged 20–29 years ATB. Animal experiments have also clearly shown that radiation exerts a greater effect at young ages, when body cells exhibit high mitotic rates[7].

Furthermore, as mentioned earlier, the cancer risk is greatest for the population aged ≤ 10 years ATB; in addition the heavily exposed population tends to develop cancer more quickly than the control population (i.e. a dose-dependent reduction is observed in the latency period, as in the case of leukemia). The reason for this is not clear, but could be due to highly radiosensitive individuals in the exposed population developing cancer earlier.

2. Sex

The relative cancer risk at various sites following a dose of 1 Gy is shown in Table 3 according to sex. No difference is observed between the sexes with respect to leukemia, but for all other cancers the relative risk from radiation exposure is higher for females than for males, except for myelomas, where the reverse holds true. This tendency is especially marked in the case of cancer of the esophagus and lung cancer, reflecting the fact that the natural cancer mortality rate at these sites is greater for men than for women. For lung cancer, when the data is adjusted to take account of smoking customs the difference between the sexes in terms of relative risk due to radiation disappears[3,14]. This shows that although there is no difference between the sexes in sensitivity to radiation itself, a difference in risk according to sex may arise depending on the amount of other carcinogenic factors such as smoking, alcohol consumption and hormones.

3. The Relationship Between Radiation and Other Carcinogenic Factors such as Smoking

Besides radiation, the atomic bomb survivors were naturally exposed to various other carcinogenic factors such as smoking, carcinogens in food, and hormones etc.

Table 3   Risk coefficient by sex (shielded kerma)[3]

Cancer site	Relative risk at 1 Gy				Number of excess deaths per 10,000 person years			
	Male	Female	Male/Female ratio	Significance	Male	Female	Male/Female ratio	Significance
Leukemia	4.96	4.92	1.00		3.14	1.80	1.74	*
All cancers except leukemia	1.17	1.44	0.81	**	5.76	8.78	0.66	
Esophagus	1.19	2.99	0.40	*	0.30	0.40	0.75	
Stomach	1.15	1.36	0.85		2.01	2.18	0.92	
Colon	1.45	1.67	0.87		0.60	0.51	1.18	
Lung	1.26	1.86	0.68	*	1.07	1.47	0.73	
Bladder	2.00	2.15	0.93		0.81	0.42	1.93	
Multiple myeloma	5.29	2.32	2.28		0.23	0.21	1.10	

*: $p < 0.05$ **: $p < 0.01$

It is therefore extremely difficult to estimate the risk due to radiation in relation to whether or not interactions occurred between the radiation and other carcinogenic factors that affect the mechanism by which cancer developed in the atomic bomb survivors. It can be considered that in the absence of interactions, the factors would act in an additive manner, whereas the presence of interactive mechanisms would be related to factors acting in a multiplicative fashion. An examination of the relationship between radiation and smoking reveals that for both smokers and non-smokers the lung cancer mortality rate is higher for the heavily exposed population than for the control population (0 Gy), and that the rates for both smokers and non-smokers increase relative to the controls by approximately the same margin (Fig. 5), i.e. the radiation and smoking interact in an additive manner. The results of a case-control study involving atomic bomb survivors[15], as well as data concerning people other than the atomic bomb survivors, have to the present time yielded virtually no data positively indicating a multiplicative effect.

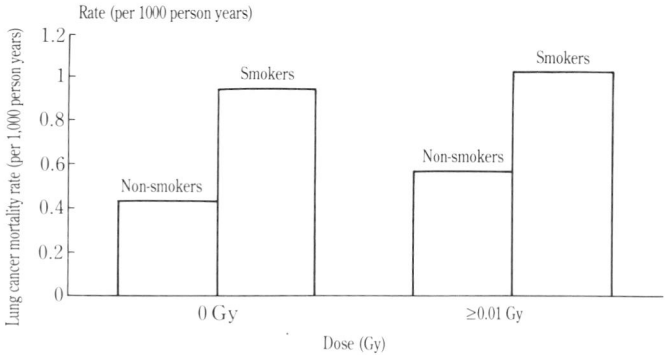

Figure 5 Combined effect of radiation and smoking on age and sex-adjusted lung cancer mortality[3]

E. The Dose-Response Relationship

Figure 6 shows the dose-response relationship for organ doses. For leukemia, the most appropriate model for comparatively low doses (< 2 Gy) is the linear quadratic (LQ) model, but for total doses and high doses greater than 2 Gy the LQ-K model, which includes cell killing, is the most suitable. For solid cancers, when the dose is < 2 Gy, the linear (L) model is appropriate. As shown in Fig. 6, each model assumes that even an extremely small dose of radiation results in a very low rate of cancer development (i.e. there is no threshold value). However, in a recent cancer mortality study, examination of the lowest dose range for which a statistically significant high cancer mortality rate occurs relative to the control group (0 Gy) (which in practice can be referred to as the threshold value), reveals that the shielded kerma values of such a threshold dose are 0.2–0.49 Gy for lung cancer and all solid cancers, 0.5–0.99 Gy for leukemia and breast cancer, 1.0–1.9 Gy for gastric cancer, and ⩾ 2 Gy for colon cancer.

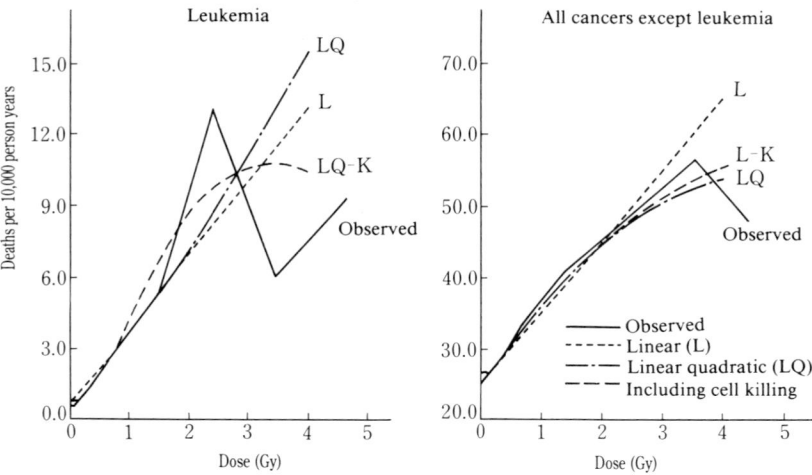

Dose categories used in plots for observed dose response curves are 0, 0.01–0.05, 0.06–0.09, 0.10–0.19, 0.20–0.49, 0.50–0.99, 1.0–1.9, 2.0–2.9, 3.0–3.9, ≥ 4.0 Gy.

Figure 6   Observed and estimated organ dose-reponse relationships for both leukemia and all cancers except leukemia[3]

Although not shown in Fig. 6, the difference in the dose-response curves for Hiroshima and Nagasaki (for an identical dose the mortality rate for Hiroshima is greater than for Nagasaki) is less than that observed using T65 dosimetry, with the difference between the two cities ceasing to be statistically significant[2]. In addition, the neutron dose for Hiroshima became extremely small using DS86 dosimetry, thus making it impossible in the present mortality data analysis to estimate the relative biological effect (RBE, i.e. the value that indicates how many times greater the effect of neutrons is relative to the effect of gamma radiation)[2].

F. The Degree to which Atomic Bomb Radiation is Responsible for Cancer Deaths amongst Atomic Bomb Survivors (The Attributable Risk)

The atomic bomb survivors were exposed to carcinogenic factors other than the atomic bomb, such as tobacco and food etc., and thus not all of the cancer deaths in this population will have been caused by radiation from the bomb. It is therefore important to ascertain what percentage of the cancer deaths among atomic bomb survivors was radiation-induced. For 42,000 people exposed to ≥ 0.01 Gy of radiation (with an average dose of 0.30 Gy), Fig. 7 shows a comparison between the expected number of excess cancer deaths during 1950–1985 and the number actually observed during that period (the attributable risk), assuming a linear dose-response relationship. The expected number of excess deaths due to leukemia was approximately 80, which was 55% of the actually observed total of 144. In other words, for this group, 55% of the observed leukemia deaths could be attributed to radiation. Similarly, the number of excess deaths from all cancers except leukemia was 260,

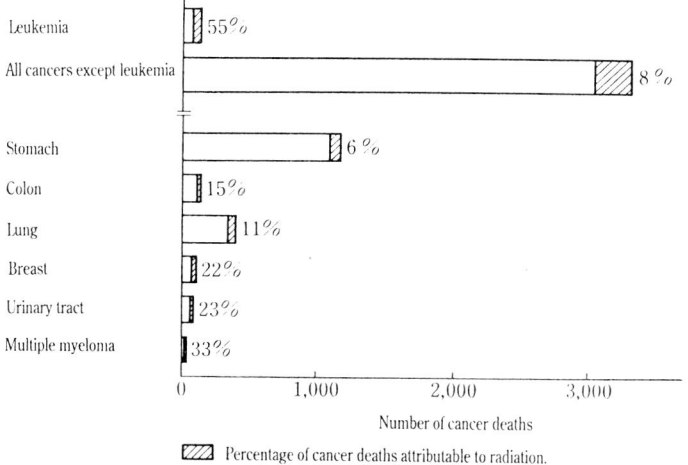

Figure 7   Estimated percentages of deaths attributable to atomic bomb radiation by cancer site[3]

which corresponded to a mere 8% of the 3,291 solid cancer deaths observed in this cohort. Furthermore, when the figures are examined by cancer site, the percentage of cancer that can be attributed to radiation ranges from 6% for gastric cancer to 33% for multiple myeloma.

G. Estimation of Lifetime Risk

The risk coefficient obtained from data on the atomic bomb survivors is widely used as the basis for estimating the lifetime cancer risk due to radiation, e.g. a report by the United Nations Scientific Committee on the Effects of Atomic Radiation (UNSCEAR)[10] and a Biological Effects of Ionizing Radiation (BEIR) report by the American National Research Council[13]. In addition, the estimated lifetime risks are used by the International Commission on Radiological Protection (ICRP) for determining radiation protection standards.

Using the fixed population in Japan in 1985 and taking the 1985 cancer mortality rate in Japan as the standard mortality rate, the lifetime cancer risk in Japan was estimated for both leukemia and all solid cancers; these values were then compared with the estimated values of other international agencies (Table 4).

The lifetime leukemia risk was calculated by assuming the additive model for changes with respect to time, taking the minimum latency period to be two years, and assuming the dose-response curve to be linear and linear quadratic. For all solid cancers, the lifetime risk was computed by assuming the multiplicative model for changes with respect to time, taking the minimum latency period to be ten years, and assuming the dose-response curve to be linear.

In the 1988 report by the United Nations (UNSCEAR) the subject population and the standard cancer mortality rate were different, but since the risk coefficients used the same data, the values were approximately equal to those obtained in the

Table 4   Estimated lifetime risk (Number of excess deaths per 1,000 persons for single exposure to 0.1 Sv)

	Leukemia	All cancers except leukemia
UNSCEAR 1977[16]	0.2	1
BEIR III[11]	0.5 (0.2)	5
UNSCEAR 1988[10]	1	10
BEIR V[13]	(1.0)	7
Life Span Study (11th report)[3]	1.1 (0.7)	10

N.B. Values were determined on the assumption that the dose-response relationship was linear (L), but values obtained by assuming a linear-quadratic (LQ) relationship are indicated in parentheses.

preliminary calculations performed at the Radiation Effects Research Foundation (RERF).

Besides using the United States values for population and standard cancer mortality rate, the 1990 BEIR-V report[13] used the multiplicative model (in which the relative risk decreases with age) as a model for the changes with respect to time for all solid cancers, yielding values lower than those reported by RERF and in the 1988 United Nations report. In addition, the new estimated values are higher than those in earlier publications such as the 1980 BEIR-III[11] and 1977 United Nations[16] reports. However, care is necessary in interpreting deductions made from these comparisons of estimated values. The differences observed in the estimations are not only due to changes in dosimetry calculations but also arise as a result of various other factors such as the model adopted in the estimation, the population used for the projection, and changes in the magnitude of the risk coefficient due to extension of the follow-up period.

(Hiroo Kato, Yukiko Shimizu)

REFERENCES

1. Kato H, Shigematsu I. Late effects of A-bomb radiation: Hiroshima and Nagasaki, Annex 5. In: Effects of nuclear war on health and health services. WHO 1984: 117–38.
2. Shimizu Y, Kato H, Schull WJ, *et al.* Studies of the mortality of A-bomb survivors. Report 9. Mortality, 1950–1985: Part 1. Comparison of risk coefficients for site specific cancer mortality based on the DS86 and T65DR shielded kerma and organ doses. *Radiat Res* 1989; **118**: 502–24.
3. Shimizu Y, Kato H, Schull WJ. Studies of the mortality of A-bomb survivors, 9. Mortality, 1950–1985: Part 2. Cancer mortality based on the recently revised doses (DS86). *Radiat Res* 1990; **121**: 120–41.
4. Yamamoto T, Moriyama IM, Asano M, *et al.* RERF pathology studies. Report 4. Autopsy program and the Life Span Study. Hiroshima and Nagasaki. January 1961–December 1975. RERF TR 18–78, 1978.
5. Ichimaru M, Ishimaru T, Belsky JL. Incidence of leukemia in atomic bomb survivors, Hiroshima and Nagasaki 1959–71 by radiation dose, years after exposure, age and type of leukemia. *J Radiat Res* 1978; **19**: 262–82.
6. Wakabayashi T, Kato H, Ikeda T, Schull WJ. Studies of the mortality of A-bomb survivors, Report 7. Part 3. Incidence of cancer in 1950–1978, based on the tumor registry. *Nagasaki Radiat Res* 1983; **93**: 112–46.

7. Yokoro K, Seyama T, Yanagihara K. Experimental radiation carcinogenesis in rodents. *GANN Monograph on Cancer Res* 1986; **32**: 89–112.
8. Yokoro K, Nakano M, Ito A, *et al.* Role of prolactin in rat mammary carcinogenesis: detection of carcinogenecity of low-dose carcinogens and persisting dormant cancer cells. *J Natl Cancer Inst* 1977; **58**: 1777–83.
9. Clifton KH. Thyroid cancer: reevaluation of an experimental model for radiogenic endocrine carcinogenesis. In: Upton AC, Albert RE, Burns FJ, Shore RE, editors. Radiation carcinogenesis. New York: Elsevier, 1986: 181–98.
10. United Nations Scientific Committee on the Effects of Atomic Radiation, 1988 Report. Annex F: Radiation carcinogenesis in man. VII. Risk projections. New York: United Nations, 1988: 481–532.
11. Committee on the Biological Effects of Ionizing Radiation. Effects on populations of exposure to low levels of ionizing radiation (BEIR-III). National Academy of Sciences-National Research Council. Washington, DC: National Academy Press, 1980.
12. Darby SC, Doll R, Gill SK, *et al.* Long term mortality after a single treatment course with X-rays in patients treated for ankylosing spondylitis. *Br J Cancer* 1987; **55**: 179–90.
13. Committee on the Biological Effects of Ionizing Radiation. Commission on Life Science. Health effects of exposure to low levels of ionizing radiation (BEIR-V). National Academy of Sciences-National Research Council. Washington, DC: National Academy Press, 1990: 176–82.
14. Kopecky KJ, Nakashima E, Yamamoto T, *et al.* Lung cancer, radiation and smoking among A-bomb survivors. RERF TR 13–86, 1986.
15. Blot WJ, Akiba S, Kato H. Ionizing radiation and lung cancer: a review including preliminary results from a case control study among A-bomb survivors. In: Prentice RL, Thompson DJ, editors. Atomic bomb survivor data: utilization and analysis. Philadelphia: Siam, 1984: 235–48.
16. United Nations Scientific Committee on the Effects of Atomic Radiation. Sources and effects of ionizing radiation. New York: United Nations, 1977.

1.2 LEUKEMIA

a. INCIDENCE AND RISK

INTRODUCTION

Radiation is widely recognized as a cause of leukemia in humans and experimental animals. In animals the type of leukemia developed and the incidence depend on the species concerned; in humans variations are presumed to depend on such factors as age at the time of bombing and sex etc. In addition, the risk of developing leukemia varies with the type of radiation, dose received, dose rate, and the site undergoing irradiation[1].

Characteristics of the atomic bomb survivors are that they covered a large age range and were externally exposed to a single dose of mostly gamma radiation. Amongst the many late effects of the atomic bombing, leukemia was the first malignancy to be observed[2].

1. LEUKEMIA REGISTRY AND POPULATIONS STUDIED

Research into the epidemiological and hematologic aspects of leukemia and the development of other hematopoietic organ tumors caused by the atomic bombing has been vigorously pursued for many years, much of this being the result of the leukemia registry. This registry, the objectives of which are the detection and diagnostic confirmation of leukemia and related hematologic disorders occurring in Hiroshima and Nagasaki, was started in 1948 as a joint research project between the Radiation Effects Research Institute, RERF (the former Atomic Bomb Casualty Commission, ABCC); the Research Institute for Nuclear Medicine and Biology, Hiroshima University; and the Atomic Bomb Disease Institute, Nagasaki University School of Medicine. At a later date the Hiroshima Red Cross Hospital and Atomic Bomb Hospital also participated, and continue to do so today. With the registry, and through a close communications network involving regional hospitals and other medical institutions and university hospitals, it has been possible to investigate leukemia in not only Hiroshima and Nagasaki, but also in other regions. Moreover, the examination of data and blood samples etc. from both Hiroshima and Nagasaki has permitted agreement between hematologists from the two cities with regard to the diagnostic confirmation of leukemia and related disorders.

In the latter half of the 1950s regional tumor registries were established in both Hiroshima and Nagasaki, and a tissue registry centered on pathologists begun in the first half of the 1970s. These registries have also been used in the detection and confirmation of leukemia and related disorders.

The leukemia registry has been compiled over many years for the regional residents (the "open" population) and the RERF cohort (i.e. the Life Span Study sample). The latter population, based on the 1950 national census, consists of approximately 120,000 individuals, including the atomic bomb survivors. In order to evaluate the late effects of the atomic bombing, national follow-up mortality studies have been carried out since that time on the subjects in this sample. Meanwhile, DS86 dosimetry has provided estimates of individual doses of atomic bomb radiation. These follow-up studies have led to the establishment of standards for risk estimations concerning the development of cancer and other radiation-caused diseases.

2. LEUKEMIA INCIDENCE

Amongst the proximally exposed Hiroshima and Nagasaki survivors, leukemia related to the atomic bombing was first reported in Nagasaki in 1947 and in Hiroshima in 1948[3]. However, it is not possible to accurately estimate the leukemia risk prior to the establishment of the above cohort in 1950 since accurate data is unavailable. Nevertheless, it is clear that the leukemia incidence began to increase before 1950[4]. The leukemia incidence in the fixed Life Span Study cohort reached a maximum during 1950–1954, after which it has gradually decreased[3].

Much has been learned about risk patterns from past analyses of leukemia incidence, but numerous unresolved problems remain. Although, as previously mentioned, the leukemia risk gradually decreased from a maximum in the early 1950s, has the risk been increasing again in recent years? Although the leukemia risk is known to be high amongst young bomb victims, to what extent does the age at the time of bombing affect temporal changes in the risk? Also, is there some difference between Hiroshima and Nagasaki in the leukemia risk attributable to radiation? Moreover, to what degree do differences in the risk due to radiation from the bomb, and in changes in the risk with respect to time, actually depend on the particular type of leukemia? In order to answer such questions, it is necessary to employ sophisticated statistical techniques. At the present time, leukemia data is being analyzed using the new DS86 dosimetry system and the application of the latest analytical methods.

The risk involved is indicated by the relative risk, in which the leukemia risk for the non-survivor population (for whom the radiation dose from the bomb can be ignored) is taken to be one. As can be seen from Fig. 1, the relative leukemia risk is directly proportional to the bone marrow dose[5]. The dose-dependent increase in relative risk is particularly striking for chronic myelogenous leukemia (CML) and acute lymphocytic leukemia (ALL), indicating the great likelihood that these forms of leukemia are induced by radiation. Following that, radiation exposure was strongly associated with acute myelogenous leukemia (AML). Two other forms of leukemia that are found are chronic lymphocytic leukemia (CLL), which is not common in Japan, and adult T-cell leukemia (ATL); however, there is no evidence to suggest that the incidence of these two types of leukemia increased as a result of the atomic explosion.

The age at the time of bombing (ATB) is one of the most important factors affecting not only the radiation-related leukemia risk but also the changes in the risk with respect to time. Figures 2 and 3 respectively show the changes with respect to time in excess leukemia risk (the increased risk of developing leukemia following

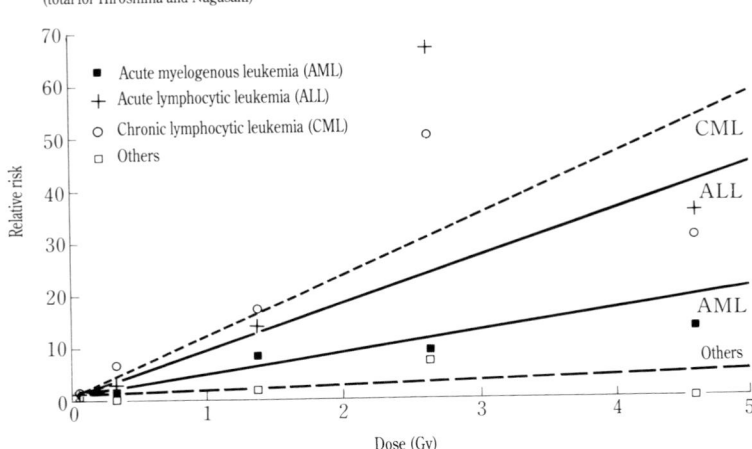

(total for Hiroshima and Nagasaki)

Figure 1   Relative risks of different forms of leukemia

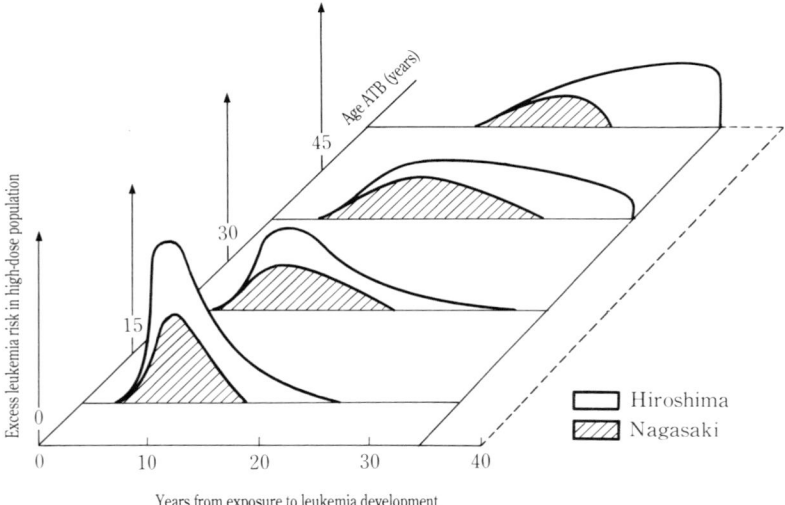

Figure 2   Excess leukemia risk due to radiation by age at the time of bombing (ATB) and years from exposure to leukemia development (latency period)

exposure to 1 Gy) and in the excess relative risk. From Fig. 2 it can be seen that of the leukemia cases occurring between 1950 and 1978, for heavily exposed individuals exposed to a ⩾ 1.0 Gy total kerma dose a difference exists between the two cities with respect to the induction of leukemia in age ATB and in the time from exposure to development of leukemia. Also, for those cases included in the total of all leukemias that developed between 1950 and 1987 for whom the DS86 method yields a clear individual dose estimate, Fig. 3 shows the excess relative risk with respect to

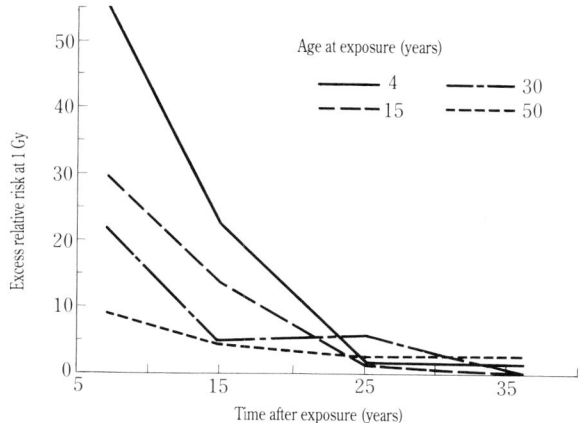

Figure 3   Excess relative risk for all types of leukemia, 1950–1987

age ATB and length of time after exposure. The results from Figs. 2 and 3 show that the leukemia risk increases with a decrease in age ATB, and that survivors exposed at young ages exhibit a maximum risk at 5 to 10 years after exposure, after which the risk decreases rapidly.

Conversely, as the age ATB increases, the increase in the short-term risk becomes less, and the tendency to decrease is gradual. At approximately 30 years after exposure, the difference in excess relative risk due to age ATB is almost negligible, with the excess relative risks for young and old survivors being approximately equal. This kind of change with respect to time in the effect of age ATB is especially striking in the case of ALL[3]. The excess relative risks of CML and AML appear to decrease with time after exposure for all age groups.

Another important factor to consider in a discussion on the incidence of leukemia in atomic bomb survivors is the frequency with which leukemia occurs naturally (the "background" frequency). By analyzing the leukemia incidence in the non-exposed population, it is possible to determine the background frequencies according to region, age, and generation. Significant observations revealed by an analysis of background data are that the CML incidence in Hiroshima is approximately three times that in Nagasaki; that the AML incidence increases with age, and moreover has been increasing in recent years; and that the incidence of ALL is lower than for AML but similarly increases in the aged and has exhibited an increase in recent years.

The previously mentioned relative risk is demonstrated by a comparison with the incidence and risk in the non-exposed population. Therefore even if the relative risk is high, if the background frequency is low, then the number of cases may be small; conversely, even if the relative risk is low, if the background frequency is high, then the number of cases observed may be high. For example, although there is no difference between Hiroshima and Nagasaki in the relative CML risk, since the background frequency in Nagasaki is low, a marked difference is believed to exist between the two cities with regard to the number of cases observed amongst the atomic bomb survivors. The absolute risk can be considered equal to the relative risk multiplied by the background frequency. It was previously believed that the CML incidence in Hiroshima amongst the proximally exposed survivors is greater than in Nagasaki, but this was a result yielded by analyses employing the excess risk model[6].

At the present time, approximately a half century after the bombing, interest is focused on the question of what percentage of leukemia is due to the atomic bomb. It appears from recent data currently being analyzed that the excess leukemia risk has not yet completely disappeared[5]. Moreover, since the background frequency is expected to rise with the aging of the young atomic bomb survivors, it is necessary to continue to closely monitor future trends in leukemia risk.

(Kiyohiko Mabuchi, Shizuyo Kusumi)

REFERENCES

1. Committee on the Biological Effects of Ionizing Radiation. Commission on Life Science. Health effects of exposure to low levels of ionizing radiation (BEIR-V). National Academy of Sciences-National Research Council. Washington, DC: National Academy Press, 1990: 421.
2. Folley JH, Borges W, Yamasaki T. Incidence of leukemia in the atomic bomb survivors of Hiroshima and Nagasaki, Japan. *Am J Med* 1952; **13**: 311–21.
3. Ishimaru T, Hoshino T, Ichimaru M, *et al.* Leukemia in atomic bomb survivors in ABCC master sample, Hiroshima and Nagasaki 1 October 1950 to 30 September 1966. ABCC TR 25–69, 1969.
4. Lange RD, Moloney WC, Yamawaki T. Leukemia in atomic bomb survivors. ABCC TR 25–59, 1959.
5. Kusumi S, Matsuo T. *Nagasaki Igakkai Zasshi* 1990; 65(Suppl): 501–6. (*In Japanese*)
6. Ichimaru M, Ishimaru T, Mikami M, *et al.* Incidence of leukemia in a fixed cohort of atomic bomb survivors and controls, Hiroshima and Nagasaki. October 1950–December 1978. RERF TR 13–81, 1981.

1.2   LEUKEMIA

b.   CHROMOSOMAL ABERRATIONS AND CLINICAL CHARACTERISTICS

INTRODUCTION

As mentioned in the general introduction and the previous chapter, leukemia was frequently observed among atomic bomb survivors, who were exposed to a single large dose of radiation. When speculating about the mechanism by which radiation causes leukemia it is extremely important to consider whether atomic bomb-related leukemia exhibits characteristic clinical features and cytogenetic findings.

Research into human chromosomes has been carried out since around 1900. In 1956 it was reported that normal human cells contain 46 chromosomes[1]; the discovery that chromosomal aberrations are present in human leukemia was made in 1960[2]. Chromosome techniques were applied to the study of leukemia cases among the Hiroshima atomic bomb survivors, and abnormalities were detected in 1962[3]. Chromosomal analysis first became possible during the period in which the leukemia incidence in Hiroshima was on the decline, but valuable data has been obtained from the later accumulation of cases. This chapter deals with chromosomal aberrations and clinical characteristics of atomic bomb-related leukemia.

There are three main clinical characteristics of atomic bomb-related leukemia. First, due to the twice-yearly examinations undergone by the atomic bomb survivors, the illness can be monitored in detail prior to actual manifestation. Second, a comparison of clinical data between exposed and non-exposed individuals at the time of the initial diagnosis of acute leukemia reveals different characteristics, with the exposed population exhibiting many characteristics of aleukemic leukemia and the leukemia observed in aged patients. Third, relative to the non-exposed, a higher frequency (and greater complexity) of chromosomal aberrations is observed in the leukemic cells of atomic bomb-related leukemia cases.

1. THE PRE-LEUKEMIC STAGE

A. Acute Leukemia

Many atomic bomb survivors exhibited long-term normocytic anemia and leuko-penia, with a considerable number developing leukemia. Figure 1 shows the case of a woman exposed to a T65D dose of 4.83 Gy at a distance of 800 meters from the hypocenter. Approximately 15 years before developing leukemia she exhibited leukopenia, followed by anemia with a hemoglobin (Hb) level below 11 g/dl; bone marrow cell instability was observed 16 years prior to onset of leukemia, and finally she developed erythroleukemia[4]. Figure 2 shows various hematologic abnormalities in 6 pre-leukemic stage cases who later developed acute leukemia[5], the abnormalities observed being refractory anemia, hypoplastic anemia, sideroblastic anemia, leuko-penia, and monocytosis. The arrows in Fig. 2 pointing up towards the base line

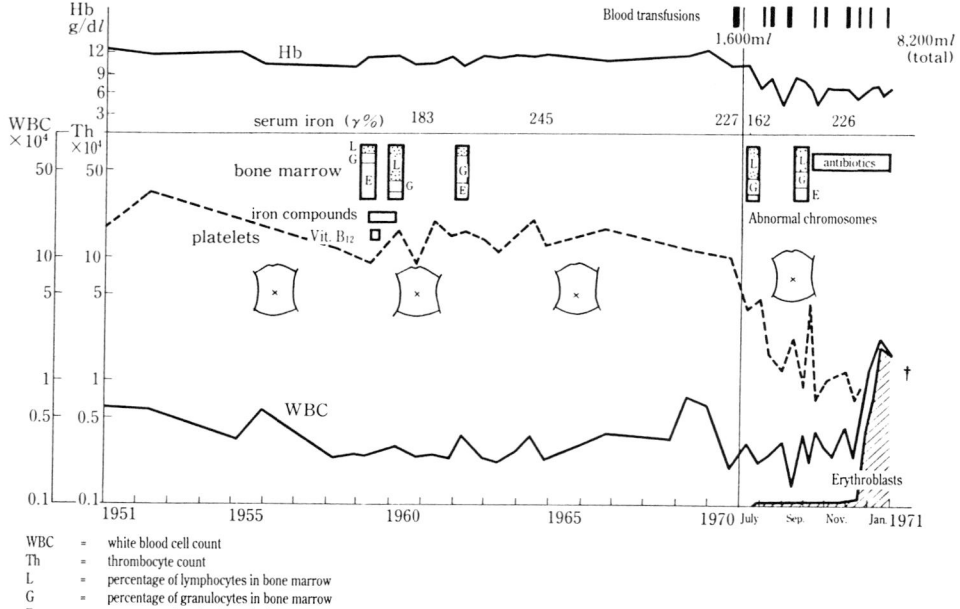

WBC   =   white blood cell count
Th   =   thrombocyte count
L   =   percentage of lymphocytes in bone marrow
G   =   percentage of granulocytes in bone marrow
E   =   percentage of erythroblasts in bone marrow

Figure 1   Clinical course of a 61 year old female with AML (acute myelogenous leukemia).
The patient had been exposed to atomic bomb radiation at 800 meters from the hypocenter, and remained in a preleukemic state for a long period of time.

Case number	Age (years)	Sex	Distance from hypocenter (Km)	Estimated radiation dose (Gy)
1	49	Female	3.1 km	0
2	54	Female	1.0	3.50
3	59	Male	Early entrant	0
4	61	Female	0.8	4.83
5	48	Female	0.9	3.64
6	73	Male	1.8	0.25

Refractory anemia (13 yrs)   ☐ AMoL
☆

Leukopenia (11 yrs)   ⊿ Eryth.L.
☆ ↑

Hypoplastic anemia (10 yrs)   ☐ Eryth.L.
↑

Leukopenia (13 yrs)   ⊿ Eryth.L.
☆ Mastectomy   ↑

Monocytosis (5 yrs)   ⊿ AMoL
⇩

Sideroblastic anemia (2 yrs)   ⊿ AGL
☆↑

1950   1955   1960   1965   1970   1975

AMol = acute monocytic leukemia
Eryth. L. = erythroleukemia
AGL = acute granulocytic leukemia

Figure 2   Pre-leukemia stage in atomic-bomb related leukemia
☆ = Time at which cells exhibited morphological abnormalities
↑ = Time at which chromosomal aberrations were observed

indicate the time at which chromosomal aberrations were detected in bone marrow cells, with chromosomal aberrations in some cases observed several years prior to the onset of leukemia. Morphological abnormalities in the bone marrow cells can be observed 2–11 years before leukemia develops, with abnormalities in bone marrow cells occurring in two or three of the following: granulocytes, erythroblasts, and megakaryocytes (platelets).

B. Chronic Myelocytic Leukemia

Hematologic abnormalities occurring prior to onset of leukemia have also been closely monitored in 28 atomic bomb survivors suffering from chronic myelocytic leukemia[6]. Figure 3 shows the changes with time in the hemograms of an atomic bomb survivor exposed at 800 meters from the hypocenter who developed leukemia 35 years after exposure[7]; Fig. 4 shows the changes for a survivor exposed at 1,800 m who developed leukemia 22 years after exposure[8]. Although detailed blood tests were carried out prior to development of leukemia, both cases showed a normal leukocyte count of 8,000, with an already apparent increase in basophils, which is characteristic of the illness (shown in the diagram as "Ba," a normal basophil count would be under 2.0%). Along with a gradual increase in leukocytes, the neutrophil alkaline phosphatase (AP) score decreases (indicated as "N-AP score," with a normal minimum of 180), the immature granulocytes (shown as "immature gr.") increase, vitamin B_{12} increases, and splenomegaly clearly occurs when the leukocyte count rises above 50,000. The detailed regular examinations undergone by the atomic

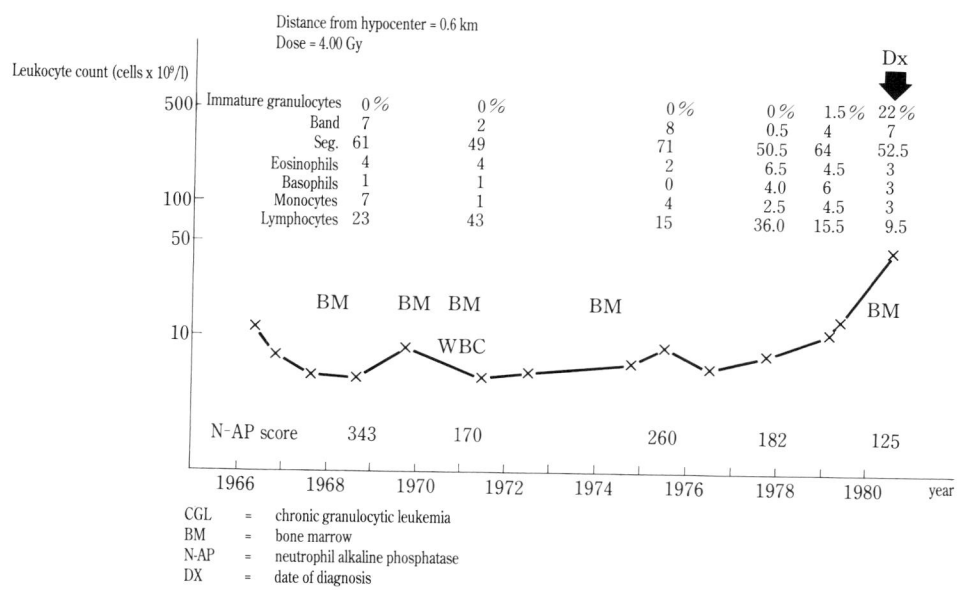

Figure 3   Blood data prior to CML development, case #1

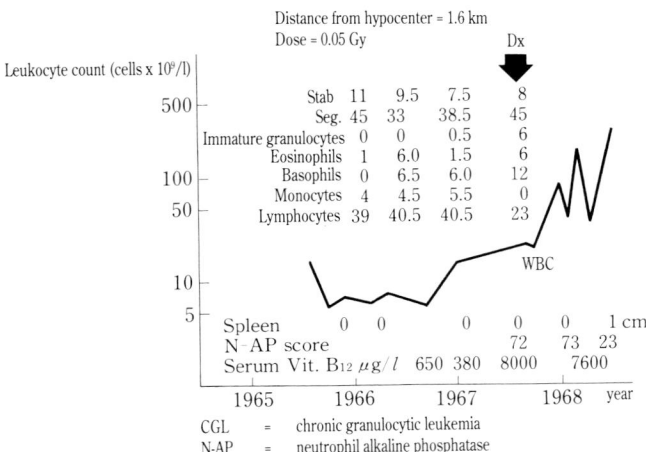

Figure 4   Blood data prior to CGL development, case #2

bomb survivors have thus clearly revealed the process by which chronic myelocytic leukemia develops and have proved extremely useful in permitting early diagnosis of this illness.

2. CLINICAL CHARACTERISTICS OF ATOMIC BOMB-RELATED LEUKEMIA

A. Acute Leukemia

When considering the process by which leukemia is initiated by radiation, an extremely important question is whether or not the clinical patterns observed are the same as those in naturally occurring leukemia. In a multivariate discriminant analysis, 31 survivors who were directly exposed within 2.5 km of the hypocenter and who developed acute myelocytic leukemia at over 35 years of age were compared with 51 leukemia cases whose situation was the same except that they had not been exposed to the bomb. Differences were found between the exposed and non-exposed leukemia populations in seven categories, as shown in Fig. 5[9]. That is, compared with the non-exposed population, the atomic bomb-related leukemia was characterized by a reduced number of leukemic cells in the peripheral blood; leukemic cells were present in the bone marrow, but tended to appear in only very small amounts in peripheral blood. In addition, the leukemia of atomic bomb survivors under 55 years of age exhibited many of the characteristics observed in non-exposed leukemia patients aged 55 and over.

B. Chronic Myelocytic Leukemia

Since 1950 the Atomic Bomb Casualty Commission, ABCC (the present-day Radiation Effects Research Foundation, RERF) has carried out regular screening of some

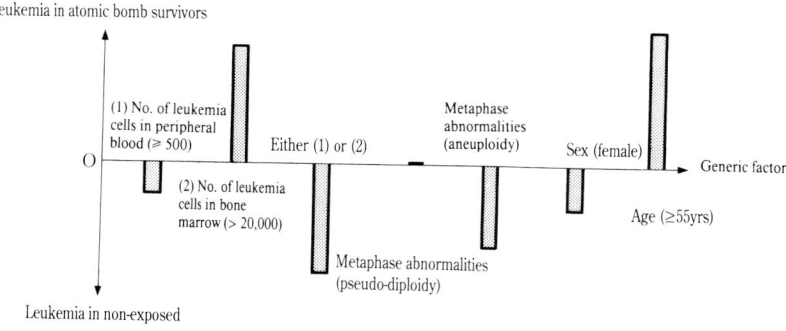

Figure 5 Comparison of leukemia in atomic bomb survivors and the non-exposed with respect to the relative importance of various generic factors (determined by discriminant analysis)

members of a cohort, while the Hiroshima Atomic Bomb Survivors Health Clinic has performed regular screening of all atomic bomb survivors since 1961. Consequently, in a considerable number of cases early detection of chronic myelocytic leukemia has been achieved in Hiroshima since this time[3,10]. As will be mentioned later, a characteristic of chronic myelocytic leukemia, the Philadelphia (Ph$_1$) chromosome, was present in all the survivors with this affliction, and apart from the mildness of the symptoms resulting from early detection such as leukocyte count and degree of splenomegaly[11,12], no clinical difference could be discerned between this population and non-exposed leukemia patients. Comparisons of survival times have not yet clarified whether the slightly extended survival period of the atomic bomb survivor population is due to the effect of early treatment, simply because of the extended period of observation accompanying early detection, or as a result of the leukemic cells in atomic bomb leukemia victims having a characteristically long cell cycle. The periodic examinations at both the governmental and private levels have recently been improved and greater opportunities for early detection have also become available to non-exposed individuals. It may now become possible to perform comparisons of leukemic conditions between exposed and non-exposed individuals.

3. CHROMOSOMAL CHANGES IN ATOMIC BOMB-RELATED LEUKEMIA

Chromosomal analysis of leukemia cases among Hiroshima atomic bomb survivors began relatively early, when chromosomal testing of leukemic cells became technologically possible. Chromosome analyses were performed on 75 atomic bomb survivors with acute leukemia and on 55 with chronic myelocytic leukemia (including both chronic and acute blastic phases).

A. Acute Leukemia

It has already been clarified that the healthy bone marrow cells of atomic bomb survivors who were exposed within 1,000 meters of the hypocenter but who did not exhibit sickness actually possess complex chromosomal aberrations which are directly proportional to the dose of radiation received[7]. However, very little is yet known about the relationship between these chromosomal aberrations and the development of leukemia[13,14]. In order to clarify this, it is possible to consider the significance of chromosome aberrations from a completely different angle, i.e. by an analysis of those cases in which leukemia had already developed. The relationship between chromosomal aberrations in the leukemic cells and radiation dose was investigated for 331 cases born before August 1945 who developed leukemia between September 1962 and March 1989[15]. Atomic bomb survivors accounted for 75 of these cases, and were divided into groups according to the DS86 bone marrow dose, i.e. ≥ 1.0 Gy (16 cases), 0.01–0.99 Gy (11 cases), and 0 Gy (25 cases), with all these being directly exposed within 1–2 km of the hypocenter. Although no dose estimate was performed for the remaining 23 cases, they were included in the 0.01–0.99 Gy population during the statistical calculations since the dose they received was believed to fall within this range. This total of 75 cases was then compared with 261 cases of naturally occurring leukemia, and an analysis was performed concerning both the frequency and complexity of chromosomal aberrations. Table 1 shows the distribution of leukemia subtypes according to the French-American-British (FAB) classification. Not a single case of acute promyelocytic leukemia (FAB M3, i.e. type M3 in the FAB classification) was observed in the ≥ 1.0 Gy population; on the other hand, the frequency of erythroleukemia (FAB M6) development was relatively high. Classification of the cases in this population by chromosomal mode (Table 2) revealed that all had chromosomal aberrations, with 4 in or below mode 45, 9 exhibiting abnormal metaphase in mode 46, and 3 in mode 47 and above. In comparison with the ≥ 1.0 Gy population, in which the chromosomal aberration rate was 100%, the frequency of chromosomal abnormalities in the other populations (0.01–0.99 Gy, 0 Gy, and the non-exposed) ranged between 52.9% and 60.9%. The heavily exposed population (≥ 1.0 Gy) thus showed a clearly greater frequency of aberration (p < 0.01).

Table 1   Distribution of leukemia subtypes by FAB classification[1,2]

Bone marrow dose (Gy) (DS86)	M1	M2	M3	M4	M5	M6	MDS	Total
1.0 ~	2	4	0	1	1	5	3	16
0.1 ~ 0.99 and unknown doses[3]	8	7	3	2	2	3	9	34
0	11	6	0	1	3	3	1	25
Non-exposed	62	72	25	24	13	30	35	261

1) Study period = Sep. 1962–March 1989.
2) Even in cases where onset of illness was prior to 1980, FAB classifications were performed on the basis of bone marrow samples.
3) Survivors exposed at 1.0 ~ 2.0 km; total includes 25 survivors for whom DS86 dose estimates were not performed.
4) MDS = myelodysplastic syndrome

Table 2   Atomic bomb-related leukemia by chromosome mode

Bone marrow dose (Gy) (DS86)	Chromosome mode										Percentage of cases with chromosomal aberrations (%)
	42	43	44	45	46 (Normal)	46 (Pseudodiploidy)	47	48	≥49	Total	
1.0 ~	2			2		9		2	1	16	100[2)]
0.1 ~ 0.99 and unknown doses[1]				4	16	10	4			34	52.9
0			2	3	11	6	2		1	25	56.0
Non-exposed	2	4	8	34	102	71	26	6	8	261	60.9

*$p < 0.001$

1) Survivors exposed at 1.0 ~ 2.0 km; total includes 25 survivors for whom 0586 estimates were not performed.

2) $p < 0.001$

When computing the number of aberrations in a typical metaphase in each of the cases, each trisomy (e.g. + 8, + 9), each monosomy (e.g. – 8, – 9), and each deletion (e.g. del)[5] was treated as a single abnormality; however, each translocation (e.g. t)[11,19], each inversion and each interstitial deletion was treated as two abnormalities. As can be seen in Table 3, in the ≥ 1.0 Gy population the number of cases exhibiting 3 or more chromosomal aberrations (i.e. those included in the categories of 3–4, 5–6, or more than 9 aberrations) accounted for 75% of the total (p < 0.05), and it is clear that the karyotype abnormalities are more complex than in the other populations.

Chromosomal aberrations were thus observed in the leukemic cells of all the leukemia cases in which the atomic bomb survivor received a bone marrow dose in excess of 1 Gy, with the karyotype abnormalities (including the aberrations in the No.5 and No.7 chromosomes) being more complex than in individuals receiving smaller doses. The significance and relevance of this becomes clear by referring to the results of the chromosome analyses carried out on healthy survivors who had not

Table 3   Frequency of various totals of chromosomal aberrations

Bone marrow dose (Gy) (DS86)	Number of metaphases with chromosomal aberrations							Percentage of cases with 3 or more chromosomal aberrations (%)
	0	1–2	3–4	5–6	7–8	9–10	11–	
1.0–	0	4	8	2	0	1	1	75*
0.1–0.99 and unknown doses[1]	16	14	3	1	0	0	0	11.7
0	11	8	2	0	0	2	2	24.0
Non-exposed	102	90	38	8	6	8	11	26.4

*$p < 0.05$

1) Survivors exposed at 1.0 ~ 2.0 km; total includes 25 survivors for whom DS86 estimates were not performed.

developed leukemia. That is, for 30 of the 31 healthy survivors exposed within 500 meters of the hypocenter (96.8%), an average of 23.6% of cells exhibited various chromosomal aberrations (it can probably be assumed that the majority of these survivors were exposed to ≥ 1 Gy); 7 of the healthy survivors possessed abnormal clones. Taking all these chromosomal aberrations into consideration, it is likely that the bone marrow stem cells in the leukemia cases in the ≥ 1.0 Gy population developed abnormalities as a result of the atomic bomb radiation, passing through various bone marrow conditions. That is, the complex abnormal metaphase observed in the leukemic cells is believed to have been caused by the atomic bomb.

B. Chronic Myelocytic Leukemia

Between 1962 and March 1985 chromosome analyses were carried out on 55 atomic bomb survivors with atomic bomb-related chronic myelocytic leukemia (36 chronic phase cases, and 19 acute blastic phase cases)[15]. By estimated T65D doses, 7 had been exposed to 2 Gy (airborne dose), 28 to 0.01–2.0 Gy, and 20 to under 0.01 Gy; these were compared to 167 non-exposed individuals (Table 4). Regardless of whether or not the patients had been exposed, in all the chronic myelocytic leukemia cases the presence of the chromosome specific to this disease, Philadelphia (Ph[1]) chromosome, [translocation between chromosomes 9 and 22; t(9; 22) (q34; q11)] was detected. Except for the presence of the Ph[1] chromosome, no difference in chromosomal aberrations was observed between the two populations, both having figures of 20% for the chronic cases and nearly 80% for the acute blastic phase cases. However, this leaves the question of why complex karyotype abnormalities are not observed in chronic myelocytic leukemia, whereas they are in acute leukemia and myelodysplastic syndrome (MDS). There is also the problem of why, although various abnormalities can be seen in bone marrow cells when the subject is in good health, only Ph[1] chromosome aberrations (specific to this illness) are observed when chronic myelocytic leukemia appears. This suggests a difference in the mechanism of leukemogenesis between acute leukemia and chronic myelocytic leukemia. In the latter disease, the cells that have suffered radiation damage do not themselves undergo leukemogenesis; however, it is the translocation between the No. 9 and No. 22 chromosomes in the bone marrow that can be considered the most important change, irrespective of the presence of damaged or non-damaged cells. The mechanism by which radiation-damaged cells undergo a malignant transformation has not yet been fully clarified, and is a major problem in the field of molecular biology requiring further thorough investigation.

Table 4   Chronic myelocytic leukemia cases[1]

Dose[2] (Gy)	Chronic phase cases	Acute blastic phase cases	Total
> 20	4	3	7
0.01–2.0	18	10	28
< 0.01	14	6	20
Non-exposed	111	56	167

CONCLUSION

As described in the previous chapter, it is common knowledge that atomic bomb survivors frequently developed leukemia; however, a major question is whether atomic bomb-related leukemia has any special clinical characteristics. Even if each individual case were examined in detail, it would be difficult to detect any direct difference from non-exposed leukemia sufferers; however, the significance of the dose-response relationship and individual observations is made clear when statistical methods are applied to the many leukemia cases in the two populations. The pre-leukemic state mentioned at the beginning is certainly not a special characteristic of atomic bomb survivors; however, intermittent regular screening was only performed on special populations, such as the atomic bomb survivors and the mustard gas workers on Ohkuno island in Hiroshima prefecture, and with the atomic bomb survivors there were numerous opportunities for hematologic abnormalities to be detected prior to the development of leukemia. Next, the multivariate analysis of clinical observations of acute myelocytic leukemia revealed clearly that the exposed leukemia patients exhibited many characteristics of aleukemic leukemia and the leukemia found among aged subjects, which was confirmed when individual cases were reexamined. Finally, with regard to chromosomal aberrations, as has been described in this chapter, various observations are needed in order to clarify the mechanism by which leukemia is initiated, and detailed study of the accumulation of future cases together with the application of molecular biology techniques is a major task that needs to be performed.

(Nanao Kamada)

REFERENCES

1. Tjio JH, Levan A. The chromosome of man. *Hereditas* 1956; **42**: 1–4.
2. Nowell PC, Hungerford DA. Chromosome studies on normal and leukemia human leukocytes. *J Natl Cancer Inst* 1960; **25**: 85–109.
3. Tanaka N, Ito K, Kamada N, *et al.* A case of atomic bomb survivor with chronic granulocytic leukemia in the early stage. *J Kyushu Hematol Society* 1963; **13**: 124–8.
4. Uchino H, Kamada N. Detection of preleukemic state. *J Jap Med Ass* 1972; **67**: 1415–38. (*In Japanese*)
5. Kamada N, Uchino H. Preleukemic states in atomic bomb survivors in Japan. *Blood Cells* 1976; **2**: 57–65.
6. Ohtaki M, Kamada N, Kamioka H, *et al.* Quantitative analysis of the clinical data on leukemia. IV. Variation of WBC at preclinical stage in CML of A-bomb survivors. *Proceedings of 23rd Late Effects of Atomic Bomb*; 1982 June 6; Nagasaki. *The Late Effects of Radiation*, 1983: 77–82. (*In Japanese*)
7. Kamada N, Tanaka K. Cytogenetic studies of hematological disorders in atomic bomb survivors. In: Ishihara T, Sasaki M, editors. Radiation induced chromosome damage in man. New York: Alan R Liss, 1983: 455–74.
8. Kamada N, Oguma N, Tanaka R, *et al.* Clinical picture of chronic granulocytic leukemia in the early stage. —A retrospective analysis from atomic bomb survivors—*Nagasaki Med J* 1976; **51**: 175–9. (*In Japanese*)
9. Kamada M, Ohtaki M, Kamioka Y, *et al.* Quantitative analysis of the clinical data on leukemia. III. Analysis of clinical features of acute non-lymphocytic leukemia in atomic bomb survivors by means of discriminant function. *J Hiroshima Med Ass* 1982; **35**: 450–4. (*In Japanese*)

10. Moloney WC, Lange RD. Leukemia in atomic bomb survivors. II. Observations on the early phase of leukemia. *Blood* 1954; **9**: 663–85.

11. Kamada N, Okada K, Ito T, *et al.* Chromosome aberrations and neutrophil alkaline phosphatase in forty-three cases of leukemia, including fourteen cases of leukemia in atomic bomb survivors. *J Kyushu Hematol Society* 1967; **17**: 115–42.

12. Tsuchimoto T, Kamada N, Ishii Y, *et al.* A study of chronic granulocytic leukemia with special reference to atomic bomb survivors. *Proc RINMB* Hiroshima Univ 1970: 132–7.

13. Tanaka K, Kamada N. Leukemogenesis and chromosome aberrations: *de novo* leukemia in humans —with special reference to atomic bomb survivors. *Acta Haemat Jpn* 1985; **48**: 1830–43.

14. Kamada N, Tanaka K, Hasegawa A. Chromosome aberrations and transforming genes in leukemia and non-leukemia patients with a history of atomic bomb exposure. In: Miller RW, editor. Unusual occurrences as clues to cancer etiology. Tokyo: Japan Sci Soc Press, 1988: 125–34.

15. Kamada N, Tanaka K, Oguma N, *et al.* Cytogenetic and molecular biological studies on atomic bomb-related leukemia. *Nagasaki Med J* 1990; **65**: 513–9. (*In Japanese*)

1.3 GASTRIC CANCER

INTRODUCTION

Malignant tumors are an important late effect of the atomic bombing. Great interest surrounds the effect of atomic bomb radiation on the incidence of gastric cancer, which is the most common form of cancer amongst Japanese people. The relationship between radiation and gastric cancer attracted attention after Court Brown and Doll[1] reported in 1965 that gastric cancer increased among patients undergoing radiotherapy for ankylosing spondylitis. Following a report by Radford et al[2] in 1977 that no increase in gastric cancer was observed among ankylosing spondylitis patients not given X-ray treatment, it became evident that a relationship existed between X-ray irradiation and the development of gastric cancer.

Animal experiments have also been performed in an attempt to induce gastric carcinomas by X-rays[3-6], with Hirose[3,4] demonstrating the development of gastric cancer in rats and mice. Histologically, however, these were well-differentiated adenocarcinomas, and differed in histologic type from the cancers in atomic bomb survivors, which will be discussed later. Nowell et al[5,6] also observed a tendency for an increased gastric cancer incidence following irradiation of mice with X-rays or neutrons. Since the natural incidence of gastric cancer in experimental animals is extremely low, these results indicate the possibility of gastric cancer induction by radiation exposure, even though the results are not directly applicable to human beings.

The mucous membrane of the human stomach and intestines is extremely sensitive to radiation, with acute radiation effects observed as damage to these organs; this has been clearly shown by e.g. abnormalities in the mucous membrane of the stomach and intestines observed at autopsy in patients who died shortly after the bombing. A very important question is whether or not gastric carcinomas are a late manifestation of this damage. This chapter will focus on the reports that have so far appeared in the literature concerning the relationship between the development of gastric cancer and atomic bomb radiation, and will also consider the histological characteristics.

1. INCIDENCE OF GASTRIC CANCER

In order to investigate the relationship between the gastric cancer incidence and atomic bomb radiation, a stomach mass-screening vehicle was used between 1964 and 1970 for testing the 45,930 atomic bomb survivors over the age of 40 who were resident in Hiroshima at the time of bombing. Ito et al[7] reported in 1973 that the number of people actually tested was 15,288 and that the incidence of gastric cancer among the population directly exposed within 1.9 km of the hypocenter (0.56%) was significantly greater than that observed among the early entrants (i.e. individuals who entered the area shortly after the bombing), first aid workers, fallout victims and those directly exposed at $\geqslant$ 4.0 km (Table 1). Even though this analysis covered a low proportion of the people concerned (33.3%) and exposure conditions were defined by distance from the hypocenter etc., leading to some slight problems regarding the accuracy relative to analyses using radiation doses, this report nevertheless was the first to use the results of mass screening to demonstrate the high rate of gastric cancer

Table 1   Observed and estimated gastric cancer detection rates[7]

Exposure status	Age (yrs)	No. of examinees	Percentage undergoing detailed examination	No. of gastric cancer cases	Estimated gastric cancer cases	Detection rate (%)	Estimated detection rate (%)
Direct exposure within 1.9 km	40–49	1,324	73.4	2	2.7	0.15	0.21
	50–59	1,451	76.5	7	9.2	0.48	0.63
	60–69	1,589	72.7	8	11.0	0.50	0.69
	50–	978	69.1	5	7.2	0.51	0.74
	Total	5,342	73.2	22	30.1	0.41	0.56
Direct exposure at 2.0 – 3.9 km	40–49	1,375	72.2	1	1.4	0.07	0.10
	50–59	1,577	77.8	3	3.9	0.19	0.24
	60–69	1,777	76.3	6	7.9	0.34	0.44
	50–	1,135	70.5	5	7.1	0.44	0.62
	Total	5,864	74.6	15	20.1	0.26	0.34
Early entry to city, etc.	40–49	1,034	82.2	0	0	0	0
	50–59	1,301	80.5	3	3.7	0.23	0.29
	60–69	1,170	89.9	3	3.7	0.25	0.31
	50–	576	74.7	1	1.3	0.17	0.23
	Total	4,082	80.5	7	8.7	0.17	0.21

among proximally exposed atomic bomb survivors. A report comparing the results of mass stomach screening between 1972 and 1982 with gastric cancer rates classified according to the T65DR atomic bomb dose revealed that the rate increased dose-dependently for both males and females, and also that the rate in the ≥ 1.0 Gy population was significantly higher than in the 0 Gy population (Table 2)[8]. The relative risk for the ≥ 1.0 Gy population was 4.29 times that for the 0 Gy population in the case of males, and 4.02 times in the case of females. The rate of gastric cancer among people aged 34 years or less at the time of bombing (ATB) tended to be higher than among those aged 35 or older.

Table 2   Gastric cancer incidence by dose[8]

Sex	Male			Female			Total		
	No. of examinees	Gastric cancer cases		No. of examinees	Gastric cancer cases		No. of examinees	Gastric cancer cases	
Estimated dose (Gy)		No. of cases	Percentage (%)		No. of cases	Percentage (%)		No. of cases	Percentage (%)
0	1,329	10	0.75	2,914	9	0.31	4,243	19	0.45
0.01 ~ 0.09	377	3	0.80	783	2	0.26	1,160	5	0.43
0.10 ~ 0.49	339	6	1.77	793	3	0.38	1,132	9	0.80
0.50 ~ 0.99	77	2	2.60	204	1	0.49	281	3	1.07
1.00 ~	127	4	3.15**	244	3	1.23*	371	7	1.89***
Total	2,249	25	1.11	4,938	18	0.36	7,187	43	0.60

*$p < 0.05$, **$p < 0.01$, ***$p < 0.005$, for ≥ 1 Gy vs. 0 Gy

The use of death certificates to investigate the rate of gastric cancer enables the collection of an extensive range of data; the accuracy of hospital diagnoses[9] was comparatively high. However, because of factors such as the early detection of gastric cancer due to advances in medicine and the expansion of mass screening programs, the rate of complete recovery from gastric cancer is rising and the use of analyses based on death certificates is gradually approaching the limit of usefulness. Analyses using tumor and tissue registries will become important in the future.

Prior to the 1977 reports by Beebe et al[10] and Nakamura[11], analyses based on death certificates showed a negative correlation between gastric cancer mortality and atomic bomb radiation[12,13]. However, in a study covering the period 1950–73, Nakamura[11] performed an analysis on approximately 80,000 individuals in a fixed population surveyed by the Atomic Bomb Casualty Commission (ABCC), and found an increased gastric cancer mortality rate among the heavily exposed population in Hiroshima.

The relationship with radioactivity first became apparent when gastric cancer incidence increased as the atomic bomb survivors reached the age at which cancer frequently occurs. According to the analysis by Shimizu et al[14] using DS86 dosimetry, classification by year of the relative gastric cancer risk for exposure to 1 Gy of radiation reveals an increased risk since 1976, with the figures being 1.45 for the period 1976–1980, 1.45 for 1981–1985, and 1.63 for 1983–85 (Table 3). Also, the lowest dose of radiation observed to lead to a significantly high cancer mortality rate relative to the 0 Gy population was calculated to be 1 Gy shielded kerma and 0.5 Gy organ dose.

As mentioned above, the reports published up until the first half of 1970 that used death certificates showed a negative correlation with radiation, but similar analyses published afterwards clearly showed high gastric cancer mortality rates for heavily exposed individuals[10,11,14].

2. HISTOLOGICAL CHARACTERISTICS OF GASTRIC CANCER

Reports concerning the histologic type of gastric cancer amongst atomic bomb survivors are scarce, but by studying autopsy cases, resected specimens, and biopsy specimens during the period 1950–1977, Sekine et al[15] demonstrated a tendency for a high rate of poorly differentiated adenocarcinomas amongst the heavily exposed atomic bomb survivors (Table 4). Yamamoto and Nakajima[16] also reported similar findings. Kato et al[17] analyzed 241 new cases of gastric cancer detected between

Table 3 Relative risk of gastric cancer at 1 Gy (shielded kerma) by period of observation[14]

Period	Deaths	Relative risk	Period	Deaths	Relative risk
1950–55	218	1.22	1971–75	330	1.11
1956–60	281	1.01	1976–80	303	1.45
1961–65	297	1.28	1981–85	256	1.45
1966–70	322	1.17	(1983–85)	145	1.63

Table 4   Histlogic type of gastric cancer by radiation dose[15]

| | Total | \multicolumn{4}{c}{T65R dose (Gy)} | | | |
		0	0.01–0.99	1.00–1.99	≥ 2.00
	1,345 (100)	386 (100)	519 (100)	41 (100)	53 (100)
Well to moderately differentiated	612 (45.5)	191 (49.5)	249 (48.0)	8 (19.5)	16 (30.2)
Poorly differentiated	474 (35.2)	123 (31.9)	187 (36.0)	19 (46.3)	22 (41.5)
Mucinous	80 (5.9)	28 (7.3)	21 (4.0)	4 (9.8)	4 (9.4)
Other	12 (0.9)	3 (0.8)	4 (0.8)	0 (0.0)	1 (1.9)
Uknown	167 (12.4)	41 (10.6)	58 (11.2)	10 (24.4)	9 (17.0)

(   ) Parentheses indicate percentage of totals.

1972 and 1982, and found that the incidence of poorly differentiated adenocarcinomas in the population directly exposed and within 1.9 km of the hypocenter was significantly higher than among early entrants (i.e. individuals who entered the city soon after the bombing) and other populations.

Problems occur in pathohistological investigations concerning the standardization of histological diagnoses and specimens (i.e. whether biopsy or resection specimens are used). Ito *et al*[18] collected pathological samples from hospitals in Hiroshima and analyzed the relationship between histologic type and exposure to radiation for the 231 cases for whom DS86 stomach doses were available out of 600 cases diagnosed by the same pathologist. As shown in Table 5, a regression coefficient of 0.319 was obtained between poorly differentiated adenocarcinomas (poorly differentiated adenocarcinomas and signet ring cell carcinoma) and the dose of radiation; a significantly higher incidence ($p > 0.05$) of poorly differentiated adenocarcinoma was found among the population exposed to ≥ 0.01 Gy (with an average organ dose of 0.306 Gy). Based on the above, the increased risk of poorly differentiated adenocarcinoma relative to an unexposed individual was 1.4 times for a DS86 stomach dose of 0.5 Gy, and 1.8 times for 1.0 Gy. Also, survivors aged under 30 ATB tended to have a higher rate of poorly differentiated adenocarcinoma.

There have been few studies on the relationships between radiation dose and stromal type, mode of invasion, and depth of invasion. Sekine *et al*[15] found that for both well-to-moderately differentiated and poorly differentiated adenocarcinomas the population exposed to a T65DR dose ≥ 2.0 Gy tended to exhibit an increased tumor interstitial volume, but that no difference was observed in the relationship between dose and mode of invasion, depth of invasion, and lymph vessel and venous invasion (Table 6). An analysis by Ito *et al*[18] using DS86 organ doses found that with

Table 5   Relative risk of poorly differentiated adenocarcinoma and regression coefficients (0 Gy vs. ≥ 0.01 Gy) with respect to percentage of cancers accounted for by poorly differentiated adenocarcinoma[15]

No. of cases	Regression coefficients			
	$\widehat{\alpha_0}$ ($\times$ 10)	$\widehat{\alpha_S}$ ($\times$ 10)	$\widehat{\alpha_a}$ ($\times$ 10)	$\widehat{\beta_d}$ ($\times$ 10)
231	4.717 (0.983)	0.263 (0.428)	-0.796Δ (0.449)	0.319 (0.315)

α_0 = intercept; α_2, α_a, and β_d = regression coefficients according to sex, age and dose respectively.
( ) Parentheses indicate standard error, $\Delta p < 0.10$, $*p < 0.05$

Relative risks

DS86 stomach dose (Gy)	0	0.01	0.20	0.50	1.00
Relative risks	1	1	1.2	1.4	1.8

Table 6   Relationship between stromal type, mode of invasion and depth of invasion (0 Gy vs. ≥ 0.01 Gy)[18]

Stromal type and mode of invasion		Regression coefficients			
		$\widehat{\alpha_0}$ ($\times$ 10)	$\widehat{\alpha_s}$ ($\times$ 10)	$\widehat{\alpha_a}$ ($\times$ 10)	$\widehat{\beta_d}$ ($\times$ 10)
Stromal type	Medullary type	4.377 (1.177)	0.675 (0.530)	0.195 (0.553)	$-0.323*$ (0.153)
	Intermediate type	2.942 (4.997)	-0.327 (0.225)	0.117 (0.235)	0.028 (0.065)
$n = 194$	Scirrhous type	2.682 (0.949)	-0.348 (0.427)	-0.312 (0.446)	0.294* (0.123)
Mode of invasion	INFα	0.462 (0.886)	0.527 (0.399)	0.885 (0.416)	-0.117 (0.115)
	INFβ	5.098 (0.799)	-0.539 (0.359)	0.001 (0.376)	-0.012 (0.104)
$n = 194$	INFγ	4.440 (1.411)	0.013 (0.635)	-0.884 (0.664)	0.189 (0.184)
Early cancer		5.039 (1.129)	-0.064 (0.051)	-0.691 (0.532)	-0.253Δ (0.152)

$*p < 0.05$, $\Delta p < 0.01$
α_S, α_a, and β_d = regression coefficients by sex, age and dose respectively.
$\gamma\alpha_0$ = intercept.
( ) Parentheses indicate standard error.

regard to stromal type, an increase in radiation dose led to a decrease in medullary type and an increase in scirrhous type (Table 7). The frequency of early cancer decreased with decreasing dose.

Table 7   Stromal type by histologic type of gastric cancer and radiation dose[15]

	T65DR dose (Gy)	No. of cases	Medullary type	Histologic type Intermediate type	Scirrhous type
Well, to moderately differentiated	0	187 (100.0)	65 (34.8)	117 (62.6)	5 (2.7)
	0.01 ~ 0.99	236 (100.0)	99 (41.9)	128 (54.2)	9 (3.8)
	1.00 ~ 1.99	7 (100.0)	4 (57.1)	3 (42.9)	0 (0.0)
	> 2.00	14 (100.0)	2 (14.3)	12 (85.7)	0 (0.0)
Poorly differentiated	0	120 (100.0)	22 (18.3)	50 (41.7)	48 (40.0)
	0.01 ~ 0.99	180 (100.0)	31 (17.2)	70 (38.9)	79 (43.9)
	1.00 ~ 1.99	19 (100.0)	3 (15.8)	10 (52.6)	6 (31.6)
	> 2.00	21 (100.0)	3 (14.3)	5 (23.8)	13 (61.9)

( ) Parentheses indicate percentages

CONCLUSION

The relationship between radiation dose and the development of gastric cancer and the pathohistological characteristics can at present be summarized as follows:

1)   The gastric cancer incidence among proximally exposed atomic bomb survivors was first clearly shown to be high in a 1973 report that used the results of mass stomach screening. Subsequent analyses employing T65DR doses also showed that both males and females in the ≥ 1.0 Gy population exhibited a clearly higher gastric cancer incidence than the 0 Gy population.

2)   The gastric cancer mortality rate obtained from death certificates increased after approximately 1976. The minimum shielded kerma dose producing a significantly high gastric cancer mortality rate relative to the 0 Gy population (DS86 dosimetry) was calculated to be 1 Gy, with the figure being 0.5 Gy in the case of organ doses.

3)   Pathohistological findings showed that poorly differentiated adenocarcinomas increased with dose, and with regard to stromal type, an increased dose led to a decrease in medullary type and an increase in scirrhous type. No difference was observed in terms of mode of invasion.

(Chikako Ito)

REFERENCES

1.   Court Brown WM, Doll R. Mortality from cancer and other causes after radiotherapy for ankylosing spondylitis. *Brit Med J* 1965; **2**: 1327–32.

2.   Radford EP, Doll R, Smith PB. Mortality among patients with ankylosing spondylitis not given X-ray therapy. *N Engl J Med* 1977; **297**: 572–6.

3.   Hirose F. Experimental induction of carcinoma in the glandular stomach by localized X-irradiation of gastric region. In: Experimental carcinoma of the glandular stomach. Japanese Cancer Association. *GANN Monograph on Cancer Res* 1969; **8**: 75–113.

4.   Hirose, F. Induction of gastric adenocarcinoma in mice by localized X-irradiation. *GANN* 1969; **60**: 253–60.

5. Nowell PC, Cole, LJ. Late effects of fast neutrons versus X-rays in mice, nephrosclerosis, tumors, longevity. *Radiat Res* 1959; **11**: 545–50.
6. Nowell PC, Cole LJ, Ellis ME. Neoplasms of the glandular stomach in mice irradiated with X-rays or fast neutrons. *Cancer Res* 1958; **18**: 257–60.
7. Ito C, Kumasawa T, Matsusaka Y. Investigation of stomach diseases in atomic bomb survivors. *J Hiroshima Med Ass* 1973; **26**: 43–53. (*In Japanese*)
8. Ito C, Hasegawa K, Kumasawa T. Incidence of gastric cancer in atomic bomb survivors residing the Hiroshima area. *Hiroshima J Med Sci* 1984; **33**: 47–52.
9. Steer A, Moriyama I, Shimizu K. ABCC-JNIH pathology studies, Hiroshima and Nagasaki, Report 3. ABCC TR 16–73, 1973.
10. Beebe GW, Kato H, Land CE. Life Span Study. Report 8. Mortality experience of atomic bomb survivors, 1950–74. RERF TR1–77, 1977.
11. Nakamura K. Stomach cancer in the atomic bomb survivors. RERF TR 8–77, 1977.
12. Murphy ES, Yasuda A. A carcinoma of the stomach in Hiroshima, Japan. *Am J Pathol* 1958; **34**: 531–42.
13. Yamamoto T, Kato H. Two major histological types of gastric carcinoma in a fixed population of Hiroshima and Nagasaki. *GANN* 1971; **62**: 381–7.
14. Shimizu Y, Kato H, Shull W. Life Span Study. Report 11. Part 2. Cancer mortality in the years 1950–85 based on the recently revised doses (DS86). RERF TR 5–88, 1988.
15. Sekine I, Nishimori I, Matsuura H, *et al.* Pathological and epidemiological studies of gastric cancer in atomic bomb survivors (1950–1977, Hiroshima and Nagasaki). *Proceedings of the 23rd Late A-bomb Effects Research Meeting*; June, 1981; Hiroshima. Hiroshima: Hiroshima Atomic Bomb Casualty Council, 1982: 105–112. (*In Japanese*)
16. Yamamoto T, Nakajima E. Histological type of cancer among A-bomb survivors. *J Hiroshima Med Ass* 1984; **37**: 448–51. (*In Japanese*)
17. Kato M, Mito K, Kumasawa T, *et al.* Pathological investigations on gastric cancer amongst atomic bomb survivors. *J Hiroshima Med Ass* 1986; **39**: 378–82. (*In Japanese*)
18. Ito C, Kato M, Yamamoto T, *et al.* Study of stomach cancer in atomic bomb survivors. Report 1. Histological findings and prognosis. *J Rad Res* 1989; **30**: 164–75.

1.4   LUNG CANCER

INTRODUCTION

Numerous reports have appeared on radiation-induced lung cancer in miners, including an old report on the Schneeberg mine in Germany[1], and others on the Joachimisthal mine in Czechoslovakia[2], a fluorspar mine in Newfoundland[3], and a uranium mine in Colorado[4] etc. As regards trials aimed at reproducing the growth of pulmonary tumors in experimental animals, some studies have involved airway inhalation of such radioactive materials as $^{144}CeO_2$ fumes, $Cr^{31}PO_4$, and $^{210}Po(NO_3)_2$etc.[5–7]; others have involved internal irradiation by intrapulmonary implantation of radioactive materials such as ^{90}Sr, ^{60}Co, and ^{106}Ru etc.[8–10]; and others have involved external irradiation[11,12].

1. LUNG CANCER INCIDENCE

The first notable report on the development of atomic bomb-related lung cancer was in 1956 by Oho[13], who classified 11,453 death certificates issued in Hiroshima between 1951 and 1955 according to whether or not the individual had been exposed to the atomic bomb, and then surveyed mortality rates due to malignant neoplasms. The number of deaths among the atomic bomb survivors due to malignant neoplasms of the digestive system, respiratory system, lymphatic tissue, and hematopoietic tissue were found to be above the national average, leading to speculation about the extent of the role played in the development of the malignant neoplasms by the primary and secondary radioactivity emanating from the atomic bomb (Table 1). In 1960 Shimizu[14–16] examined the population shifts and death certificates for Hiroshima over the period 1957–60 and found an increase in lung cancer deaths among males possessing atomic bomb survivors' health handbooks in comparison with both unregistered persons and the national average. In 1961 the Research Committee on Tumor Statistics of the Hiroshima City Medical Association[17] investigated documents relating to 1,750 malignant tumor cases registered over a 20-month period from 1957 to 1958. By comparing the expected and actually observed numbers of malignant neoplasms at various sites, the frequencies of cancer of the stomach, lung, breast, and ovary in atomic bomb survivors exposed within 1,500 meters of the hypocenter were found to be significantly higher than the expected values, and in the case of lung cancer 4.31 times the expected rate. In 1967 Fujimoto[18] reported on 50 patients confirmed as having lung cancer by cytologic diagnoses, surgery and autopsies at the Hiroshima Atomic Bomb Hospital during the 10-year period from 1956 to 1965. Twenty-six of the 50 cases had been within 2 km of the explosion, and since no difference was observed between the numbers of males and females within this cohort (a male : female ratio of 0.9 : 1.0) it was inferred that the lung cancer developed by the atomic bomb survivors was caused by the radioactivity released by the atomic bomb.

In 1968 Mansur *et al*[19] investigated the 200 cases of lung cancer included in 1,576 autopsies performed at the Atomic Bomb Casualty Commission (ABCC) in Hiroshima and Nagasaki during the 15-year period from 1950 to 1964, and found that

Table 1 Comparison of adjusted atomic bomb survivor mortality rates by type of malignant neoplasm with all-Japan figure (per 100,000 of total 1951 population)[13]

Disease type / Population	Oral cavity and pharynx		Digestive tract organs and peritoneum		Respiratory tract organs		Breasts	Uterus and other female organs	Male organs	Urinary organs		Lymphatic tissue and hematopoietic tissue		Others (including unknown sites)	
	Male	Female	Male	Female	Male	Female	Female	Female	Male	Male	Female	Male	Female	Male	Female
All Japan (1951)	1.0	0.5	68.2	43.9	4.2	2.0	3.3	19.9	0.7	1.1	0.7	3.1	2.0	3.2	3.1
Atomic bomb survivors (1951–55)	0.2	0.4	83.1	37.6	7.8	3.6	3.4	19.8	1.2	1.4	0.7	9.7	8.7	1.9	3.0

the relative frequency of each histologic type was similar to the results obtained in foreign studies. Radiation doses were estimated for 63 lung cancer cases in the ABCC Life Span Study sample autopsied during 1961–64. A significantly increased lung cancer risk was found for individuals exposed to ≥ 1.28 Gy relative to the low-dose population, including those distally exposed at over 2,000 meters from the hypocenter. In 1969 Tahara et al[20] reported on 60 autopsies carried out during the 8-year period between 1960 and 1967 on atomic bomb survivors who had died of lung cancer, and discovered that they were older than the idiopathic cases, that many of them had been within 2,000 meters of the bomb and, moreover, that the number of epidermoid cancer cases among the group within 2 km of the explosion was exceedingly high. It was reported that the primary lesion was frequently in the middle lung field, and that in comparison with the number of idiopathic lung cancer patients both men and women exhibited a high frequency of undifferentiated small cell carcinoma. In 1972 Cihak et al[21] surveyed the approximately 100,000-strong ABCC Life Span Study sample; 10,412 deaths occurred during the 10-year period 1961–1970, with 204 of the 3,778 cases autopsied recorded as having lung cancer. The prevalence of lung cancer amongst the survivors exposed to ≥ 2.0 Gy of atomic bomb radiation was double that for survivors exposed to ≤ 0.01 Gy. For atomic bomb survivors exposed to ≥ 2.0 Gy, a significant increase was found only for undifferentiated small cell carcinoma. Furthermore, all the three cases estimated to have received ≥ 4.0 Gy developed undifferentiated small cell carcinoma (Table 2).

In 1974 Hamada and Ishida[22] investigated the 650 malignant tumor cases included in the 1,037 autopsies performed at the Hiroshima Atomic Bomb Hospital and the Hiroshima Red Cross Hospital during the 16-year period between 1957 and 1972. Of these, 197 cases of malignant neoplasm were found in survivors exposed within 2 km of the hypocenter, with lung cancer predominant (39 cases). The number of autopsies on the proximally exposed lung cancer victims formed 13.4% of the total number of autopsies, and 19.8% of the number involving malignant neoplasms. These rates were double those recorded over a 5-year period by the "Annual of the Pathological Autopsy Cases in Japan" (edited by the Japan Pathological Society), which found that the national ratio of lung cancer cases to the total number of autopsies performed in Japan was 6.1% and that the ratio to total neoplasia cases autopsied in Japan was 10.4%. For every atomic bomb survivor population the lung cancer rate was inversely proportional to distance from the hypocenter, indicating a relationship with atomic bomb radiation.

In 1983 Sasaki et al[23] performed a comparative study of 138 atomic bomb survivors who developed lung cancer, and 226 lung cancers in non-exposed individuals who had been diagnosed at the Hiroshima Atomic Bomb Survivors Health Clinic and the Second Department of Internal Medicine at Hiroshima University during the 9-year period from 1972 to 1981; a significant increase in adenocarcinomas was observed among the male atomic bomb survivors. Also, in comparison with the non-exposed cases, the lung cancer victims who had been directly exposed within 2 km of the hypocenter exhibited a significantly lower frequency of squamous cell carcinomas, but a significantly higher frequency of adenocarcinomas (Tables 3 and 4). In 1987 Nishimoto et al[24] compared 206 atomic bomb survivors who were

Table 2 Crude prevalence rate for lung cancer in Life Span Study autopsy series by histologic type and dose, Hiroshima and Nagasaki, 1961–70[21]

Histologic type		Total dose (Gy)				Not in city	Total	Prevalence test
		No estimate	≥ 2.00	0.01 ~ 1.99	0.01			
Autopsies		58	127	1573	1196	824	3378	
Epidermoid	Number	2	3	30	17	13	65	
	Rate	34.5	23.6	19.1	14.2	15.8	17.2	P > .10
	Relative risk	2.4	1.7	1.3	1.0	—		
Small cell carcinoma	Number	0	5	14	12	8	39	
	Rate	—	39.4	8.9	10.0	9.7	10.3	P < .05
	Relative risk		3.9	0.9	1.0	—		
Bronchogenic adenocarcinoma	Number	2	4	21	19	13	59	
	Rate	34.5	31.5	13.4	15.9	15.8	15.6	P < .10
	Relative risk	2.2	2.0	0.8	1.0	—		
Bronchiolo-alveolar adenocarcinoma	Number	0	0	11	6	2	19	
	Rate	—	—	7.0	5.0	2.4	5.0	
	Relative risk	—	—	1.4	1.0	—	—	
Large cell carcinoma	Number	0	0	3	3	1	7	
	Rate	—	—	1.9	2.5	1.2	1.9	
	Relative risk	—	—	0.8	1.0	—	—	
Combined and unclassified	Number	0	1	5	4	5	15	
	Rate	—	7.9	3.2	3.3	6.1	4.0	
	Relative risk	—	2.4	1.0	1.0	—	—	

Table 3 Classification by histologic type[23]

Histologic type	Atomic bomb survivors						Non-exposed					
	Male		Female		Total		Male		Female		Total	
	No. of cases	%	No. of cases	%	No. of cases	%	No. of cases	%	No. of cases	%	No. of cases	%
Squamous cell carcinoma	3.1	40.0	5	23.8	39	36.8	91	52.9	8	22.9	99	47.8
Adenocarcinoma	33	38.8	14	66.7	47	44.3	37	21.5	24	68.6	61	29.5
Large cell carcinoma	5	5.9	1	4.8	6	5.7	9	5.2	1	2.9	10	4.8
Small cell carcinoma	11	12.9	1	4.8	12	11.3	31	18.0	2	5.7	33	15.9
Others	2	2.1	0	0	2	1.9	4	2.3	0	0	4	1.9
Total	85	100	21	100	106	100	172	100	35	100	207	100

hospitalized and receiving treatment for lung cancer during the 9-year period 1975–83 at five institutions (Second Department of Internal Medicine, Hiroshima University School of Medicine; Hiroshima Byoin National Sanatorium; Kure

Table 4   Histologic type and exposure status[23]

Histologic type	Atomic bomb survivors				Non-exposed	
	Direct exposure within 2.0 km		Others			
	No. of cases	%	No. of cases	%	No. of cases	%
Squamous cell carcinoma	9	30.0	30	39.5	99	48.7
Adenocarcinoma	16	53.3	31	40.8	61	29.5
Large cell carcinoma	2	6.7	4	5.3	10	4.8
Small cell carcinoma	3	10.9	9	11.8	33	15.9
Others	0	0	2	2.6	4	1.9
Total	30	100	76	100	207	100

National Hospital; Hiroshima City Hospital; and Asa City Hospital) with 317 non-exposed lung cancer patients admitted to the Second Department of Internal Medicine at Hiroshima University over the same period. The frequency of squamous cell carcinomas tended to be high amongst the non-exposed group, whereas adenocarcinomas tended to have a rather high incidence amongst atomic bomb survivors. Also, an examination of histologic type with reference to distance from the hypocenter in 101 directly exposed cases revealed that of those proximally exposed within 2 km, 23 developed adenocarcinoma (42.6%), which was more than the number who developed squamous cell carcinoma (16 cases, 29.6%); in contrast, however, in the distally exposed ($\geqslant$ 2 km) atomic bomb survivors, squamous cell carcinoma was predominant (22 cases, 46.8%), followed by the number with adenocarcinoma (12 cases, 25.5%) (Table 5). In 1989 Nanbu et al[25] studied 161 lung cancer cases autopsied at the Hiroshima Atomic Bomb Hospital during the 32 year period 1956–1987. The frequency by histologic type was adenocarcinoma (67 cases, 41.6%), squamous cell carcinoma (47 cases, 29.2%), undifferentiated small cell

Table 5   Histologic type and distance from hypocenter[24]

Histologic type	No. of survivors within 2.0 km	No. of survivors at $\geqslant$ 2.1 km	Total
Squamous cell carcinoma	16 (29.6)	22 (46.8)	88 (37.6)
Adenocarcinoma	23 (42.6)	12 (25.5)	35 (34.7)
Small cell carcinoma	10 (18.5)	8 (17.0)	18 (17.8)
Large cell carcinoma	4 (7.4)	4 (8.5)	8 (7.9)
Others	1 (1.9)	2 (2.2)	2 (2.0)
Total	54 (100.0)	47 (100.0)	101 (100.0)

( ) Parentheses indicate the percentage of total cases for each period

Table 6   Changes with time in frequency and number of cases by number of lung cancer autopsies and histologic type[25]

Time period	1 1957–1962	2 1963–1967	3 1968–1972	4 1973–1977	5 1978–1982	6 1983–1987
No. of cases	16	28	30	31	38	18
Average age	61.4	65.9	69.7	69.0	72.4	71.2
Average age at time of bombing	46.8	44.9	44.7	39.0	37.3	31.2
Adenocarcinoma	4 (25.0)	9 (32.1)	12 (40.0)	14 (45.1)	19 (50.0)	9 (50.0)
Squamous cell carcinoma	8 (50.0)	7 (25.0)	11 (36.6)	7 (22.5)	10 (26.3)	4 (22.2)
Small cell carcinoma	3 (18.7)	10 (35.7)	7 (23.3)	5 (16.1)	5 (13.1)	2 (11.1)
Large cell carcinoma	1 (6.2)	2 (7.1)		4 (12.9)	2 (5.2)	2 (11.1)
Adenosquamous cell carcinoma				1 (3.2)	2 (5.2)	1 (5.5)

( ) Parentheses indicate the percentage of total cases for each period.

carcinoma (32 cases, 19.9%), undifferentiated large cell carcinoma (11 cases, 6.8%), and adenosquamous cell carcinoma (4 cases, 2.5%). In order to investigate changes in the frequency of different histologic types with respect to time, the above carcinomas were classified by date of development into 6 separate time periods; the first period covered the six years between 1957 and 1962, with periods 2 to 6 respectively covering the following five consecutive 5-year intervals beginning with 1963–67 (Table 6). During the first period (1957–62) adenocarcinomas accounted for 25% of the cases, but after that gradually increased and accounted for 50% of the total in the fifth period. Conversely, squamous cell carcinoma accounted for 50% in the first period, but after that varied within the 22–37% range, with the figure in the sixth period falling to 22.2%. Also, undifferentiated small cell carcinoma exhibited a higher frequency of 35.7% in the second period, but then gradually decreased to 11.1% in the sixth period.

CONCLUSION

The high lung cancer risk faced by atomic bomb survivors relative to non-exposed individuals has been indicated by death certificates, statistical studies on tumors and clinical data, and also autopsy results since approximately ten years after the atomic bomb was dropped. With regard to the histologic characteristics of lung cancer in atomic bomb survivors, reports prior to approximately 1970 showed that relative to the non-exposed, survivors exhibited a higher frequency of undifferentiated small cell carcinoma and squamous cell carcinoma, but reports after 1970 indicated that the frequency of squamous cell carcinoma decreased while that of adenocarcinoma increased; all these tendencies were marked among the proximally exposed. However, the reasons for the changes in the frequency of the different histologic types are as yet unknown, and require further study.

(*Hideao Sasaki*)

REFERENCES

1. Arnstein A. Sozialhygienische Untersuchungen über die Bergleute in den Schneeberger Kobaltgruben, insbesondere über das Vorkommen des sogenanten "Schneeberger Lungenkrebses". San Wes Wiem 1913; 25: 64–83.
2. Löwy J. Über die Joachimstarer Bergkrankheit; Vorlaufige Mittelung. *Med Klinik* 1929; **25**: 141–2.
3. de Villiers AJ, Windish JP. Lung cancer in a fluorspar mining community: 1. Radiation, dust and mortality experience. *Brit J Ind Med* 1964; **21**: 94–109.
4. Wagoner JK, Archer VE, Lundin FE, *et al.* Radiation as the cause of lung cancer among uranium miners. *New Engl J Med* 1965; **273**: 181–8.
5. Lisco H, Finkel MP. Observations on lung pathology following the inhalation of radioactive cerium. *(Abstract) Fed Proc* 1949; **8**: 360–1.
6. Kotschetkowa TA, Awrunia G. Veranderungen in den Lungen und in anderen Organen bei intratrachealer Einfuhrung einiger Radioisotope (^{24}Na, ^{32}P, ^{198}Au). *Arch Gewrbepath Gewerbehyg* 1957; **16**: 24.
7. Scott JK, Thomas R. Polonium: induction of pulmonary tumors following intratracheal injection. Univ of Rochester Atomic Energy Project Quarterly Review. 1957; July–Sept.
8. Watanabe S, Yokoro K. Somatic effects of radiation. In: Kayama T, Tabuchi A, Watanabe S, editors. *Genshi Igaku* (Nuclear Medicine). Tokyo: Kanehara Shuppan, 1963: 287–316. (*In Japanese*)
9. Gates O, Warren S. The production of bronchial carcinomas in mice. *Am J Path* 1960; **36**: 653–71.
10. Kuschner M, Laskin S, Nelson N, *et al.* Radiation-induced bronchogenic carcinoma in rats. *Sci Proc Am J Path* 1958; **34**: 554.
11. de Villiers AJ, Gross P. Morphological changes induced in the lungs of hamsters and rats by external radiation (X-rays)—a study in experimental carcinogenesis. *Cancer* 1966; **19**: 1933–410.
12. Kodama T. Pathological studies on carcinoma of the lung in rats induced by external X-ray irradiation. *Med J Hiroshima Univ.* 1978; **26**: 289–329. (*In Japanese*)
13. Obo G. Statistical observations of deaths due to malignant neoplasms among atomic bomb survivors. *Japan Med J* 1956; **1686**: 8–19. (*In Japanese*)
14. Shisui K. A tendency of cancer death in Hiroshima City. Part 1. On the comparison of survivors' health cards between issued and non-issued persons. *J Hiroshima Med Ass* 1960; **13**: 885–8. (*In Japanese*)
15. Shisui K. A tendency of cancer death in Hiroshima City. Part 2. The death tendency of authorized patients in atomic bomb diseases. *J Hiroshima Med Ass* 1960; **13**: 956–60. (*In Japanese*)
16. Shisui K. A tendency of cancer death in Hiroshima City. Part 3. On the comparison of survivors' health cards between issued and non-issued persons in 1960 and 1958–1960. *J Hiroshima Med Ass* 1961; **14**: 578–83. (*In Japanese*)
17. Hiroshima Medical Association Tumor Statistics Committee. Epidemiological observations on malignant neoplasms in Hiroshima atomic bomb survivors (1st report). *J Hiroshima Med Ass* 1961; **14**: 347–56. (*In Japanese*)
18. Fujimoto Y. Lung cancer among Hiroshima atomic bomb survivors. *J Hiroshima Med Ass* 1967; **20**: 360–7. (*In Japanese*)
19. Mansur GP, Keehn RJ, Hiramoto T, *et al.* Lung cancer among atomic bomb survivors Hiroshima-Nagasaki 1950–64. ABCC TR 19–68,1968.
20. Tahara E, Yamada A. Autopsy studies on lung cancer among Hiroshima atomic bomb survivors. *Haigan* (Lung Cancer) 1969; **9**: 68–9. (*In Japanese*)
21. Cihak RW, Ishimaru T, Steer A, *et al.* Lung cancer in autopsy atomic bomb survivors and controls, Hiroshima and Nagasaki 1961–70. 1. Autopsy findings and relation to radiation. ABCC TR32–72, 1972.

22. Hamada T, Ishida T. Lung cancer among atomic bomb survivors-study of 114 autopsy cases, 1957–72. *J Hiroshima Med Ass* 1974; **27**: 558–69. (*In Japanese*)

23. Sasaki H, Ito C, Mitsuyama T, *et al.* Clinical studies of lung cancer of A-bomb survivors. Report 1. Investigation of histological types. *Proceedings of the 23rd Meeting of the Research Society for Late Effects of Atomic Bomb*; 1982 June 6; Nagasaki. The Late Effects of Radiation 1983: 113–8. (*In Japanese*)

24. Nishimoto Y, Katsuta S, Mochizuki K, *et al.* The clinical studies of lung cancer among A-bomb survivors. *Genbaku shougaishou chousa kenkyuuhan houkokusho* (1986 report) 1987; **63**: 692–700. (*In Japanese*)

25. Kusube S, Akagi H, Kuramoto K, Hamada T. Pathological review of lung cancer among A-bomb survivors at Hiroshima Atomic-Bomb Hospital. *Nagasaki Med J* 1989; **63**: 692–700. (*In Japanese*)

1.5   THYROID CANCER

INTRODUCTION

Since Duffy and Fitzgerald[1] reported in 1950 that thyroid cancer developed in patients who underwent thymal irradiation while young, several similar reports have appeared, establishing the theory that thyroid cancer is induced by radiation. Predictably, thyroid cancer is today considered the second most common late effect of the atomic bombs among atomic bomb survivors, after leukemia. This chapter reviews the literature pertaining to thyroid cancer and radiation exposure.

It is first necessary to classify thyroid cancer into clinically-detected cancer and autopsy-detected minute cancer. Among the clinically-detected thyroid cancers, it is not unusual for the minute cancer to be detected during surgery for benign thyroid disease. This is essentially the same as autopsy-detected minute cancer, with a biological character completely different from clinically detected cancer. Minute cancers are 1.0–1.5 cm or less, and are believed to remain as minute cancers throughout the lifetime without developing clinical manifestations of cancer. Although differences are observed depending on the method of examination, the frequency is of the order of several per cent, which is several thousand times the rate of development of clinically detected cancer. Since the biological characters of the two are different, and as there is a large difference in frequency, these two forms of disease will be considered separately.

1.   CLINICALLY DETECTED CANCER

There have long been reports concerning thyroid cancer in atomic bomb survivors, but the first serious statistical study was by Socolow et al[2]. In alternate years, the Atomic Bomb Casualty Commission (ABCC) (the present-day Radiation Effects Research Foundation, RERF) screens a population of approximately 20,000 atomic bomb survivors from Hiroshima and Nagasaki (the Adult Health Study sample). Analyses were performed with respect to age and sex after classification into the following four categories: (1) survivors exposed within 0–1,999 meters of the hypocenter who exhibited acute radiation illness, (2) survivors exposed within 0–1,999 m of the hypocenter who did not exhibit acute radiation illness, (3) survivors exposed within 3,000–3,499 m of the Hiroshima bomb or 3,000–3,999 m of the Nagasaki bomb (these different distances reflecting differences in the types of bombs), and (4) survivors exposed at distances greater than 10,000 m. Between 1958 and 1961, 21 cases of thyroid cancer were observed, with 10 appearing among survivors in category (1), which was a greater number than in the more distally exposed populations ($0.02 < p < 0.05$); however, when the 4 cases diagnosed at other hospitals are excluded, the statistically significant difference in frequency with the distally exposed populations disappears ($p > 0.30$). In addition, 42% of the cases occurred among the population aged 30–39 years.

Following this, Wood et al[3] studied one 2-year cycle of examinations of the Adult Health Study sample (December 1963–December 1965), and discovered 39 thyroid cancer cases. However, comparison with other findings is difficult since this figure includes autopsy-detected minute cancer. A high rate of development was observed among proximally exposed female atomic bomb survivors (p < 0.01), but although such a tendency was found among males, there was no statistical significance due to the low number of cases. A high rate was also seen among those aged ≤ 40 (aged ≤ 20 at the time of bombing, ATB). The male : female ratio deserves emphasis, since the ratio for all survivors is approximately 1 : 3, whereas this difference disappears for survivors aged ≤ 40.

Ezaki et al[4,5] investigated the percentage of thyroid disease cases accounted for by atomic bomb survivors; the study population consisted of patients born on and after August 6th 1945 who were examined at the Second Department of Surgery of Hiroshima University Medical School and the Department of Surgery of the Research Institute for Nuclear Medicine and Biology, Hiroshima University, during the period 1951–63.

Atomic bomb survivors accounted for 14.1% of all thyroid disease patients, with the figures for the various diseases being thyroid cancer 27.9%, nodular goiter 20.5%, chronic thyroiditis 18.3%, diffuse goiter 11.5%, and hyperthyroidism 8.6% (Fig. 1). Among outpatients, thyroid cancer was observed in 34 out of 1,509 atomic bomb survivors (2.25%), high in comparison with the 58 cases observed among the 13,211 non-exposed patients (0.44%) (p < 0.01). Chronologically, the rate of development increased from around 1960. With regard to age at diagnosis, the rate in the non-exposed population was approximately uniform in patients aged between their 30s and 50s, whereas for the atomic bomb survivor population with thyroid cancer almost half developed the disease in their 30s (after which it decreased gradually), with the estimated age at onset extremely high for ages 30–34. That is, the figure was high for survivors exposed while young. Six of the 38 thyroid cancer cases among the atomic bomb survivors (15.8%) occurred among the population exposed within 999 m of the hypocenter, whereas only 7 of the 213 non-cancer thyroid disease cases (3.2%) occurred among the same population; thus the rate of thyroid cancer development was high among the proximally exposed (p < 0.01). However, the statistical significance is no longer found for survivors exposed within 1,999 m. A supplementary study using data from the national health insurance scheme administered by Hiroshima city and covering the 17-month period from August 1960 to December 1961 examined thyroid cancer diagnoses according to whether

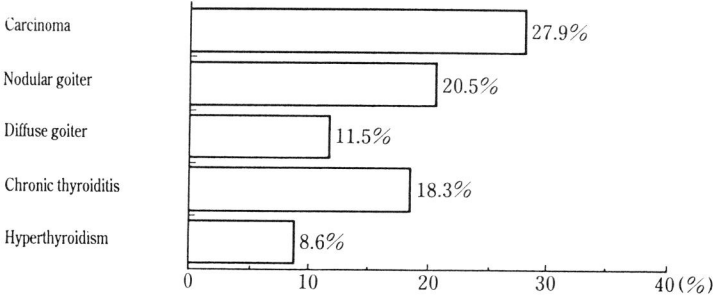

Figure 1   Percentage of thyroid disease patients accounted for by atomic bomb survivors (adapted from Ref. 4)

the individual had been exposed to the atomic bomb. Six cases were observed among 22,386 atomic bomb survivors (a rate of 26.8 per 100,000 population), and 6 cases observed among 114,262 non-exposed patients (a rate of 5.25 per 100,000 population); the frequency among the atomic bomb survivor population was thus greater than among the non-exposed population (p < 0.01).

Continuing the work of Socolow, Parker *et al*[6] analyzed 74 thyroid cancer cases detected among the Adult Health Study sample during the 14-year period 1958–71, of which 40 were clinically detected cancer cases. The population exposed to a dose of ≥ 0.50 Gy (T65D doses estimated on the basis of distance from the hypocenter and shielding conditions) were compared with a control population exposed to > 1 Gy. The rate of thyroid cancer development was high, the relative risks being 5.0 for females (p > 0.01) and 9.4 for males (p $\simeq$ 0.04). The rate among females was high for those aged < 20 at exposure, but results for males are unclear due to the low number of cases.

Manabe *et al*[7] continued the work of Parker *et al* for a further 5 years, and analyzed the data for 1958–76 using thyroid doses, which had become available. This study also included autopsy-detected minute cancer and thus a mention of clinically detected cancer only will be made. Nine additional cases were considered, giving a total of 49 cases. The conclusions did not differ greatly from those of Parker *et al*, with the rate of development increasing with dose. The rate of development of clinically evident cancer among females was high in comparison with autopsy-detected minute cancer. It should also be emphasized that even at this time the frequency of thyroid cancer was high.

Although every study demonstrated an accelerated occurrence of atomic bomb-related thyroid cancer, the ABCC Adult Health Study sample (which had been selected for its statistical appropriateness as a subject population) exhibited only 49 clinical thyroid cancer cases during a 19-year period; it is impossible to avoid criticism regarding the small number of cases, thus rendering a detailed analysis of the various factors inappropriate. Conversely, use of hospital statistics such as those at Hiroshima University Hospital allows consideration of 92 cases, but this introduces the difficult problem of bias.

Ezaki *et al*[8-10] considered the above points in a study on the expanded Life Span Study sample at the Radiation Effects Research Foundation (RERF). Since this population was originally selected with the objective of studying the life span of atomic bomb survivors, it was a fixed population designed to accommodate sex and age differences. Unlike the afore-mentioned Adult Health Study sample, the subjects did not undergo examinations, but the population was large (over 76,700, all of whom were in Hiroshima; Nagasaki survivors were not included), and the institute was informed of deaths etc. When added to the Hiroshima University Hospital data, an examination of each case during the 22-year period 1958–79 produces a total of 136 clinical thyroid cancer cases; tissue specimens were procured in 103 cases, and 32 cases diagnosed on the basis of records from medical treatment institutions etc, with 1 case presumed to be thyroid cancer on the basis of the death certificate alone. Minute cancer was omitted from the survey. This study suffers from the dispersal of the subjects throughout the country and the consequent gaps in data, and also from the difficulty of acquiring accurate records for the individual subjects. As a result, the researchers restricted their activities to Hiroshima atomic bomb survivors, for whom records were readily available. Excluding the 11 cases for whom radiation dose estimates were not available or who were known to have had thyroid cancer prior to January 1958, analyses were performed on 125 cases (15 males, 110 females). The crude annual incidences per 100,000 population were found to be 2.7 for males and 12.4 for females, the rate rising with increasing dose (Fig. 2). The increase among females is marked, but not so among heavily exposed males, a result due to the low number of cases; nevertheless, the tendencies are the same as for women. There is a distinct tendency for the rate among females exposed to the atomic bomb while young to rise with increasing dose. An examination by dose of the ratio of observed and expected numbers of thyroid cancer cases (the O/E ratio) for both all subjects and for females reveals a rise in thyroid cancer with increasing dose (Fig. 3), with this linear increase statistically significant for both all subjects and for females only

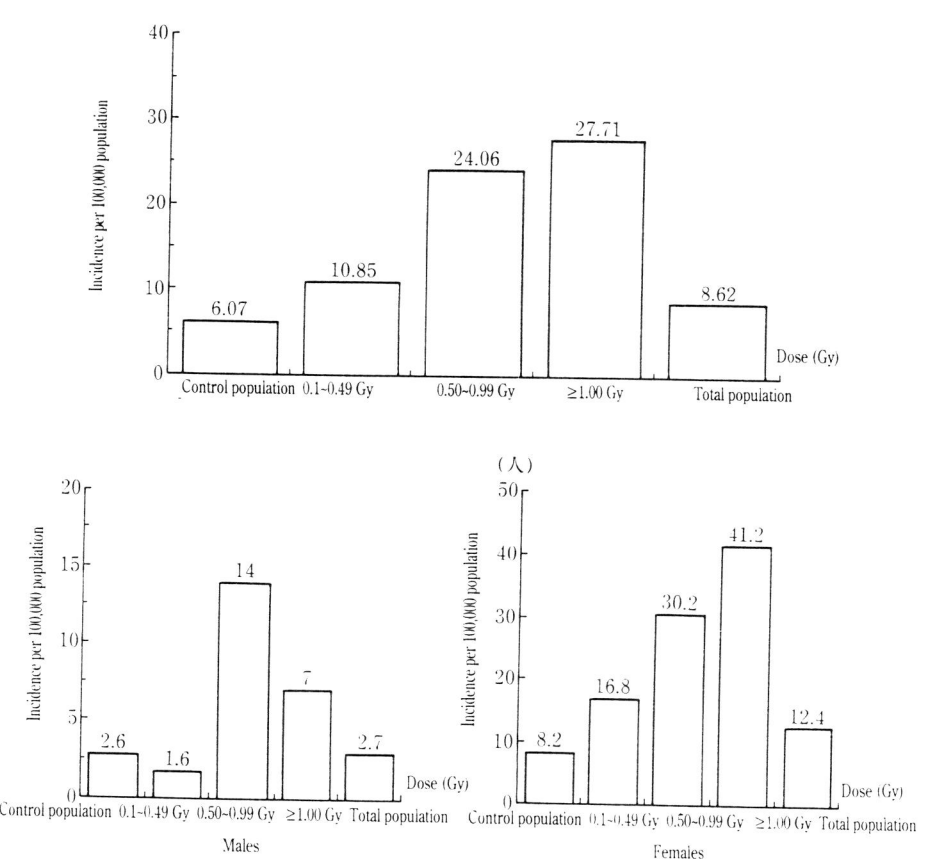

Figure 2   Crude annual incidence of thyroid cancer per 100,000 population by sex and dose (adapted from Ref. 8)

(p < 0.01); for males alone there was a tendency to increase, but it was not significant (p > 0.10). As shown in Fig. 3, the results by dose show a statistical significance for survivors aged < 20 ATB (p < 0.01), a suggested but unconfirmed significance for those aged 20–39 ATB (0.05 < p < 0.01), but no statistical significance among survivors aged ≥ 40 years ATB. Compared to the < 0.01 Gy population, the relative risk for the 0.50–0.99 Gy population was approximately 4.2, the value being similar for both males and females. However, with respect to age ATB, the relative risk was 7.9 (p < 0.01) for survivors aged < 20 ATB, and 2.8 (p < 0.01) for the 20–39 and ≤ 40 populations combined. The statistically significant regression coefficient obtained for females aged < 20 ATB showed the increased risk per 0.01 Gy to be equivalent to an annual incidence of 3.4 cases per 1 million population. Recently, Akiba et al[11] investigated the thyroid cancer risk using the combined data for Hiroshima and Nagasaki for the period 1958–79 and obtained results virtually the same as those described above.

2. AUTOPSY-DETECTED MINUTE CANCER

Since minute cancer may not be detected until autopsy, the frequency rises with finer dissection. This section will therefore separately consider the findings of Sampson

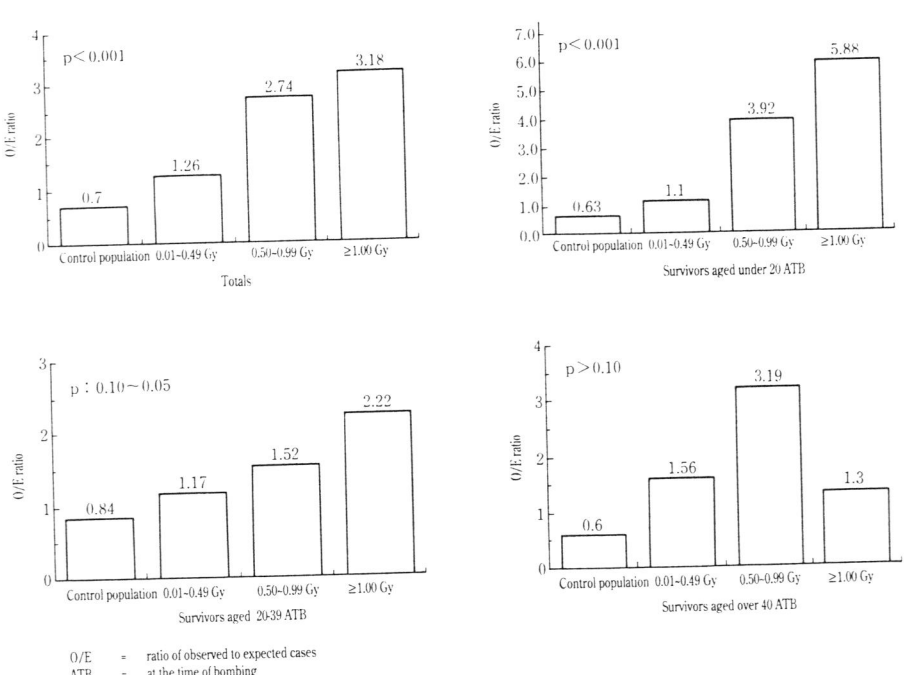

O/E = ratio of observed to expected cases
ATB = at the time of bombing

Figure 3   Ratio of observed to expected number of cases by age at the time of bombing (adapted from Ref. 7)

and his co-workers, who made a special effort to detect minute cancer, and the other studies which investigated minute cancer detected by general autopsy.

A. The Findings of Sampson *et al.*

1. *Prevalence of Autopsy-Detected Minute Cancer*[12,13]

Examinations were performed on 2,327 cases autopsied at Hiroshima between January 1957 and February 1968, and on 740 cases autopsied in Nagasaki between January 1951 and September 1967, i.e. a total of 3,067 cases. The thyroids were cut into sections 2–3 mm thick, and the presence of nodules investigated; histologic examination led to the detection of 536 thyroid cancer cases. The prevalencies were 402 out of 2,327 in Hiroshima (17.3%), and 134 out of 740 in Nagasaki (18.1%). With respect to sex, the rate for males was 254/1,614 (15.7%) and for females 282/1,453 (19.4%); the rate was therefore higher among females ($p < 0.01$). Unlike general cancer, there was no clear tendency for the frequency to increase with increasing age at autopsy. Thyroid cancer was listed as the cause of death in 5 cases, undifferentiated cancer in 2 cases, and papillary adenocarcinoma with whole body metastasis in 3 cases, the sizes of the primary lesions being respectively 1.5, 1.8 and 3.0 cm; the latter 2 cases were too large to be termed minute cancer. Of the 536 cases, 525 (98%) were papillary carcinomas, with 518 of the 536 (97%) having tumors 1.5 cm or less. Compared to the 0 Gy population, the ⩾ 0.50 Gy population (T65D dose) exhibited a high frequency ($p < 0.01$), with a relative risk of 1.41 and an attributable risk of 6.7%; in other words, the ⩾ 0.50 Gy faced an excess thyroid cancer risk of 6.5%.

2. *Number and Size of Autopsy-Detected Minute Cancers with Respect to Sex*[14]

The presence of two or more papillary adenocarcinoma lesions was observed in 170/525 cases (32%), and 6 or more lesions in 12/525 cases (2.3%). In multiple tumor cases involving the thyroid, lesions were observed in only one lobe (including the isthmus) in 52/129 cases (41%), which was less frequent than bilateral lesions (76/129 cases, 51%). Females tended to have smaller tumors with increasing age, but this was not observed in males. For females, tumor size was greater among the ⩾ 0.50 Gy population than in the low-dose population ($p = 0.05$), whereas for males it was smaller ($p = 0.16$). Irrespective of radiation exposure, females generally exhibited a greater tumor size ($p < 0.01$). Thus the difference between males and females is likely to be due to a sex-related factor in addition to radiation exposure.

3. *Autopsy-Detected Minute Cancer and Age*[15]

The prevalence of minute cancer is high among the ⩾ 0.50 Gy population. This population was classified into 3 categories according to age ATB (< 20, 20–45, and ⩾ 46), and the dose-prevalence relationship examined for the youngest and oldest populations. In the population aged ⩾ 46 (which included numerous cases) the prevalence of autopsy-detected minute cancer increased with dose, with a significant difference observed between the 0 Gy and the $\geqslant 0.50$ Gy populations ($p < 0.05$). In the population aged < 20 ATB, the rate increased with dose, although the difference between the 0 Gy and the $\geqslant 0.50$ Gy populations was not significant ($0.05 < p < 0.14$), which may be attributable to the low number of cases.

4. *Autopsy-Detected Minute Cancer and Lymph Node Metastasis* [16]

In the above study, examination of the cervical lymph nodes was possible in 128 cases, revealing metastasis in 20 cases (16%). These 20 cases plus an additional 25 cases found to have metastasis during general autopsy (i.e. a total of 45 cases) were compared with 108 cases in which lymph node metastasis was absent. In the vast majority of cases the primary lesion occurred in the thyroid ipsilaterally to the metastasis, but in 3 cases it only appeared on the contralateral side. In addition these 3 cases also exhibited metastasis in the mediastinal lymph nodes. The frequency of metastasis increased with increasing size of the primary lesion, but metastasis was observed even with lesions of $\geqslant 1$ cm. The frequency of metastasis was greater among males (12 out of 48 cases, 29.2%) than among females (8 out of 79 cases, 10.1%) ($p < 0.05$). Other factors frequently causing metastasis were multiple primary lesions, infiltration of the primary lesion into the surrounding tissue or invasion of the blood vessels, extension over 50% or more of the papillary region, and the presence of psammoma bodies. It should be noted that no correlation existed between the frequency of metastasis and exposure to atomic bomb radiation. Although 1 death resulted from whole-body metastasis despite the primary lesion being a minute cancer, in other cases death occurred without knowledge of the existence of thyroid cancer, even when lymph node metastasis was present.

B. Studies Involving Detection of Minute Cancer During General Autopsy

Studying the Adult Health Study sample over the period 1964–65, Wood *et al*[3] found that even though thyroid cancer (including clinically detected cancer and autopsy-detected minute cancer) was frequently observed in the populations either exposed within 1,400 m of the hypocenter or aged under 20 ATB, not even one case of occult sclerosing carcinoma was observed among the population aged under 20, irrespective of distance from the hypocenter.

Parker *et al*[6] analyzed autopsy cases among the Adult Health Study sample for the period 1958–71, finding 34 minute cancer cases. In comparison to the atomic bomb survivors exposed to < 0.01 Gy, the relative risk of minute thyroid cancer in the $\geqslant 0.50$ Gy population was high for females at 3.1 ($p \approx 0.02$), but not high for males at 0.75. Furthermore, a high rate was not observed among survivors exposed while young. As previously mentioned, Manabe *et al*[7] continued the work of Parker *et al.* and investigated the development of thyroid cancer in the Adult Health Study sample for the period 1958–76. Of the cases detected by autopsy, 42 cases of minute cancer were detected during this period, with no difference in frequency observed between males and females, and an increase in frequency with increasing dose observed only in females.

Ezaki[8] analyzed clinical thyroid cancer data for the Life Span Study sample over the period 1958–79, and in a supplementary study examined the autopsy data for 4,425 cases among this population for whom the received radiation dose was known; analyses were performed on 155 cases of autopsy-detected minute cancer (a frequency of 3.5%). Compared to a frequency of 82 out of 2,495 cases (3.3%) in the < 0.01 Gy population, the frequency in the ≥ 0.50 Gy population (21 out of 341 cases, 6.2%) was high (p < 0.05). The ratio between observed and expected numbers of minute cancer cases (the O/E ratio) for the above atomic bomb survivor population and the controls was 1.6 for males and 1.8 for females, revealing a statistical significance for females only. The frequencies by sex were 56 out of 2,233 cases for males (2.5%) and 99 out of 2,192 cases for females (4.5%), the figure for females thus being 1.8 times greater than for males. For subjects who died aged 50 or less, almost no difference was observed between the sexes, which was an extremely low ratio in comparison with the male : female ratio of 4.6 : 1 that was observed with clinically detected cancer. Also, it should be pointed out that the frequency did not vary with age at the time of death. In other words, minute cancer appears to develop at 50 years of age or less, but does not increase after that.

Ezaki et al[10] studied 4,834 cases among the autopsies performed at the Radiation Effects Research Foundation in Hiroshima between October 1950 and December 1985 for whom a DS86 dose estimate was available, and investigated the prevalence of minute cancer, thyroid adenoma, nodular goiter, and chronic thyroiditis. In order to exclude clinically detected thyroid cancer, a total of 22 cases were omitted from the study because they had either died from thyroid cancer, had been diagnosed as having thyroid cancer whilst still alive, or had thyroid cancer with a maximum tumor diameter of ≥ 1.6 cm and for whom a pre-death diagnosis could have been anticipated. Of the 4,812 remaining cases, minute cancer was detected in 132. From Fig. 4, it is immediately evident that the prevalence rises with increasing thyroid dose. Furthermore, the 132 cases consisted of 51 males (an overall prevalence of 51/2,411, i.e. 2.1%) and 81 females (an overall prevalence of 81/2,371, i.e. 3.4%), the figure for females thus being 1.63 times greater than for males. The population not present in the city at the time of bombing was excluded from an analysis of the effects of radiation dose. A logistical model was employed to consider separately to

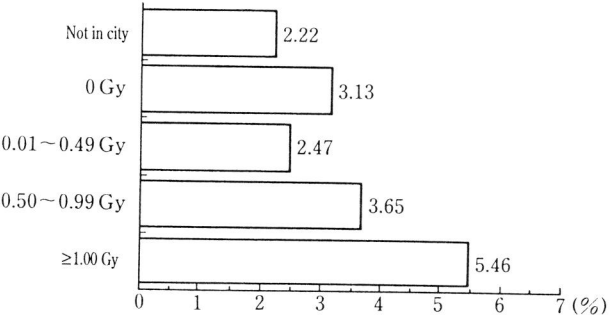

Figure 4   Frequency of minute thyroid cancer by dose

atomic bomb radiation the effects of date of autopsy, sex, age at death, and whether non-thyroid cancer was the cause of death. The prevalence was found to increase with increasing dose (p < 0.01). Next, the data was classified according to the effects with respect to dose for both sex and age ATB (< 30, 30–50, ⩾ 60). A comparison of individual data revealed a rather low significance (p = 0.049) for all ages, with no difference in the O/E ratios between the various ages ATB.

The prevalence of other thyroid diseases studied at the same time can be summarized briefly. The thyroid adenoma prevalence rose with increasing radiation dose, the tendency being distinct among females and survivors aged under 30. In contrast, no relationship with received dose was discerned for nodular goiter (colloid nodules and adenomatous goiter) and chronic thyroiditis. Another point of great interest is that the frequency of thyroid diseases other than autopsy-detected minute cancer rose with increasing age at death, whereas autopsy-detected minute cancer did not exhibit such a distinct age dependence.

CONCLUSION

Despite differences in the populations studied and the techniques adopted, similar conclusions were arrived at with respect to the atomic bomb and the development of thyroid cancer. All studies on clinically detected cancer found that the rate of development increased with dose. The risk was statistically significant among females only; a similar tendency was observed among males, although significance could not be deduced due to the small number of cases. A clear dose-response relationship was observed among the young (⩾ 20 years). Even for autopsy-detected minute cancer, the frequency increased significantly with increasing dose, with the tendency being clear among females, but not among males even though the number of minute cancer cases was not small in comparison to clinically detected cancer. In addition, the difference in prevalence with age ATB among autopsy cases was also small. It is believed that one reason for this was the low number of survivors aged < 20 ATB when classification was made by autopsy results. In general the frequency of clinically detected cancer was much greater among females than in males; for autopsy-detected minute cancer, however, female cases were more numerous, but the difference was small. Thus in analyses of the radiation effects it is important to distinguish between clinically evident minute cancer and autopsy-detected minute cancer.

(*Haruo Ezaki*)

REFERENCES

1.   Duffy BJ, Fitzgerald PJ. Thyroid cancer in childhood and adolescence. A report on twenty-eight cases. *Cancer* 1950; **3**: 1018–32.
2.   Socolow EL, Hashizume A, Neriishi S, *et al.* Thyroid carcinoma in man after exposure to ionizing radiation. A summary of the findings in Hiroshima and Nagasaki. *New Engl J Med* 1963; **268**: 406–10.

3. Wood JW, Tamagaki H, Neriishi S, *et al.* Thyroid carcinoma in atomic bomb survivors, Hiroshima and Nagasaki. *Am J Epid* 1969; **89**: 4–14.

4. Ezaki H, Shigemitsu T. Studies on thyroid cancer induced by A-bomb exposure, and its clinical significance. *J Hiroshima Med Ass* 1967; **20** Suppl: 336–47. (*In Japanese*)

5. Ezaki H, Shigemitsu T. Studies on thyroid cancer induced by A-bomb exposure. *Proc Hiroshima Univ RINMB* 1970; *11*: 166–8.

6. Parker LN, Belsky JL, Yamamoto T, *et al.* Thyroid carcinoma after exposure to atomic radiation. A continuing survey of a fixed population, Hiroshima and Nagasaki, 1958–1971. *Ann Int Med* 1974; **80**: 600–4.

7. Manabe Y, Toyota E, Yamamoto T. Thyroid carcinoma in the atomic bomb survivors of Hiroshima and Nagasaki, 1958–1976. *Hiroshima J Med Ass* 1978; **31**: 421–23. (*In Japanese*)

8. Ezaki H. Thyroid carcinoma induced by A-bomb exposure in Hiroshima A-bomb survivors. *J Jap Clin Surg* 1985; **4**: 1127–37. (*In Japanese*)

9. Ezaki H, Ishimaru T, Hayashi Y, *et al.* Cancer of the thyroid and salivary gland. *GANN Monograph on Cancer Res* 1986; **32**: 129–42.

10. Ezaki H, Takeichi N, Yoshimoto Y. Thyroid cancer. Epidemiological study of thyroid cancer in A-bomb survivors from extended Life Span Study cohort in Hiroshima. *J Radiat Res* 1991; (Suppl); 193–200.

11. Akiba S, Lubin J, Ezaki H, *et al.* Thyroid cancer incidence among atomic bomb survivors in Hiroshima and Nagasaki, 1958–79. RERF TR 5–91, 1991.

12. Sampson RJ, Key CR, Buncher CR, *et al.* Prevalence of thyroid carcinoma at autopsy, Hiroshima 1957–68, Nagasaki 1951–67. ABCC TR 25–68, 1968.

13. Sampson RJ, Key CR, Buncher CR, *et al.* Thyroid carcinoma in Hiroshima and Nagasaki. *JAMA* 1969; **209**: 65–70.

14. Sampson RJ, Key CR, Buncher CR, *et al.* Papillary carcinoma of the thyroid gland, sex and size related feature. A study of 525 cases diagnosed at Hiroshima and Nagasaki. ABCC TR 8–69, 1969.

15. Sampson RJ, Key CR, Buncher CR, *et al.* The age factor in radiation carcinogenesis of the human thyroid. A study of 536 cases of thyroid carcinoma. ABCC TR 7–69, 1969.

16. Sampson RJ, Oka H, Key CR, *et al.* Metastases from occult thyroid carcinoma. An autopsy study from Hiroshima and Nagasaki, Japan. *Cancer* 1970; **25**: 803–11.

1.6 MULTIPLE MYELOMA

INTRODUCTION

Multiple myeloma is a disease that affects the whole body since the plasma cells (probably of B-cell lineage), which produce immunoglobulins, undergo a malignant transformation, and proliferate as monoclonal plasma cells.

Clinical characteristics of the illness are monoclonal hyper-gamma-globulinemia, an increased number of myeloma cells in the bone marrow, the occurrence of Bence-Jones proteinuria, nephropathy, punched out bone lesions, hypercalcemia, and susceptibility to infection etc. The disease tends to appear from late middle age onwards, at an average age in the 60s and 70s, and a relatively higher frequency among men. Consequently, with the increasing average age of Japanese society, this disease is one of the hematologic malignancies that will probably tend to increase. Even the atomic bomb survivors are becoming old, and it can now be expected that patterns of illness will change, necessitating counter-measures against this and other related illnesses. On the other hand, a high frequency of leukemia was observed among atomic bomb survivors, and since multiple myeloma is a bone marrow hematologic malignancy, consideration must be given to the possibility that the development of multiple myeloma is a late effect of radiation among atomic bomb survivors. This was supported by a study by Lewis[1], who in 1963 reported a high myeloma mortality rate among American radiologists, and another study in 1977 that reported a significantly increased myeloma mortality among workers engaged in the production of radioactive materials[2]. Also, in 1981 Cuzick[3] reported a statistically high myeloma frequency among a population 15 to 25 years after undergoing radiotherapy or radiologic examination. All these results suggest a causative relationship between exposure to radiation and myeloma development; it is important to investigate myeloma and related diseases in atomic bomb survivors, both from the viewpoint of the elucidation of the mechanism by which cancer is induced by radiation and also for the health management of atomic bomb survivors. Because of this, screening tests for myeloma have been conducted on exposed individuals since 1988. This chapter summarizes the findings to date pertaining to myeloma and related diseases in the atomic bomb survivors.

1. MYELOMAS IN ATOMIC BOMB SURVIVORS

Attention focused on myeloma development after the interest in leukemia, the first report on myeloma being by Anderson and Ishida[4] in 1964. According to that, an examination of the autopsy data compiled by the Atomic Bomb Casualty Commission (ABCC) during the 15-year period between 1948 and 1962 revealed that among Hiroshima atomic bomb survivors within 1400 meters of the hypocenter the frequency of multiple myeloma was only slightly higher than in the more distally exposed population; however, only one case of multiple myeloma was observed in the proximally exposed group. In 1969 Yamamoto and Wakabayashi[5] reported that data on the development of bone tumors (including multiple myelomas) among the atomic bomb survivors of Hiroshima and Nagasaki between 1950 and 1963 provided no evidence that the tumors were induced by radiation. In 1973 Nishiyama et al[6] also studied the frequency of malignant lymphoma and multiple myeloma in a fixed population of atomic bomb survivors in Hiroshima and Nagasaki, and found that even in the heavily exposed population the multiple myeloma risk was not significantly greater. Few reports prior to 1965 indicated a high frequency of multiple myeloma among exposed subjects, and most investigations in fact tended to indicate negative findings. Beginning around 1963, reports on the incidence of multiple myeloma among exposed Nagasaki survivors were published by Ichimaru et al. In 1978 they reported on a fixed population of approximately 100,000 exposed individuals in the Life Span Study performed by the Hiroshima and Nagasaki branches of the Radiation Effects Research Foundation (RERF) over the 26-year period 1950–1976, and also on the ABCC-RERF detection program aimed at identifying leukemia and other related diseases. Thirty-five multiple myeloma cases were detected, with a detailed investigation providing confirmation of the disease in 29 cases; Ichimaru et al[7] investigated the relative risk and crude incidence of multiple myeloma among this group according to the radiation dose received. Of the 29 cases, 22 were directly exposed, while 7 were non-exposed. The relative risk was 4.7 for a T65 dose of ≥ 1.0 Gy; 1.5 for a dose of 0.01–0.99 Gy; and 1.0 for a dose of < 0.01 Gy. The relative multiple myeloma risk in the heavily exposed population (i.e. exposed to ≥ 1.0 Gy) was thus between approximately 4 and 5 times greater than in the low-dose population, which represents a significant increase (Table 1). Also, the crude multiple myeloma incidence by dose per 1,000 population was 0.97 for the ≥ 1.0 Gy population, 0.3 for the 0.01–0.99 Gy population, and 0.21 for the < 0.01 Gy control population, thus demonstrating the dose-dependence of the crude multiple myeloma incidence (Table 2).

The crude annual incidence per 100,000 population was calculated to be 4.2 for the atomic bomb survivors exposed to ≥ 1.00 Gy, 1.3 for the 0.01–0.99 Gy population, and 0.9 for the controls (Table 2), with the same tendencies observed in both Hiroshima and Nagasaki. An examination of these multiple myeloma cases by age at the time of bombing (ATB) revealed that all the five cases in the high dose (≥ 1.00 Gy) population were aged 20–59 years ATB. In contrast to the previous

Table 1   Standardized relative risk of confirmed multiple myeloma cases among atomic bomb survivors, Hiroshima and Nagasaki, in the Life Span Study sample by dose, 1950–1976[T]

| T65 total dose (Gy) | Standardized relative risk (adjusted for sex, city and age ATB) | |
	Relative risk	Test of significance [+]
≥ 1.00 (3) 0.01–0.99 (2) < 0.01 (1)	4.7 1.5 1.0	Null hypothesis HO : PE = PC $(3) = (1)\ x^2[1] = 4.21$ $P < 0.05$ $(2) = (1)\ x^2[1]$ 0.27 $P < 0.05$

[+] Mantel and Haenszel's procedure[19]

Factors adjusted: sex (M, F), city (Hiroshima & Nagasaki), age at the time of bombing (ATB) (0–19, 20–39, 40–59, ≥ 60)

Table 2   Crude incidence rate per 1,000 population and crude annual incidence rate per 100,000 population of confirmed multiple myeloma among atomic bomb survivors and controls, Hiroshima and Nagasaki, in the Life Span Study sample by dose, Oct. 1950–Dec. 1976[7]

Dose (Gy)	No. of subjects	No. of cases	Crude incidence rate per 1,000 population			C.R.R.	Person years	Crude annual incidence rate (per 100,000)
			Average	90% confidence limit				
				Upper	Lower			
Unknown	1,725	0	0.00	1.33	0.00	—	38,250	0.0
≥ 1.00	5,144	5	0.97	1.81	0.47	4.6	117,924	4.2
0.01 ~ 0.99	33,069	10	0.30	0.46	0.19	1.4	751,517	1.3
< 0.01	32,864	7	0.21	0.36	0.12	1.0	745,912	0.9
NIC*	26,581**	7	—	—	—	—	587,052	1.2
Total	99,383	29	—	—	—	—	2,240,655	1.3

C.R.R. = Crude relative risk
*NIC : Not in city at the time of bombing
**14,495 subjects were selected in 1951 and 1958

reports which considered cases occurring prior to 1965, this report expanded the study to cover up to 1976, and showed a clear relationship between multiple myeloma and radiation exposure. As indicated in previous reports, there is a long latency period before clinical diagnosis of multiple myeloma, and as this study covered cases over the approximately 30-year period after the atomic bombing, it provides statistically meaningful results.

Later Ichimaru et al reanalyzed the results for the same group of subjects up to 1976[8,9,10], but no clinical differences in comparison to non-exposed multiple myeloma patients were detected. However, classification into three groups by T65DR bone marrow dose (the control population, the 0.01–0.49 Gy population, and the ≥ 0.50 Gy population), revealed that the relative risk in the ≥ 0.50 Gy population increased for both men and women; the tendency was the same in both Hiroshima and Nagasaki, with the risk being significantly higher for those aged 20–59 ATB and who also received a bone marrow dose of ≥ 0.50 Gy (Table 3). Furthermore, the estimated multiple myeloma risk for heavily exposed individuals aged 20–59 ATB was calculated as approximately 0.48 cases for a bone marrow total dose of 0.01 Gy per 10^6 person years. Figure 1 shows the crude cumulative incidence by year for the 20–59 year ATB group for all dose populations between 1950 and 1976. Relative to the other populations, the high dose population (≥ 0.50 Gy) showed a rapid increase after 1960 (Fig. 1). Consequently this was the first report in which both the incidence and relative risk of multiple myeloma among atomic bomb survivors aged 20–59 years ATB was high and dose-dependent.

Tumor statistics revealed that in Nagasaki during the 10-year period from 1973 to 1982 there were 48 cases of multiple myeloma among atomic bomb survivors and 37 cases among the non-exposed. Relative to the non-exposed population, a high rate was observed among middle-aged atomic bomb survivors (i.e. people in their 50s). A high relative risk was observed among the proximally exposed (< 2 km), but when

Table 3 Specific annual incidence of multiple myeloma (by marrow total dose, sex, city, and age) in the Life Span Study sample Oct. 1950–Dec. 1976, Hiroshima and Nagasaki

Specification	Controls	Marrow total dose (Gy)		Totals
		0.01 ~ 0.49	≥ 0.50	
Male				
Person years	517,563	322,571	53,255	893,389
No. of cases	4	3	3	10
Rate per 10,000	0.77	0.93	5.63	1.12
Crude relative risk	1.0	1.2	6.4	—
Female				
Person years	756,083	480,509	70,597	1,307,189
No. of cases	10	7	2	19
Rate per 10,000	1.32	1.46	2.83	1.45
Crude relative risk	1.0	1.1	2.1	—
Hiroshima				
Person years	1,032,403	543,374	62,572	1,638,352
No. of cases	11	6	2	19
Rate per 10,000	1.07	1.10	3.20	1.16
Crude relative risk	1.0	1.0	3.0	—
Nagasaki				
Person years	241,243	259,706	61,276	562,225
No. of cases	3	4	3	10
Rate per 10,000	1.24	1.54	4.90	1.78
Crude relative risk	1.0	1.2	4.0	—
Age ATB: 0–19				
Person years	577,303	373,998	59,606	1,010,907
No. of cases	1	0	0	1
Rate per 10,000	0.17	0.0	0.0	0.10
Crude relative risk	1.0	—	—	
Age ATB: 20–39				
Person years	391,526	228,147	37,527	657,200
No. of cases	3	2	2	7
Rate per 10,000	0.77	0.88	5.33	1.07
Crude relative risk	1.0	1.1	6.9	—
Age ATB: 40–59				
Person years	272,033	178,330	24,817	475,180
No. of cases	9	8	3	20
Rate per 10,000	3.31	4.49	12.09	4.21
Crude relative risk	1.0	1.4	3.7	—
Age ATB: ≥ 60				
Person years	32,785	22,605	1,902	57,292
No. of cases	1	0	0	1
Rate per 10,000	3.05	0.0	0.0	1.75
Crude relative risk	1.0	—	—	—

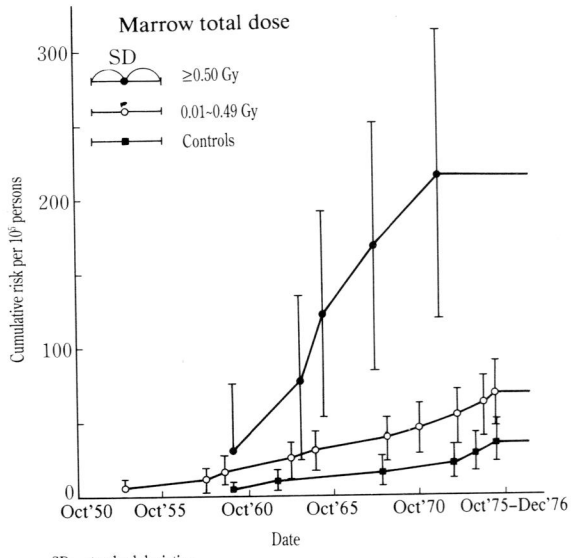

SD = standard deviation

Note: Study covered the period Oct. 1950 ~ Dec. 1976 for both Hiroshima and Nagasaki, for a control group consisting
of those not present in the cities at the time of bombing, and for those present in Oct. 1950 who had been
exposed to < 0.01 Gy of atomic bomb radiation.

Figure 1   Cumulative risk among the atomic bomb survivors (aged 20–59 at the time of bombing and the control group in the Life Span Study sample)[8,10]

the relative risks (5.34 for males, 3.05 for females) are adjusted for age (1.59 for males, 1.68 for females), no statistically significant difference is found. From a pathological viewpoint, an investigation of the annual number of multiple myeloma cases autopsied in Nagasaki between 1946 and 1988 showed that the number tended to increase after 1975, and that between 1981 and 1985 the incidence amongst atomic bomb survivors was significantly high in comparison to the control population[11].

2. MONOCLONAL GAMMOPATHY AND ATOMIC BOMB SURVIVORS

As mentioned in the previous section, following reports that the development of multiple myeloma among atomic bomb survivors was strongly affected by radiation, attention turned towards multiple myeloma when the atomic bomb survivors underwent examination and treatment. In 1980 Abe *et al*[12] compared the clinical features of 21 atomic bomb survivor multiple myeloma cases at one facility with 31 non-exposed cases, and reconfirmed the earlier results of Ichimaru *et al* that no particular difference could be observed between the two populations. However, it became apparent that early or pre-multiple myeloma could be detected from an analysis of past data for atomic bomb survivors.

Monoclonal gammopathy is usually classified into the two extreme forms, the malignant form of multiple myeloma, and the benign form, benign monoclonal gammopathy (BMG). However, the screening data suggests the detection of cases with a form intermediate between the two extremes[13]. Various forms have been recognized among these cases, ranging from conditions close to those observed in BMG to conditions close to those in multiple myeloma, which should perhaps be referred to as a pre-myeloma state; in the literature these cases have been provisionally termed either intermediate forms or lumped together as monoclonal gammopathy of undetermined significance (MGUS). In either case, advantages of screening atomic bomb survivors are that there are cases in which it is possible to analyze abnormal data by delving into the past, and also that regular follow-up examinations can be performed. Thus it is necessary in the future to use these as a technique for clinical clarification of whether the development of monoclonal gammopathy is in some way related to radiation.

In view of the above, multiple myeloma screening was incorporated into the cancer screening of atomic bomb survivors in Hiroshima in 1988[15,16]. By 1990, 52,477 atomic bomb survivors had been screened in Hiroshima, with monoclonal gammopathy detected in 344 cases (a rate of 0.66%) (Table 4)[17]. All these cases were asymptomatic, and were diagnosed for the first time by the screening tests. A conveniently determined classification of the screening results showed that the monoclonal gammopathy cases could be categorized as benign monoclonal gammopathy (BMG) (219 cases, 63.7%), pre-multiple myeloma (Pre-MM) (65 cases, 18.9%), multiple myeloma (54 cases, 15.7%), and primary macroglobulinemia (MG) (6 cases, 1.7%). No significant difference was observed in the frequency of monoclonal gammopathy with respect to distance from the hypocenter (i.e. between city entrants who entered the city after the bombing, and the groups who were directly exposed at distances of ≥ 2.1 km and < 2 km, respectively). Also, no particular difference was observed between the three populations in terms of the form of monoclonal gammopathy developed (Table 5). The incidence of monoclonal gammopathy increases with age, with a sudden increase conspicuous among people in their 70s. The incidence of BMG and pre-multiple myeloma levels off after the age of 80, but the incidence of multiple myeloma tends to increase further (Fig. 2).

Similar findings have recently been reported concerning screening results in Nagasaki[18]. Utilizing previous screening data, investigations have been performed

Table 4   Classification of monoclonal gammopathy (Hiroshima, Sep. 1989 ~ Mar. 1990)[17]

	Male	Female	Total	
Benign monoclonal gammopathy (BMG)	88	131	219	(63.7%)
Pre-multiple myeloma (Pre-MM)	26	39	65	(18.9%)
Myeloma (MM) stage I A	22	30	52 ⎤ 54	
stage II A	0	2	2 ⎦	(15.7%)
stage III	0	0	0	
Primary macroglobulinemia (MG)	6	0	6	(1.7%)
Total	142	202	344	

Table 5   Incidence (%) of monoclonal gammopathy by distance from the hypocenter (Hiroshima, Sep. 1988–Mar. 1990)[17]

Distance from hypocenter	> 2.0 km	< 2.1 km	Entered city after bombing
BMG	0.36	0.40	0.47
Pre-MM	0.14	0.12	0.11
MM + MG	0.13	0.11	0.10
Total	0.64	0.63	0.69

BMG = benign monoclonal gammopathy; Pre MM = pre-multiple myeloma; MM = multiple myeloma; MG = monoclonal gammopathy

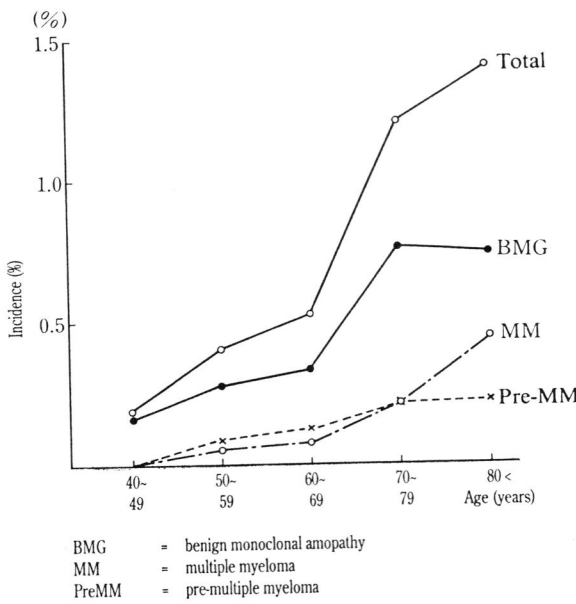

Figure 2   Incidence of monoclonal gammopathy by age group (Hiroshima, Sep. 1988–Mar. 1990)[17]

on the changes in the form of monoclonal gammopathy occurring among atomic bomb survivors[17]. It was found that there were 87 possible cases with monoclonal gammopathy even more than 5 years earlier, and 14 cases were confirmed as existing over 10 years earlier. This even included 18 cases now diagnosed as multiple myeloma but in which monoclonal gammopathy was found to have been present over 5 years earlier, suggesting that multiple myeloma develops extremely slowly among atomic bomb survivors, as is the case with non-exposed patients. An analysis of the 18 cases in which the previous form of monoclonal gammopathy could be determined revealed that, over a 5-to-10 year period, in 8 of the cases either the BMG developed into multiple myeloma or pre-multiple myeloma, or else there was a change from pre-multiple myeloma into multiple myeloma. This is of great importance in the management of monoclonal gammopathy and the clarification of changes in the type of monoclonal gammopathy in atomic bomb survivors.

Two surveys on myeloma screening were performed on subjects in the Hiroshima and Nagasaki RERF Adult Health Study sample; the first covered the years 1979–1981 and involved 8,796 persons, with the second covering the years 1985–1987 and involving 7,350 individuals[19]. The first study revealed monoclonal gammopathy in 0.38% of the population, and the second 0.94%, thus reconfirming the increasing frequency of monoclonal gammopathy (Table 6). However, multiple myeloma was not observed in the second study, and the question of whether or not the multiple myeloma incidence is decreasing remains a matter to be settled by the continuation of the screening program. The study found that among atomic bomb survivor cases exposed to an estimated DS86 bone marrow dose of $\geqslant 0.01$ Gy the relative risks of new development of BMG and MGUS were 1.3 and 2.0 respectively. Although high, these tendencies were not statistically significant (Table 7).

Table 6 Number of monoclonal gammopathy cases (1st and 2nd studies)[19]

	1st study	2nd study
No. of people examined	8,796	7,350
Average age (years)	58.3	61.9
No. of cases	33	69
Prevalence (%)	0.38	0.94

Table 7 Incidence of monoclonal gammopathy between Oct. 1979 ~ Sep. 1981 and June 1985 ~ May 1987[19]

		DS86 bone marrow dose (Gy)					
		0	0.01–0.49	0.50–0.99	$\geqslant 1.00$	$\geqslant 0.01$	Total
Number at risk		2214	1605	756	675	2361	4576
MGUS	Obs.	4	8	3	0	11	15
	Exp.	6.25	4.72	2.36	1.67	8.75	15.00
	RR	1.00	2.65	1.99	0.00	1.96	
	Estimated RR	1.00				1.96 ($p = 0.225$)	
BMG	Obs.	4	6	4	1	11	15
	Exp.	6.39	4.54	2.21	1.87	8.61	150
+	Exp.	12.64	9.26	4.56	3.53	17.36	300
BMG	RR	1.00	2.39	2.45	0.45	2.00	
	Estimated RR	1.00				1.27	($p = 0.180$)

Obs. = observed; Exp. = expected; RR = relative risk; BMG = benign monoclonal gammopathy; MGUS = monoclonal gammopathy of undetermined significance

3. THE ROLE OF INTERLEUKIN-6 IN THE DEVELOPMENT OF MYELOMA IN ATOMIC BOMB SURVIVORS.

In many cases of the disease, the malignant transformation of the plasma cells (so-called myeloma cells) results in the production of interleukin-6 (IL-6). The proliferation of myeloma cells themselves is accelerated by IL-6, and thus the myeloma cell proliferation is believed to follow the autocrine mechanism through the medium of IL-6[20]. With respect to this, and in order to investigate whether or not special radiation-related characteristics act in the development of multiple myeloma in atomic bomb survivors, a study was carried out on the myeloma cells of multiple myeloma patients, including both atomic bomb survivors and non-exposed patients. No difference was observed between the two populations in either IL-6 production or in the mRNA level in IL-6; moreover, there was no difference between the populations regarding the appearance of IL-6 receptors (the number of IL-6 receptors, the value of the dissociation constant Kd, the production of IL-6 receptor mRNA, and IL-6 receptor gene rearrangement)[21,22]. However, further research is necessary in order to elucidate the role played by cystokine in radiation-induced carcinogenesis.

CONCLUSIONS

(1) Widespread development of multiple myeloma occurred among atomic bomb survivors nearly 20 years after exposure. In cases prior to 1976 the multiple myeloma incidence was dependent on the T65DR bone marrow dose and increased in the ≥ 0.50 Gy population, and was particularly evident amongst those aged 20–59 ATB.

(2) From a pathological viewpoint, the number of multiple myeloma cases autopsied increased after 1975, reaching a significant level among atomic bomb survivors after 1981.

(3) Screening of the atomic bomb survivors revealed the presence of monoclonal gammopathy, indicating a form intermediate between multiple myeloma and benign monoclonal gammopathy (BMG).

(4) For all forms of monoclonal gammopathy, no significant difference in frequency has been observed to date with respect to distance from the hypocenter, but a change in the form of monoclonal gammopathy has been observed over a 5- to 10-year period. Therefore, the development of monoclonal gammopathy, which is representative of multiple myeloma (the malignant transformation of plasma cells, which have a relatively high radiosensitivity), can be considered a late effect of atomic bomb radiation. On the other hand, the tendency of monoclonal gammopathy to increase can be considered merely a change that occurs with advancing age. However, further screening is necessary in order to clarify whether the increasing frequency among individuals aged under 30 ATB is due to the effects of exposure exerting an influence additional to the increase caused by their reaching the age at which monoclonal gammopathy frequently appears.

(Kingo Fujimura)

REFERENCES

1. Lewis EB. Leukemia, multiple myeloma, and aplastic anemia in American radiologists. *Science* 1963; **142**: 1492–4.
2. Mancuso TF, Stewart A, Kneale, G. Radiation exposures of Hanford workers dying from cancer and other causes. *Health Physics* 1977; **33**: 369–95.
3. Cuzick J. Radiation-induced myelomatosis. *N Engl J Med* 1981; **304**: 204–10.
4. Anderson RE, Ishida K. Malignant lymphoma in survivors of the atomic bomb in Hiroshima. *Ann Intern Med* 1964; **61**: 853–62.
5. Yamamoto T, Wakabayashi T. Bone tumors among the atomic bomb survivors of Hiroshima and Nagasaki. *Acta Path Jap* 1969; **19**: 201–12.
6. Nishiyama H, Anderson RE, Ishimaru T, *et al.* The incidence of malignant lymphoma and multiple myeloma in Hiroshima and Nagasaki atomic bomb survivors, 1945–1965. *Cancer* 1973; **32**: 1301–9.
7. Ichimaru M, Ishimaru T, Mikami M, *et al.* Multiple myeloma among atomic bomb survivors. *Nagasaki Med J* 1978; **53**: 404–12.
8. Ichimaru M, Ishimaru T, Mikami M, *et al.* Multiple myeloma among atomic bomb survivors in Hiroshima and Nagasaki, 1950–76: relationship to radiation dose absorbed by marrow. *JNCI* 1982; **69**: 323–8.
9. Ichimaru M, Ohkita T, Ishimaru T. Leukemia, multiple myeloma, and malignant lymphoma. *GANN Monograph on Cancer Res* 1986; **32**: 113–27.
10. Ichimaru M, Ishimaru T, Mikami M, *et al.* Multiple myeloma among atomic bomb survivors in Hiroshima and Nagasaki, 1950–76: relationship to radiation dose absorbed by marrow. *J Hiroshima Med Ass* 1983; **36**: 1323–31.
11. Nishimori I, Kishikawa M, Iseki M, *et al.* Pathologic studies of multiple myeloma of atomic bomb survivors (Nagasaki 1946–1988). *J Hiroshima Med Ass* 1990; **43**: 402–5.
12. Abe T, Kimura A, Mizuno T, *et al.* The clinical study of 52 cases of monoclonal gammopathy (1962–1979) including 21 cases of atomic bomb survivors. *J Hiroshima Med Ass* 1980; **33**: 440–4.
13. Abe T, Doi H, Ihara A, *et al.* The clinical study of 41 cases of monoclonal gammopathy in atomic bomb survivors. *J Hiroshima Med Ass* 1982; **35**: 471–4.
14. Abe T, Takimoto Y, Maehama S, *et al.* The clinical study of monoclonal gammopathy among the atomic bomb survivors. 4. The follow up study of the intermediate type—a case of typical myeloma advanced from intermediate type. *J Hiroshima Med Ass* 1984; **37**: 484–6.
15. Fujimura K, Kimura A, Iwato K, *et al.* Clinical studies of 44 cases of monoclonal gammopathy which were detected at atomic bomb health examination in the past 3 years. *Nagasaki Med J* 1989; **63**: 678–84.
16. Fujimura K, Kimura A, Kuramoto A, *et al.* M-proteinemia in atomic bomb survivors. First report: cancer examination report in 1988. *J Hiroshima Med Ass* 1990; **43**: 406–9.
17. Fujimura K, Kawano M, Kimura A, *et al.* The study of monoclonal gammopathy which was detected at atomic bomb health examination. *Nagasaki Med J* 1990; **65**: 529–35.
18. Momita S, Atogami S, Ikeda S, *et al.* Current status of multiple myeloma examination in atomic bomb survivors, Nagasaki. *Nagasaki Med J* 1990; **65**: 611–5.
19. Neriishi K, Yoshimoto Y, Mikami M, *et al.* M-proteinemia in atomic bomb survivors in Hiroshima and Nagasaki—comparison between first and second surveys—*Nagasaki Med J* 1990; **65**: 544–51.
20. Kawano M, Hirano T, Matsuda T, *et al.* Autocrine generation and requirement of BSF-2/IL-6 for human multiple myeloma. *Nature* 1988; **332**: 83–5.
21. Kawano M, Iwato K, Asaoku H, *et al.* Cell biological study in multiple myeloma among atomic bomb survivors. 1. IL-6 production from myeloma cells. *Nagasaki Med J* 1989; 63: 782–7.
22. Ishikawa H, Tanabe O, Tanaka H, *et al.* Cell biological study in multiple myeloma among atomic bomb survivors. 3. Expression of IL-6 receptor on myeloma cells. *Nagasaki Med J* 1990; **65**: 561–7.

1.7 COLORECTAL CANCER

INTRODUCTION

The incidence of colon cancer in Japan is at present only one third to one half the level observed in Western countries, but in recent years cancers of the sigmoid colon etc have registered a rapid increase, and the incidence of colorectal cancer is expected to reach virtually the same level as in Western countries in the near future. The relationship between radiation and colorectal cancer is not as marked as with leukemia and thyroid cancer etc., but it is at least clear that the colon cancer incidence increased following exposure to atomic bomb radiation. It is anticipated that the atomic bomb survivors will exhibit a rapid increase in colorectal cancer to accompany the increased incidence in the non-exposed general population.

The following discussion examines the relationship between exposure to atomic bomb radiation and the risk of developing colorectal cancer, with separate sections dealing with the colon and the rectum.

1. COLON CANCER

An increased colon cancer risk due to exposure to atomic bomb radiation has been observed since the 1960s, but since the 1970s it has become more pronounced, with the data from the 1950–78 mortality follow-up study (the Life Span Study) performed on the atomic bomb survivors by the Radiation Effects Research Foundation (RERF) showing the increase to be statistically significant[1]. Later analysis of the Life Span Study data for regularly extended periods of observation has also confirmed an increase in colon cancer mortality due to radiation exposure[2]; analyses of incidence surveys and data from tumor registries in Hiroshima and Nagasaki have also yielded results similar to those obtained from mortality rate surveys[3,4]. No great difference is apparent between the various colon sites (Fig. 1) with respect to the relative cancer risk of developing cancer (i.e. the ratio of incidence among the exposed to the incidence among the non-exposed) and the excess relative risk (i.e. the relative risk minus one). However, since almost half the colon cancer found in Japanese develops in the sigmoid colon, when the excess incidence (incidence in the exposed minus incidence in the non-exposed) is used as an indicator of risk, the cancer risk at this site becomes greater than at other colon sites. For example, as shown in Fig. 2, when the excess incidence by site based on the 1984 Hiroshima colon cancer incidence is calculated for exposure to 1 Gy, the excess incidence of sigmoid colon cancer is greater than for other colon cancers. On the other hand, even though the rectum is continuous with the sigmoid colon and histologically quite similar, none of the RERF incidence studies reveals much increase in radiation-related cancer [2-4].

An analysis of the dose-response relationship reveals that the colon cancer risk increases in a virtually linear fashion with the atomic bomb radiation dose[5]. The increased risk associated with exposure to 1 Gy of radiation is estimated at approximately just under a factor of two and, as with other malignant tumors, is high among

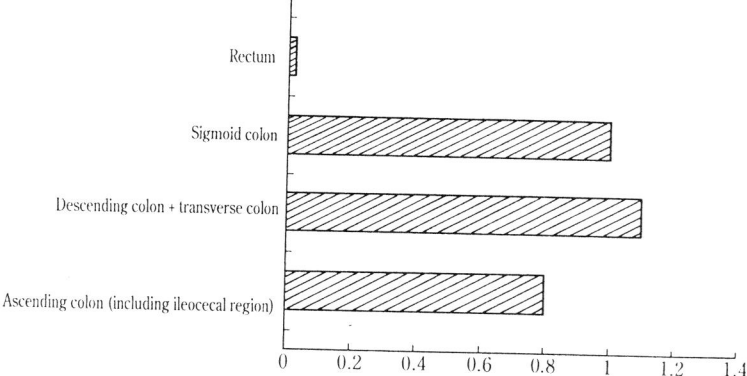

Figure 1   Colorectal cancer risk in atomic bomb survivors by site.

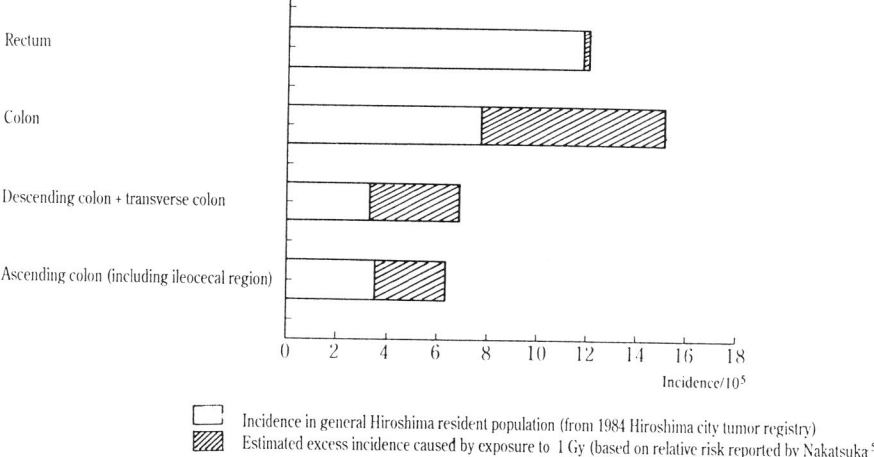

☐   Incidence in general Hiroshima resident population (from 1984 Hiroshima city tumor registry)

▨   Estimated excess incidence caused by exposure to 1 Gy (based on relative risk reported by Nakatsuka[5]

Figure 2   Estimated radiation-caused excess incidence of colorectal cancer by site.

those exposed at a young age, although the tendency is not as marked as in thyroid cancer or breast cancer. Moreover, no clear difference in radiation risk is observed between males and females, or between Hiroshima and Nagasaki. It can generally be considered that an excess number of solid tumors appears approximately 10 years after exposure to radiation[7]. However, numerous difficulties are involved in actually confirming this, and accurate values relating to colon cancer are not available.

2. RECTAL CANCER

It is unknown why the rectum, which is anatomically adjacent to the colon and histologically similar, virtually fails to exhibit any radiation-related excess incidence of malignant tumors. In some studies involving subjects other than the atomic bomb survivors, it has been reported that the cancer risk increases following localized exposure to high doses of radiation, and the possibility exists that the radiosensitivity of the rectum is somewhat different from the colon. Also, a number of the non-radiation risk factors that affect the two sites do not overlap, and thus the mechanisms of carcinogenesis at the two sites can be regarded as slightly different[8,9], a fact supported by the male : female incidence ratio being close to 1 : 1 for colon cancer, but 2–3 : 1 for rectal cancer[8].

CONCLUSION

A clear increase in colorectal cancer is observed among atomic bomb survivors, with the risk increasing as the age at the time of bombing decreases. Also, as with other solid tumors, the excess incidence due to exposure to atomic bomb radiation increases in an approximately proportional manner, as observed among non-exposed patients, and it is anticipated that from now on the excess incidence will increase rapidly as all the atomic bomb survivors become older and those who were exposed while young reach the age at which the incidence of cancer usually increases.

It is believed that colorectal cancer can to some extent be prevented by improved eating habits etc.[10], but at the present time it is unclear whether or not such actions can prevent an excess colorectal cancer incidence among atomic bomb survivors. However, due to the advances in diagnostic techniques and the improvements in therapeutic methods etc. that have occurred in recent years, early detection and early treatment is making it possible to prolong the life of cancer patients[10], and it is important to redouble efforts with regard to cancer screening of the atomic bomb survivors.

(Suminori Akiba)

REFERENCES

1. Kato H, Schull WS. Studies of the mortality of A-bomb survivors. Report 7. Mortality 1950–78: Part 1. Cancer mortality. *Radiat Res* 1982; **90**: 395–432.
2. Shimizu Y, Kato H, Schull WS. Studies of the mortality of A-bomb survivors. Report 9. Mortality, 1950–85: Part 2. Cancer mortality based on the recently revised doses (DS86). *Radiat Res* 1990; **121**: 120–41.
3. Nakatsuka H, Ezaki H. Colorectal cancer among atomic bomb survivors. *GANN Monograph on Cancer Res* 1986; **32**: 155–65.
4. Monzen T, Wakabayashi T. Tumor and tissue registries in Hiroshima and Nagasaki. *GANN Monograph on Cancer Res* 1986; **32**: 29–40.
5. Nakatsuka H, Shimizu Y, Yamamoto T, *et al.* Colorectal cancer incidence and radiation dose among atomic bomb survivors, Hiroshima and Nagasaki, 1950–1980. *J Radiat Res* 1992; **33**: 342–61.
6. Thompson DE, Mabuchi K, Ron E, *et al.* Cancer incidence in atomic bomb survivors. Part II: Solid tumors, 1958–87. *Radiat Res* 1994; **137**: S17–67.
7. Committee on the Biological Effects of Ionizing Radiation. Commission on Life Science. Health effects of exposure to low levels of ionizing radiation (BEIR-V). National Academy of Sciences-National Research Council. Washington, DC: National Academy Press, 1990: 161–241.

8. Tajima K, Kuroishi T, Tominaga S, *et al.* The recent trend of colon cancer in Japan. *Igaku no ayumi* (Advances in Medicine) 1982; **122** (5): 398–407. (*In Japanese*)

9. Schottenfeld D, Winawer SJ. Large intestine. In: Schottenfeld D, Fraumeni J, editors. Cancer epidemiology and prevention. Philadelphia: WB Saunders, 1982: 703–27.

10. Tominaga S. The possibility of chemoprevention of cancer. *Gan to Kagaku-ryohou* (Japanese Journal of Cancer and Chemotherapy) 1990; **17** (2): 173–9. (*In Japanese*)

1.8 SKIN CANCER

INTRODUCTION

It is well known that skin cancer is induced as a result of occupational exposure to radiation and radiotherapy. In atomic bomb survivors, an increase has been observed in the incidence of malignant tumors such as leukemia, thyroid cancer, breast cancer, and lung cancer etc., and a question of great interest is whether or not skin cancer is increasing in atomic bomb survivors. This chapter reviews current knowledge regarding the development of radiation-related skin cancer, considers the main findings concerning atomic bomb radiation and skin cancer which have recently drawn attention, and mentions future topics for investigation.

1. RADIATION AND SKIN CANCER

X-rays were discovered by Roentgen in the year 1895; the problem of radiation damage first arose with acute and chronic radiodermatitis. In 1902 Frieben[1] reported a case of skin cancer in the hand of an employee working in a factory making X-ray tubes which was believed to have been caused by the action of X-rays. Since that time, the development of radiation-induced skin cancer in occupationally exposed individuals such as physicians and radiologic technologists has become a social issue. Radiation was later applied therapeutically, and particularly in the early period radiation was used for not only malignant tumors but also for various benign diseases; consequently, numerous accounts of radiation-induced skin cancer appeared in the literature[2].

The incidence and histologic type of radiation-induced skin cancer is thought to vary with the radiation source, the particular disease for which radiotherapy is employed, and the site of irradiation. The International Commission on Radiological Protection (ICRP) task group summarized the situation regarding radiotherapy-induced skin cancer, stating that most studies have revealed a predominance of basal cell carcinoma, with smaller excesses of squamous cell carcinoma. The risk of radiation-induced skin cancer was high for radiotherapy to sites likely to be exposed to ultra-violet (UV) radiation (e.g. the head, face, and arms etc.), but low for sites shielded from UV-radiation (e.g. trunk, legs etc.). A marked variation has been observed in incidence rates between ethnic groups, but most studies to date have concerned increases in radiation-induced skin cancer among light-colored racial groups, and it would be expected that darker-colored groups would face a reduced risk[3]. The vast majority of the radiation-induced skin cancer reported in Japan has been squamous cell carcinoma, which has accounted for approximately 80% of the total[4]. However, Okazaki et al[5] have recently reported that since 1975 there has been an increase in basal cell carcinoma even in Japan, with the proportion of squamous cell carcinoma decreasing.

The large majority of reports concerning radiation-induced skin cancer have dealt with either continuous long-term irradiation or intermittent radiation[6]. It is believed that some cases of acute radiodermatitis occur following a single dose of radiation, which then develop into chronic radiodermatitis, but as yet no conclusions have been reached as to whether skin cancer is induced following a single dose of irradiation. Comparisons between single and multiple doses of radiation have been performed in animal experiments. Hoshino and Tanooka[7] described the skin irradiation of mice with beta rays and found that although the majority of the mice exhibited acute radiodermatitis following a single dose, no skin tumors were observed within the study period of 23 months. On the other hand, malignant and benign tumors of the skin were observed after multiple irradiation.

In many instances the radiation-induced skin cancer developed from the chronic radiodermatitis that appeared at the irradiated site. Selecting a random sample of 257 out of 2,400 patients who had received radiotherapy for benign diseases, Willem et al[8] investigated the relationship between radiodermatitis and the development of skin cancer. The severity of radiodermatitis was associated with a higher prevalence of skin cancer. In the population not exhibiting radiodermatitis the skin cancer prevalence was 1.4%, with the rates observed in the populations exhibiting light, medium and severe symptoms being 7.2%, 20.5%, and 16.6% respectively.

Concerning the late effects of nuclear tests, Conard[9] surveyed the exposed population of the Marshall islands, and reported that although cases of burns and epilation were attributable to radiation, no malignant skin tumors were observed. Caldwell[10] followed the progress over 22 years of 3,217 participants in the Nevada nuclear test program, and identified 23 non-melanotic skin cancers. The average dose received by the skin cancer cases was 2.5 mGy, whereas the remainder received an average of 4.6 mGy. Thus no relationship was observed between radiation dose and skin cancer.

2. SKIN CANCER AMONG ATOMIC BOMB SURVIVORS

Between July 1964 and August 1966 Johnson et al[11] studied the relationship between radiation and skin cancer by investigating 303 dermatologic characteristics and their severity in 10,650 subjects in the Adult Health Study sample of the Atomic Bomb Casualty Commission (ABCC) (the present-day Radiation Effects Research Foundation, RERF). The only case of skin cancer observed among the subjects was a case of Bowen's squamous cell carcinoma; in that case the dose received was much less than 0.01 Gy. Regarding the frequency of dermatologic characteristics of radiodermatitis, it was found that in comparison to the control population the atomic bomb survivors exhibited a higher frequency of atrophic scars, pigmentation and depigmentation, and showed a tendency for fine telangiectasia of the arm to increase with increasing doses. Since similarities can be observed between chronic radiodermatitis and skin changes due to aging, the relationship between radiation dose and the symptoms of skin changes due to aging was also analyzed, but it was found that associations were limited to hair graying and facial senile elastoses. The first study on skin cancer among atomic bomb survivors thus failed to find an increase in malignant skin neoplasms or skin precancerosis lesions during the 20 years following the atomic explosion.

Key[12] used the data concerning autopsies and biopsies accumulated in the period 1945–67 to investigate the relationship between radiation and skin cancer in the ABCC Life Span Study sample. Twenty skin carcinoma cases were confirmed, of whom 7 were proximally exposed; in 3 of the 20 cases the carcinoma developed at the site of lacerations or burn scars caused by the atomic explosion. However, no significant increase in skin cancer was observed among the atomic bomb survivors.

At the 28th Late A-bomb Effects Research Meeting in 1987 Sadamori et al[13] reported that a skin cancer study covering up to 1985 showed a high correlation between radiation dose and the incidence of skin cancer among the RERF Nagasaki Life Span Study sample. At the same conference Yamada et al[14,15] reported that a 1958–85 skin cancer study found a significant increase in basal cell carcinoma and squamous cell carcinoma among the RERF Hiroshima Adult Health Study sample exposed to ≥ 1 Gy (T65D doses).

Sadamori et al[16] later studied data at the Scientific Data Center of the Atomic Bomb Disaster, Nagasaki University School of Medicine, concerning the approximately 60,000 individuals who were directly exposed to the atomic bomb, and reported on the 140 skin cancer cases confirmed during the period 1961–87. According to histologic type, these consisted of basal cell carcinoma (67 cases), squamous cell carcinoma (43 cases), malignant melanoma (11 cases), Paget's disease (7 cases), skin adnexal tumors (6 cases), and skin sarcomas (6 cases). A significant correlation existed between the incidence of skin carcinoma and distance from the hypocenter, with the incidence increasing with time in recent years. In particular, a conspicuously increased incidence has been apparent since 1975 in the population exposed within 2 km of the hypocenter[16,17].

In 1991 Sadamori et al[18] employed DS86 dosimetry to investigate the relationship between ionizing radiation and the skin cancer incidence among the expanded RERF Nagasaki Life Span Study sample for the period 1958–85. The dose-response relationship for skin cancer was a linear one without a threshold value. The excess relative risk for a dose of 1 Gy was found to be 2.2 (95% confidence limit, range 0.5–5.0), a value which was highly significant.

Based on the tumor tissue registries, Mabuchi et al[19] analyzed the incidence of non-melanotic skin cancers for the period 1958–87 among the expanded RERF Life Span Study samples in Hiroshima and Nagasaki. Skin cancer was confirmed in 168 of the 79,972 individuals surveyed, with the skin cancer incidence showing a marked increase with age, and rising in recent years. The excess relative risk per 1 Sv (Sievert) was 1.0 (95% confidence limit, range 0.41–1.09), with the relative risk increasing with decreasing age at the time of bombing. An analysis of histologic type revealed that ionizing radiation had a greater effect on basal cell carcinoma than on squamous cell carcinoma.

3. THEMES FOR FUTURE INVESTIGATION

Despite the investigations on the relationship between skin cancer and atomic bomb exposure, various points remain unclear.

The damage caused by the atomic bomb was due to the effects of the bomb blast, heat and radiation, all of which affect the skin. Burns were observed in victims within 3.5 km of the hypocenter in the case of Hiroshima, and 4.0 km in the case of Nagasaki; this included both primary thermal burns due to the direct effect of heat rays from the atomic bomb on human bodies, and secondary indirect burns due to fires etc. Numerous victims suffered cuts and lacerations as a result of the bomb blast and the destruction of buildings etc. A high percentage of skin cancer (in particular squamous cell carcinoma) was found to occur at scars formed as a result of burns or lacerations[4]. It is important to carry out further investigations in order to determine whether the increase in skin cancer occurred at the sites of scars resulting from burns or lacerations caused by the atomic bomb. Thus in the case of skin cancer, unlike cancers in other organs, it is necessary to consider not only the radiation emitted by the bomb, but also the effects produced by the bomb blast and thermal radiation.

An increase in malignant tumors such as lung cancer, breast cancer and thyroid cancer has been confirmed among atomic bomb survivors, and it is believed that the number of these complaints among individuals who underwent radiotherapy for these cancers is also high in comparison with the control population. It is therefore possible that the increase in skin cancer among atomic bomb survivors is a reflection of skin cancers being induced by radiotherapy either alone or in conjunction with atomic bomb radiation.

It is also necessary to consider the extent of the roles played in skin cancer development by the important risk factor of occupational and non-occupational exposure to sunlight, and by other risk factors such as tobacco etc.

If the development of malignant tumors (including skin cancer) is accepted as being strongly connected to DNA damage caused by the effect of whole-body radiation, then molecular biological studies are likely to become important in the future.

CONCLUSION

Reports have been published on the relationship between skin cancer and exposure to ionizing radiation from the atomic bomb for the RERF Life Span Study and Adult Health Study samples, as well as for the population that was directly exposed in Nagasaki. However, various studies are still required before it can be concluded that the skin cancer risk was increased by exposure to the atomic bomb.

(Michiko Yamada)

REFERENCES

1. Frieben EA. Demonstration eines cancroids des rechten Handrückens das sich nach langdauernder Einwirkung von Röntgenstrahlen entwickelt hatte. *Fortschr Geb Röntgenstr* 1902; **6**: 106–11.
2. Okazaki M, Ogata K, Inoue S. Statistical observations on post-irradiation skin malignancies reported in Japan. *J Nagasaki Med Ass* 1989; **6**: 548–55. (*In Japanese*)
3. Fry RJM. The biological basis for dose limitation in the skin. *Annals of the ICRP* 1991; **22** (2).

4. Eguchi K, Murayama M, Tsutsumi S. Radiation-induced cancer. *Diagnosis of Skin Disease* 1986; **8** (11): 1047–50. (*In Japanese*)
5. Okazaki M, Inoue K, Ogata K. Statistical studies on radiation-induced malignant neoplasms of the skin in Japanese. *The Nishi Nihon Journal of Dermatology* 1982; **44**: 824–31. (*In Japanese*)
6. Ishihara K. Radiation-induced skin cancer and precancerous epithelial tumors. In: Yamamura Y, Kukita A, editors. An outline of contemporary dermatology. Vol. 9 Epithelial tumors. Tokyo: Nakayama Shoten, 1980: 157–66. (*In Japanese*)
7. Hoshino H, Tanooka H. Interval effect of β-irradiation and subsequent 4-nitroquinoline l-oxide painting on skin tumor induction in mice. *Cancer Res.* 1975; **35**: 3663–6.
8. van Vloten WA, Hermans J, van Daal WAJ. Radiation-induced skin cancer and radiodermatitis of the head and neck. *Cancer* 1987; **59**: 411–414.
9. Conard RA. Review of medical findings in Marshallese population 26 years after accidental exposure to radioactive fallout. Brookhaven National Laboratory, 1980. BNL 51261.
10. Caldwell G. Cancer incidence and mortality in nuclear test participants – an interim report. Quantitative risk in standards setting. Proceedings of the 16th Annual Meeting of the NCRP. Bethesda: National Council on Radiation Protection and Measurements, 1981: 159–69.
11. Johnson M-LT, Land CE, Gregory PB, *et al.* Effects of ionizing radiation on the skin, Hiroshima and Nagasaki. ABCC TR 20–69, 1969.
12. Key CR. Carcinoma of the skin. *Human Pathology* 1971; **2** (4): 529–30.
13. Sadamori N, Honda T, Mine M, *et al.* The incidence of skin cancer in Nagasaki atomic bomb survivors, 1955–1984. *J Hiroshima Med Ass* 1988; **41** (3): 424–32. (*In Japanese*)
14. Yamada M, Mabuchi K, Mizuno S, *et al.* Preliminary skin cancer survey in Hiroshima Adult Health Study. *J Hiroshima Med Ass* 1988; **41** (3): 419–23. (*In Japanese*)
15. Yamada M, Kodama K. Preliminary study of skin cancer incidence in atomic bomb survivors in Hiroshima and future research plan. *Nagasaki J Med* 1989; **63**: 542–7. (*In Japanese*)
16. Sadamori N, Mine M. Epidemiologic study of skin cancer in Nagasaki atomic bomb survivors. *Nagasaki J Med* 1989; **63**: 556–66. (*In Japanese*)
17. Sadamori N, Mine M, Hori M. Skin cancer among atomic bomb survivors. *Lancet* 1989; **3**: 1267.
18. Sadamori N, Otake M, Honda T. Incidence of skin cancer among A-bomb survivors in Nagasaki based on DS86 dosimetry system 1958–85. RERF TR 10–91, 1991.
19. Thompson D, Mabuchi K, Ron E, *et al.* Solid tumor incidence in A-bomb survivors 1958–1987. RERF TR 5–92, 1992.

1.9 BREAST CANCER

INTRODUCTION

It is well-known that the breast is a target organ for female hormones, and that the risk factors involved in the development of breast cancer are dependent on factors related to the female hormonal environment, such as age at menarche and meno-pause, and age at the first mature birth, etc. Other important risk factors include nutrition and obesity, family predisposition to cancer, and atypical proliferative breast disease etc.[1]

On the other hand, exposure to radiation is known to be an external environmen-tal factor contributing to the development of breast cancer. Research into radiation-induced breast cancer has a long history, with the early studies involving animal experiments. An association between radiation and human breast cancer was demon-strated by follow-up studies on several populations of women with a history of medical exposure during treatment for mastitis[2] or benign breast disorders[3], and on female tuberculosis patients given repeated fluoroscopic examinations following artificial pneumothorax therapy[4,5]. In addition, follow-up studies on breast cancer development among atomic bomb survivors in Hiroshima and Nagasaki have already been pursued for over 20 years, and have played a central role in research on radiation-caused breast cancer. Nevertheless, new knowledge is acquired every time the period of a follow-up study is extended or previous findings revised, and it will be necessary to carry out further long-term follow-up studies in order to clarify the true situation regarding radiation-related breast cancer.

1. BREAST CANCER STUDIES ON ATOMIC BOMB SURVIVORS

The excess breast cancer risk among atomic bomb survivors was first reported by Wanebo et al[6] in 1967, a mere two years after Mackenzie[4] had shown an association between the development of breast cancer and repeated irradiation during post-operative monitoring of tuberculosis patients who had undergone artifi-cial pneumothorax therapy at a Nova Scotia sanatorium. During the period 1950–1966, Wanebo[6] detected 27 breast cancer cases among the Adult Health Study sample of the Radiation Effects Research Foundation, RERF (the former Atomic Bomb Casualty Commission, ABCC).

McGregor et al[7] confirmed 231 cases of breast cancer when performing the first breast cancer study (1950–69) on the RERF Life Span Study sample. Later studies on breast cancer development among the same population over an extended time period were performed by Tokunaga et al for the periods 1950–74[8], 1950–80[9] and 1950–85. The data from the fourth study are still being analyzed, but although the sample sizes differ slightly, the number of confirmed breast cancer cases in the first three studies (360, 564, and 816 respectively) revealed a marked increase. The results from the second breast cancer study in 1974 show an unmistakable linear dose-response relationship between radiation dose and cancer incidence, with no difference observed between Hiroshima and Nagasaki. Also, the dose-response relationship indicated an excess risk for a dose of < 0.50 Gy. An analysis of the data with respect to age at the time of bombing (ATB) revealed no breast cancer cases among females under 10 years ATB, but a strong dose-response relationship was found among women aged 10–39 years ATB (and particularly for those aged 10–19 ATB). On the other hand, the breast cancer risk among women exposed at the age of 50 or more was extremely small, and for those aged 40–49 ATB there was even a statistically significant decrease in risk with increasing dose. A fresh finding from the third study (1980) was that females under 10 years of age ATB were at risk from radiation-related breast cancer, showing that the risk of radiation-induced breast cancer tends to decrease both relatively and absolutely with an increase in age at exposure.

2. CHARACTERISTICS OF RADIATION-RELATED BREAST CANCER

In addition to the breast cancer research conducted on atomic bomb survivors, studies have also been performed on individuals exposed to radiation during medical procedures. This accumulation of data has led to clarification of the following characteristics of radiation-related breast cancer[10]:

1. An unmistakable and virtually linear relationship relationship exists between breast tissue dose and the development of breast cancer (Fig. 1). This result is in agreement not only with previous studies on atomic bomb survivors, but also with studies on women who underwent fluoroscopy following pneumothorax therapy and radiotherapy for benign breast disease. Also, notwithstanding the qualitative differences in radiation between Hiroshima and Nagasaki, the dose-response relationships in the two cities were almost identical.

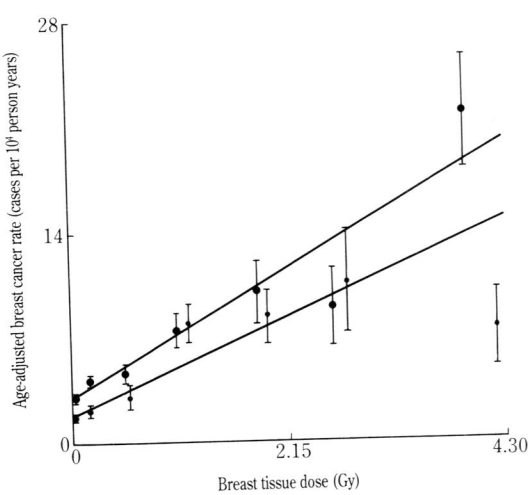

Figure 1   Age-adjusted breast cancer rates (cases/10⁴ person years) by estimated dose to breast tissue, Hiroshima (●) and Nagasaki (•), 1950–80[14]

2. The age at exposure is the most important variable in radiation-related breast cancer, with the excess breast cancer risk heavily dependent on this (Table 1). Every time the breast cancer study on atomic bomb survivors is extended, different results are obtained with regard to age at exposure. However, recent results have shown both a relative and absolute increase in the breast cancer risk with decreasing age at exposure (Fig. 2). In particular, the maximum relative risk occurs with exposure below the age of 10 (4.51 ± 2.45). Confirmation of risk among this age group was not forthcoming until 30 years after exposure. Examination of the cumulative breast cancer incidence by calendar year among females aged under 10 ATB reveals that both high and low dose populations exhibited an increased cancer incidence after 1966, with the heavily exposed population showing a dramatic increase after that date (Fig. 3).

3. The age distribution of breast cancer cases among the heavily exposed population was similar to that observed among the non-exposed and low dose populations, with no difference regarding the histologic type.

These results show that female breast tissue is highly sensitive to radiation, and that this radiosensitivity is at a maximum for immature pre-puberty breast cells. Furthermore, it is believed that other factors may be necessary before cancer develops in the irradiated breasts. That is, no evidence to date has indicated that exposure to radiation has a strong effect on either the age at which breast cancer develops or on histologic type. Furthermore, it is believed that the length of the latency period following exposure depends on other factors.

Such results agree with numerous findings concerning medically irradiated populations. Even a parallel analysis by Land et al[14] on breast cancer data for three exposed populations produced similar results, with no correlation found between the excess radiation and the risk faced by each particular population (Fig. 4). Little research has been performed on the young population exposed at under 10 years ATB, but recent reports on the breast cancer risk following radiotherapy for thymic enlargement during infancy[12] and radiation treatment for childhood cancers[15] support the findings for atomic bomb survivors, and can be considered characteristic of radiation-related breast cancer.

Table 1   Comparisons of published estimates of excess relative risk per Gy breast tissue dose from specified studies and newly computed estimates from the 1950–80 Life Span Study (LSS) series[11]

Study	Age at Irradiation	% Excess RR/Gy (95% CL or ± S.D.)	Comparable LSS Estimate[1]	Age ATB
Study Hildreth[12]	1	248 (107,517)	560 (192,1630)	0–9
Shore[2]	20–40 (mainly)	58 (± 18)	129 (78,215)	20–39
Hubec[13]	20	164 (38,382)	273 (170,439)	10–19
	20–29	40 (−31,158)	130 (67,253)	20–29
	30 +	151 (−61,651)	128 (58,282)	30–39

[1]LSS estimates were increased by 30% as a rough conversion between the T65D and DS86 dosimetries.
RR = relative risk; CL = confidence limit; SD = standard deviation; ATB = at the time of bombing

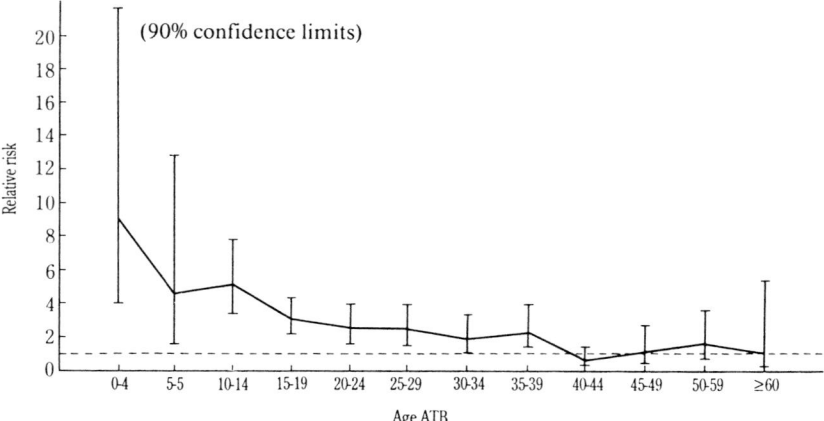

Figure 2   Relative risk of breast cancer for ⩾ 0.50Gy vs 0–.09 Gy kerma (including the not-in-city population by age at the time of bombing (ATB). Vertical bars are 90% confidence limits[9].

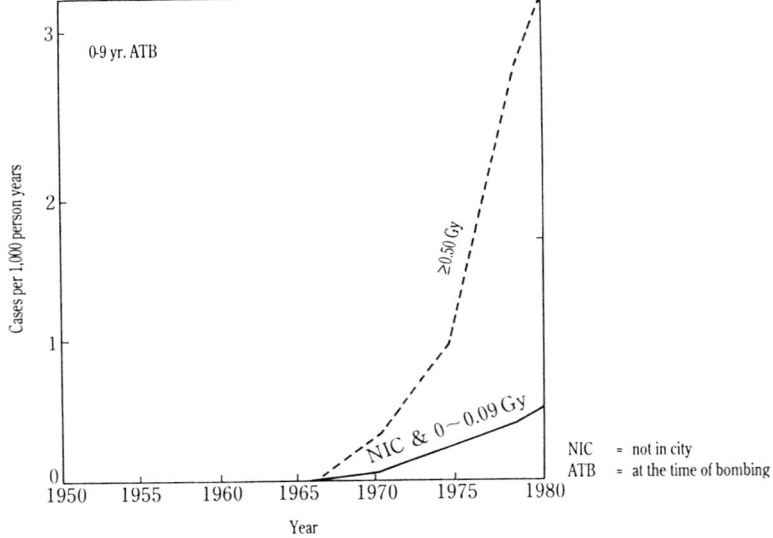

Figure 3   Cumulative breast cancer for women aged 0–9 ATB, high dose (0.5 Gy kerma)

On the other hand, although the risk of radiation-related breast cancer has been clarified for women aged under 40 ATB, the risk for women in their 40s and over 50 ATB has been found to be extremely small. Women exposed at this age have already reached middle age, and the studies performed after 1980 have produced no breast cancer cases that seem to affect the results. Consequently, it is believed that no future changes in breast cancer risk will be observed among this age bracket. This age group includes both pre- and post-menopausal women, but it is difficult to believe that the

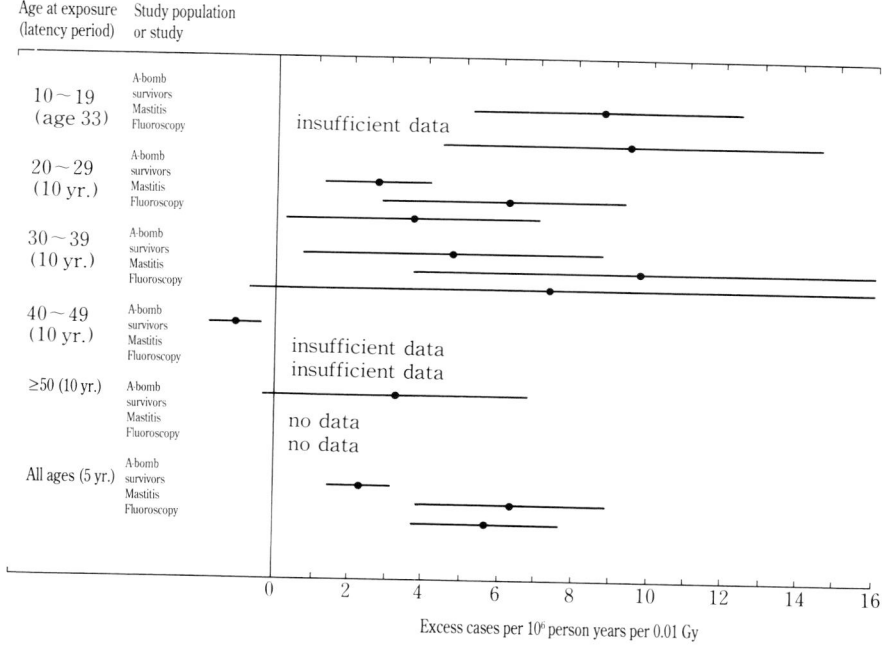

Figure 4   Excess breast cancer risk per 0.01 Gy with 90% confidence limits: parallel data was obtained from Ref. 8 analysis of three exposed populations

radiosensitivity of the mammary gland cells is the same for both the former group, whose female hormones are active, and for the latter older group. Rather, the possibility can be considered that even if the pre-menopausal women in their 40s were exposed to radiation, the time that elapsed before development of cancer was insufficient considering the other risks[16]. That is, it is believed that the endocrine hormonal environment factor does not lead to the development of cancer within 10 years of exposure, and clinical recognition of cancer in particular. Also, studies on breast tissue obtained from autopsies revealed that relative to the controls the breast tissue of heavily exposed women who were exposed while in their 40s exhibited a high rate of proliferative breast epithelial changes which were believed to be pre-cancerous lesions[17].

3. FUTURE BREAST CANCER DEVELOPMENT IN ATOMIC BOMB SURVIVORS

As previously mentioned, heavily exposed atomic bomb survivors face a high breast cancer risk, and of the various organs associated with radiation-induced cancers, the breast is clearly one of the highest risk organs. The risk is particularly high for women exposed at a young age, and since these women are now at the age when breast cancer frequently appears, it is likely that the number of breast cancer cases will continue to increase. In addition, the incidence of breast cancer in Japanese women has tended to rise in recent years, and it is necessary to observe future breast cancer incidence among the high risk group of women exposed to radiation at a young age.

Even for such women, an accurate assessment of risk has not yet proved possible for those who experienced early menarche or a late first childbirth, and especially those with a family predisposition to cancer or a past history of atypical proliferative breast disease. Nevertheless, it is anticipated that the risk will increase still further. Also, past studies indicate the possibility of a higher rate of bilateral breast cancer among heavily exposed atomic bomb survivors. Although conclusive evidence is not available due to the small number of cases so far observed, it is necessary to consider the possibility that heavily exposed women who have a history of unilateral breast cancer may also develop cancer in the contralateral breast.

It is important for these high risk women to undergo breast screening, and that they be shown how to carry out self-examinations etc. Also, the preventative application of anti-hormonal therapy has been tested in Europe and North America for high risk women such as those with a family predisposition to cancer, and it is possible that this may prevent the development of breast cancer[18,19].

(Masayoshi Tokunaga)

REFERENCES

1. Dupont WL, Page DL. Risk factors for breast cancer in women with proliferative breast disease. *N Engl J Med* 1985; **312**: 146–51.
2. Shore RE, Hildreth NG, Woodward E, *et al.* Breast cancer in women given X-ray therapy for acute postpartum mastitis. *J Natl Cancer Inst* 1986; **77**: 689–96.
3. Barel E, Larsson LE, Mattson B. Breast cancer following irradiation of the breast. *Cancer* 1977; **40**: 2905–10.
4. Mackenzie I. Breast cancer following multiple fluoroscopies. *Br J Cancer* 1965; **19**: 1–8.
5. Boice JD Jr, Monson RR. Breast cancer in women after repeated fluoroscopic examinations of the chest. *J Natl Cancer Inst* 1977; **59**: 823–32.
6. Wanebo CK, Johnson KG, Sato K, *et al.* Breast cancer after exposure to the atomic bombings of Hiroshima and Nagasaki. *N Engl J Med* 1968; **279**: 667–71.
7. McGregor DH, Land CE, Choi K, *et al.* Breast cancer incidence among atomic bomb survivors, Hiroshima and Nagasaki, 1950–69. *J Natl Cancer Inst* 1977; **59**: 799–811.
8. Tokunaga M, Norman JE, Asano M, *et al.* Malignant breast tumors among atomic bomb survivors, Hiroshima and Nagasaki, 1950–74. *J Natl Cancer Inst* 1979; **62**: 1347–59.
9. Tokunaga M, Land CE, Yamamoto T, *et al.* Incidence of female breast cancer among atomic bomb survivors, Hiroshima and Nagasaki, 1950–80. *Radiat Res* 1987; **112**: 243–72.
10. Tokunaga M, Tokuoka S, Land CE. Breast cancer in atomic bomb survivors. In: Cancer in atomic bomb survivors. *GANN Monograph on Cancer Res* 1986; **32**: 167–77.
11. Tokunaga M, Land CE, Tokuoka S. Follow-up studies of breast cancer incidence among atomic bomb survivors. *J Radiat Res* 1991; **32**: 201–11.
12. Hildreth NG, Shore RE, Dvoretsky PM. The risk of breast cancer after irradiation of the thymus in infancy. *N Engl J Med* 1989; **321**: 1281–4.
13. Hrubec Z, Boice JD Jr, Monson RR, *et al.* Breast cancer after multiple chest fluoroscopies: second follow-up of Massachusetts women with tuberculosis. *Cancer Res* 1989; **49**: 229–34.
14. Land CE, Boice JD Jr, Shore RE, *et al.* Breast cancer risk from low-dose exposures to ionizing radiation: results of parallel analysis of three exposed populations of women. *J Natl Cancer Inst* 1980; **65**: 353–76.
15. Li EP, Corkery J, Vawter G, *et al.* Breast carcinoma after cancer therapy in childhood. *Cancer* 1983; **51**: 521–3.

16. Tokunaga M, Land CE, Yamamoto T, *et al.* Breast cancer among atomic bomb survivors. In: Boice JD Jr, Fraumeni JF Jr, editors. Radiation carcinogenesis: epidemiology and biological significance. New York: Raven Press, 1984: 45–56.
17. Tokunaga M, Land CE, Page DL, *et al.* Proliferative and non-proliferative breast disease in relation to radiation dose from the atomic bombings of Hiroshima and Nagasaki. Results of a histopathology review of autopsy tissue. *Cancer* 1993; **71**: 1657–65.
18. Cuzick J, Wang DY, Bulbroof RD. The prevention of breast cancer. *Lancet* 1986; **1**: 83–6.
19. Powles TJ, Hardy JR, Ashley SE, *et al.* A pilot trial to evaluate the acute toxicity and feasibility of tamoxifen for prevention of breast cancer. *Br J Cancer* 1989; **60**: 126–31.

1.10   UTERINE CANCER

INTRODUCTION

Ovarian cancer in animals has been reported to be a radiation-related malignant neoplasm of the female reproductive organs. However, there have been few reports of radiation causing malignant neoplasms in human female reproductive organs, and only an extremely small number of reports have indicated a significant correlation. Nevertheless, the uterine cancer mortality rate among atomic bomb survivors in Hiroshima prefecture has been reported to be high in comparison with non-exposed women[1].

The following reviews current knowledge regarding the effect of atomic bomb radiation on uterine cancer in atomic bomb survivors.

1. INCIDENCE

Reports concerning uterine cancer have appeared since approximately 1960. Twenty-eight cases of utero-cervical cancer were detected between 1953 and 1957 during gynecological examinations performed at the Atomic Bomb Casualty Commission (ABCC), but no significant difference was observed between the control population and survivors exposed within 2 km of the hypocenter[2].

Studies on the atomic bomb survivors in Hiroshima and Nagasaki have utilized clinical statistics and tumor registry data, etc.[3,4], and although statistical treatment of the data was not performed, a high rate of uterine cancer was reported among atomic bomb survivors.

2. MORTALITY STATISTICS BY DOSE

In the 1970s the mortality rates by T65D dose became available for various malignant neoplasm sites.

According to a mortality rate study covering the period 1950–74 by the Radiation Effects Research Foundation (RERF, the successor to ABCC), 282 deaths were attributable to cancers of the cervix and uterine body, but a relationship to radiation dose was not confirmed.

As shown in Table 1, no relationship was observed between radiation dose and cervical cancer. Nevertheless, an investigation of cases listed in tumor registries reveals that although almost no evidence suggests a radiation effect in Nagasaki, a significant role was indicated in Hiroshima[6,7].

Later follow-up data by RERF for the period up to 1982 also failed to show any statistical significance between mortality rates and the dose-response relationship for uterine cancer[8].

According to the 11th (and most recent) RERF Life Span Study[9], observations over the period 1950–85 show that the uterine cancer mortality rate among women exposed to ≤ 1 Gy was 22% higher than in the control population (p < 0.10) (Fig. 1). This was the first report to indicate that radiation also has an effect on uterine cancer.

Table 1   Observed and expected deaths due to cancer of the cervix and uterus by city, 1950–74[5]

Cases		Total	\multicolumn{8}{c}{T65 Dose (Gy)}	Homo-geneity test	Trend test
			0	0.01–0.09	0.10–0.49	0.50–0.99	1.00–1.99	2.00–2.99	3.00–3.99	4.00 +		
\multicolumn{13}{c}{Cancer of the Cervix and Uterus (ICD 180–182)}
Total	Obs	282	105	83	66	11	9	1	2	5	0.043	0.324
	Exp		125	68.6	55.1	15.1	9.4	4.1	2.0	2.5		
City: Hiroshima	Obs	227	97	52	55	11	6	1	1	4	0.176	0.103
	Exp		113	47.8	43.7	11.3	6.0	2.3	1.2	1.5		
Nagasaki	Obs	55	8	31	11	0	3	0	1	1	0.095	0.824
	Exp		12.1	20.8	11.4	3.8	3.5	1.7	0.7	1.0		

Obs. = observed; Exp. = expected; ICD = International Classification of Diseases (World Health Organization)

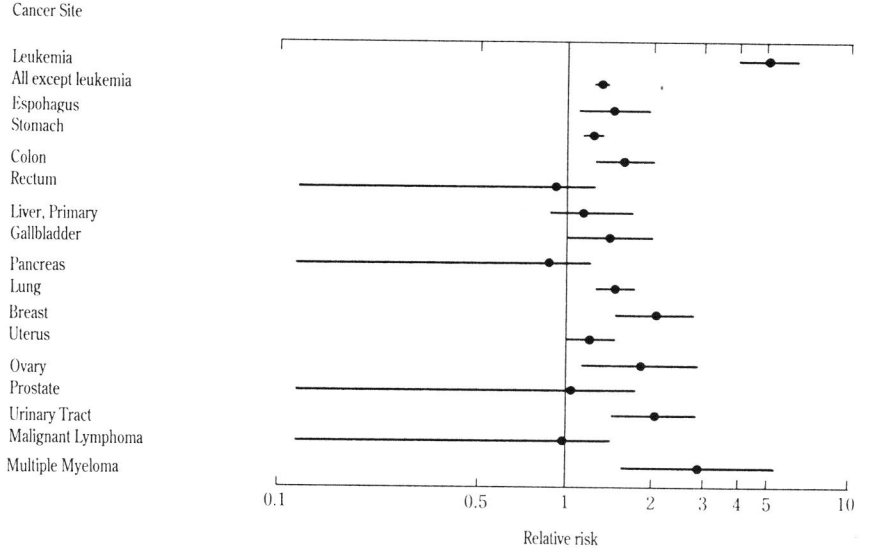

Cancer Site

Leukemia
All except leukemia
Esophagus
Stomach
Colon
Rectum
Liver, Primary
Gallbladder
Pancreas
Lung
Breast
Uterus
Ovary
Prostate
Urinary Tract
Malignant Lymphoma
Multiple Myeloma

0.1   0.5   1   2   3 4 5   10

Relative risk

Figure 1   Relative risk and 90% confidence limits for specific cancer sites at 1 Gy shielded kerma, 1950–1985[9]

3. MORTALITY STATISTICS AT HIROSHIMA UNIVERSITY

Since 1965, the Research Institute for Nuclear Medicine and Biology, Hiroshima University, has continued to observe Hiroshima atomic bomb survivors resident in Hiroshima prefecture. Unlike the RERF sample, this population did not exist solely of directly exposed survivors but also included early entrants (i.e. those individuals who entered the city within 3 days of the atomic explosion), people who handled the corpses, and nurses etc. Observations were therefore performed on populations classified according to conditions of exposure, the three categories being survivors directly exposed within approximately 2 km of the hypocenter; early entrants who were less than approximately 2 km from the hypocenter; and other survivors.

A. Changes in Uterine Cancer Mortality Rates

Mortality statistics covering all survivors show that relative to non-exposed women in Hiroshima prefecture, the uterine cancer mortality rate among the above Hiroshima University populations was 19% higher during the 5-year period 1968–72. The figure for directly and proximally exposed women (i.e. those exposed within approx. 2 km) was slightly less than 30% higher, although this was not statistically significant. The cervical cancer mortality rate for directly and proximally exposed women was 1.8 times greater than for non-exposed women[10].

For the 5-year period 1973–1977, the mortality rate for uterine cancer among all atomic bomb survivors was 1.4 times that among the non-exposed population, with the figure being 1.6 and 1.35 respectively for women directly exposed within approximately 2 km of the hypocenter and for early entrants. However, the cervical cancer mortality rate tended to be higher among the total survivor population and early entrants than among the non-exposed[11].

During the 5-year period 1978–82, the number of uterine cancer deaths was 41% higher among the directly and proximally exposed population, but no statistical significant differences were reported in the other populations. A statistically significant high mortality rate was also reported for utero-cervical cancer, the figure being approximately double that for the non-exposed population.

With regard to changes with time, the national uterine cancer mortality rate showed a yearly decline, whereas it increased among Hiroshima atomic bomb survivors.

Since 5-yearly observations of mortality rates can lead to haphazard variations, a study was performed for the 15-year period from 1968 to 1982[1]. The mortality rate among all atomic bomb survivors was found to be 1.2 times greater than in the non-exposed population, and among those directly and proximally exposed the rate was 1.4 times greater, both figures being statistically significant; among early entrants the mortality rate tended to increase (1.1 times greater) (Fig. 2).

B. Mortality Rates by Place of Residence

Since the residences of the atomic bomb survivors included both urban and rural communities, and as it was felt possible that atomic bomb survivors could be influenced by their daily living environment, Hayakawa et al[1] compared residents in the city of Hiroshima and those living in other parts of the prefecture. As shown in Fig. 3, it was found that the uterine cancer mortality rate for all atomic bomb survivors among non-city residents was 1.3 times greater than among the non-exposed population. Among the population directly exposed in Hiroshima city within 2 km, the rate was 1.3 times greater, and for both the early entrants and other exposed groups living in other parts of the prefecture the rate was also 1.3 times greater.

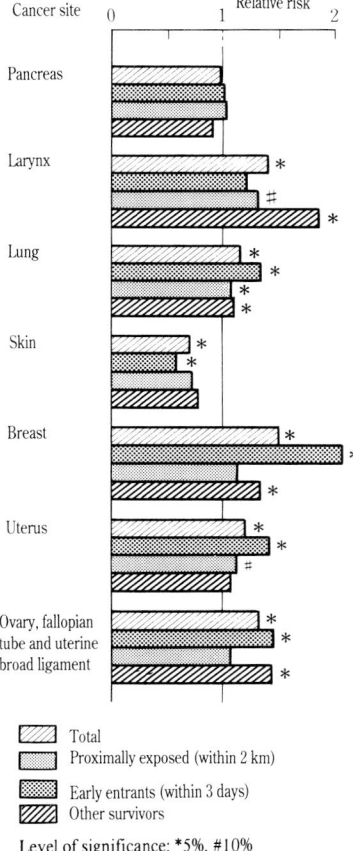

Figure 2 Standardized mortality ratios for atomic bomb survivors compared to the non-exposed population for specific malignant sites as a function of exposure

C. Mortality Rates by Period after Issuance of A-bomb Survivor's Health Handbook

The atomic bomb survivors have now entered old age, and due to various health conditions some people have applied on the basis of the A-bomb Survivors' Medical Treatment Law to be issued with atomic bomb survivors health handbooks. Since there could be a relationship with mortality rates Hayakawa et al[1] examined these with respect to time elapsed after issuance of the handbooks, and found that the mortality rate was at a maximum within one year of official certification and equal to 1.4 times greater than among the non-exposed population (Fig. 4); the figure stood at 1.6 times for the 1–2 year period. With respect to distance from the hypocenter, for the directly and proximally exposed population the mortality rate within 1 year of being granted official certification was 8.4 times greater than for the non-exposed population, and in the 1–2 year period was 6.9 times greater. Even for early entrants,

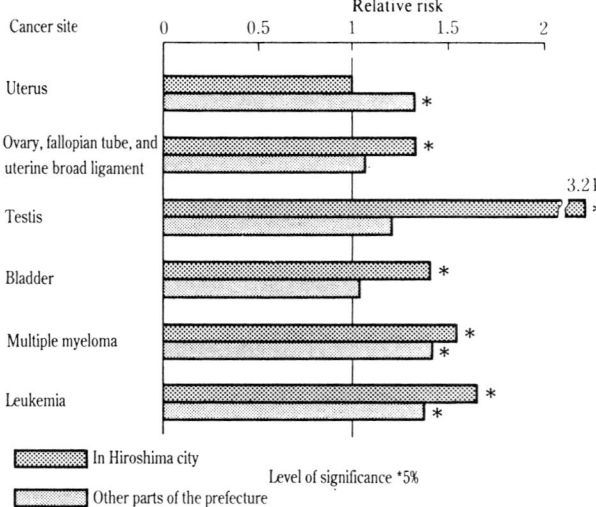

Figure 3   Standardized mortality ratios for atomic bomb survivors compared to the non-exposed population for specific malignant sites as a function of residential location

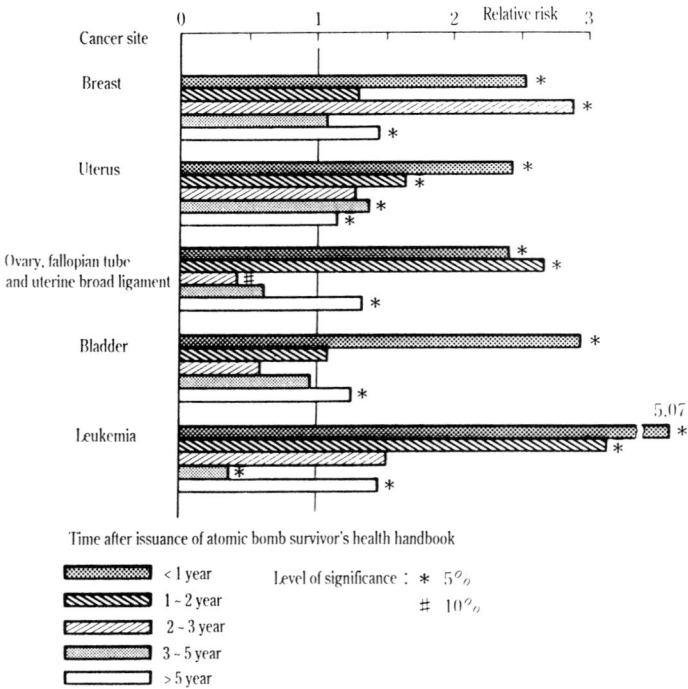

Figure 4   Standardized mortality ratios for atomic bomb survivors compared to the non-exposed population for specific neoplasms as a function of time elapsed after issuance of atomic bomb survivor's health handbook

the mortality rate within 1 year of certification was 3 times greater. This shows that many handbooks were issued after worsening of bodily condition.

D. Other Factors

Besides radiation, socioeconomic factors are also important, with a clue being given by a report examining the degree of family destruction[1]. As can be seen from Fig. 5, the uterine mortality rate among families suffering severe destruction was 1.4 times greater than in families experiencing slight destruction.

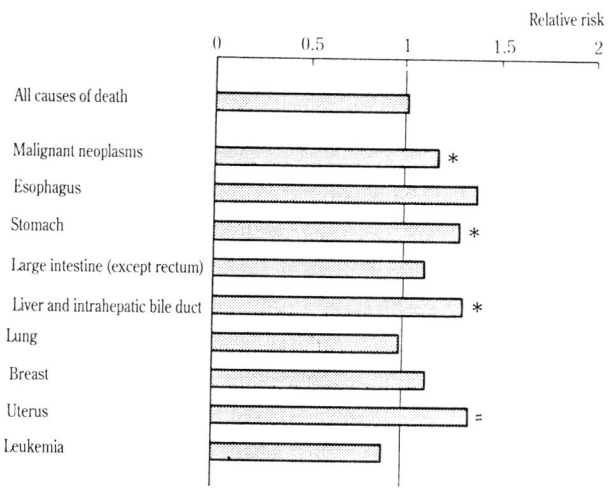

Level of significance: *5%, #10%

The level of family destruction produced by the atomic bomb was classified as severe when any of the following criteria were met:
1) Death of the head of the household due to the bombing
2) Death of either the father or mother due to the bombing when the individual was younger than 20 years of age
3) Death of the husband due to the bombing
4) Death of the first son due to the bombing when the individual was more than 45 years of age
5) Death of at least one-third of the family members due to the bombing
Family destruction was classified as slight when none of these criteria were met.
(Deaths deemed as due to the bombing were deaths occurring by the end of October 1945 dollowing direct exposure to the bomb).

Figure 5   Comparison of standardized mortality ratios for persons suffering "severe" family destruction with those suffering "slight" family destruction

CONCLUSION

Uterine cancer has until now been regarded as having almost no relationship with radiation, but an analysis using the revised DS86 dose estimates shows that a difference with the control population also exists with uterine cancer deaths among atomic bomb survivors exposed to ≥ 1 Gy. Furthermore, the mortality statistics for Hiroshima indicate that atomic bomb survivors suffer a higher uterine cancer mortality rate than the non-exposed population. With the aging of the atomic bomb survivors, those who were exposed during puberty have now reached the age at which cancer frequently develops, and it is important to monitor the situation with great care, even for those types of cancer assumed to be unrelated to radiation.

(Norihiko Hayakawa)

REFERENCES

1. Hayakawa N, Ohtaki M, Ueoka H, *et al.* Mortality statistics of major causes of death among atomic bomb survivors in Hiroshima prefecture from 1986 to 1982. *Hiroshima J Med Sci* 1989; **38**: 53–67.
2. Sawada H. Evaluation of gynecological tumors in the atomic bomb survivors. Hiroshima J Med Sci 1958; 7: 187–97.
3. Mitani Y, Mori S. Statistical study on neoplasm-related deaths among Nagasaki A-bomb survivors. *Nagasaki Med J* 1961; **36**: 724–31. (*In Japanese*)
4. Harada T, Ouchi G, Ishida M. Neoplasms among bomb survivors in Hiroshima city. *J Hiroshima Med Ass* 1961; **14**: 347–56. (*In Japanese*)
5. Beebe GW, Kato H, Land CE. Studies of mortality of A-bomb survivors. 6. Mortality and radiation dose, 1950–74. *J Hiroshima Med Ass* 1979; **32**: 842–61. (*In Japanese*)
6. Wakabayashi T, Kato H, Ikeda T, *et al.* Studies of the mortality of A-bomb survivors, report 7. Incidence of cancer in 1959–1978, based on the tumor registry, Nagasaki. *J Hiroshima Med Ass* 1983; **36**: 1011–23. (*In Japanese*)
7. Kato H, Schull WJ. Studies of the mortality of A-bomb survivors, report 7. Mortality, 1950–1978, Part 1. Cancer mortality. *Radiat Res* 1982; **90**: 395–432.
8. Preston DL, Kato H, Kopecky KJ, *et al.* Studies of the mortality of A-bomb survivors, report 8. Cancer mortality, 1950–1982. *Radiat Res* 1987; **111**: 151–78.
9. Shimizu Y, Kato H, Schull WJ. Life span study report 11. Part 2. Cancer mortality in the years 1950–85 based on the recently revised doses (DS86). Hiroshima (Japan): Radiation Effects Research Foundation; 1988. Report No.: RERF TR 5–88. (*In Japanese*)
10. Kurihara M, Munaka M, Hayakawa N, *et al.* Mortality statistics among A-bomb survivors in Hiroshima prefecture, 1968–1972. *Proc Hiroshima Univ RINMB* 1981; **22**: 235–55. (*In Japanese*)
11. Hayakawa N, Munaka M, Kurihara M, *et al.* Mortality statistics by causes of death among A-bomb survivors in Hiroshima prefecture, 1973–1977. *Proc Hiroshima Univ RINMB* 1985; **26**: 1134–47. (*In Japanese*)

1.11 NON-THYROID ENDOCRINE TUMORS

INTRODUCTION

The histologic changes occurring in the endocrine and gonadal glands directly after exposure have been well documented by Iijima *et al*[1]. Concern has naturally arisen over the development of non-thyroid endocrine and gonadal tumors as a late effect of radiation. However, the data available to date from animal experiments and cases of post-irradiation tumor development in humans have suggested the existence of a long latency period, and few reports have appeared concerning atomic bomb survivors other than for thyroid and ovarian cancers. In order to more accuately comprehend the tendencies among atomic bomb survivors with non-thyroid endocrine tumors, both autopsy cases and clinical reports are discussed here.

Out of the pathological study population of 74,355 selected from Hiroshima residents surviving on October 1st 1950, the Hiroshima Radiation Effects Research Foundation (RERF) conducted autopsies on 4,136 of the 15,619 individuals who died during the period 1961–77[2]. Doses were calculated according to the tentative 1965 dosimetry (T65D) system[3]. Also, the clinical cases consisted of those undergoing surgery at Hiroshima University and those registered between 1974 and 1987 in the Hiroshima prefectural tumor tissue registry (cases based on histopathological diagnoses made following surgery or biopsy).

1. PARATHYROID TUMORS

Two case studies of giant functioning parathyroid tumor with marked fractures and renal calculi were reported among the RERF autopsies on atomic bomb survivors[4,5]. As with other endocrine glands, it is difficult to differentiate between cancer and adenoma, and between adenoma and hyperplasia, and pathological follow-up on the parathyroid tumors is necessary. Table 1 shows the relationship between radiation dose and parathyroid classification in the autopsy cases. Parathyroid tumors were observed in 13 cases (accompanied by hyperparathyroidism, HPT, in 3 cases); and

Table 1 Parathyroid diseases in autopsy cases of ABCC-RERF pathology study in Hiroshima, 1961–77

Dose (Gy) (T65D)	No. of cases			
	Adenoma	Hyperplasia	Cyst	Total
NIC	0	16	1	17
0	3	20	4	27
0.01–0.49	5 (1)	18	3	26
⩾ 50	5 (2)	4	0	9
Total	13 (3)	58	8	79

( ): Cases exhibiting primary hyperparathyroidism
NIC: not in city at the time of bombing

although the number of cases was small an increase with dose was suggested. Furthermore, the relative risk for the ≥ 0.50 Gy population (5 cases) was 5.1 times greater than in the 0 Gy population (3 cases)[6,7].

In addition, even among the 15 parathyroid tumor cases treated at Hiroshima University between 1956 and 1989, 7 cases (46.7%) were atomic bomb survivors, and a relationship with the atomic bomb cannot be discounted[8]. Furthermore, since there were many cases of secondary hyperplasia accompanying renal insufficiency, care is necessary when discussing the relationship with exposure.

Figure 1a shows the relationship with exposure for 18 parathyroid tumor cases based on data in the Hiroshima prefectural tumor tissue registry for 1974–1987 (excluding individuals born after the atomic bombing). The cases were classified into 3 groups according to exposure status (proximally exposed within 2 km of the hypocenter, other exposed, and non-exposed), the number of tumors developed, the standardized incidence per 100,000 population, and the relative risk with respect to the non-exposed population were presented. The relative risk in comparison with the non-exposed was 5.6 times for the total exposed population and 16.2 times for the proximally exposed; in addition, the number of tumors tended to increase with dose. As shown in Fig. 1b, the 12 cases of functioning parathyroid tumor accompanied by hyperparathyroidism showed the same tendencies[9,10]. Serum calcium levels must be measured for the detection of hyperparathyroidism, and in recent years measurements of serum calcium and parathyroid hormone (PTH) have been simplified, and these are expected to be included in future examinations of atomic bomb survivors. Cases of surgery on parathyroid tumors with HPT have been increasing since 1980[9].

2. ADRENAL GLAND TUMORS

The autopsies performed at RERF revealed 23 cases of adrenal gland tumors among those not in the city at the time of bombing (NIC) and the 0 Gy population, and an equal number in atomic bomb survivors exposed to ≥ 0.01 Gy, thus showing no relationship with exposure.

Investigations on 123 adrenal gland tumor cases in the Hiroshima prefectural tumor tissue registry during the 13-year period 1975–87 revealed 66 adrenocortical tumors; studies on 47 of these (excluding the 19 cases developed among individuals born after the atomic bombing) found that atomic bomb survivors accounted for 15 cases (31.5%)[11]. It was noteworthy that atomic bomb survivors accounted for a high percentage (6 cases, 54.5%) of the 11 adrenal Cushing's syndrome cases. During the same period 24 cases of adrenal pheochromocytoma in the adrenal medulla were found; no study was conducted, however, since only 1 case occurred in an atomic bomb survivor. It is necessary to undertake detailed histologic studies into the relationship between adrenal gland tumors and radiation exposure.

3. PITUITARY GLAND TUMORS

In a study on exposure to radioactive fallout following the 1954 hydrogen bomb tests in the Marshall Islands, Adams et al[12] reported the development of 2 cases of

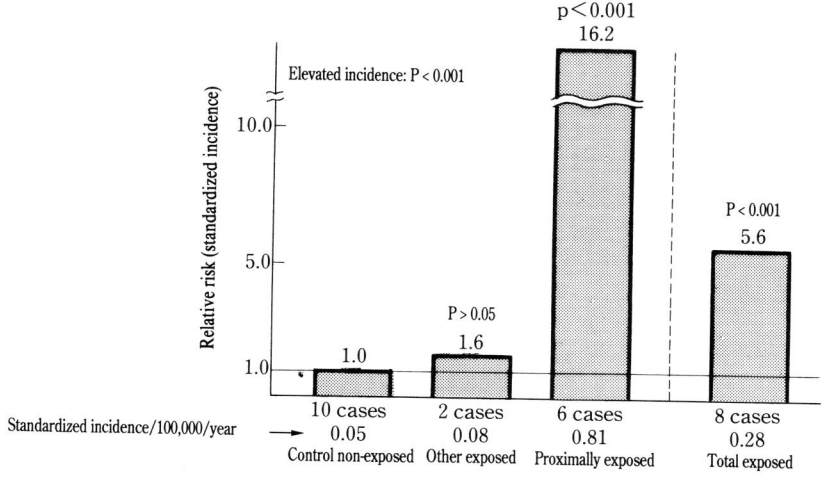

a

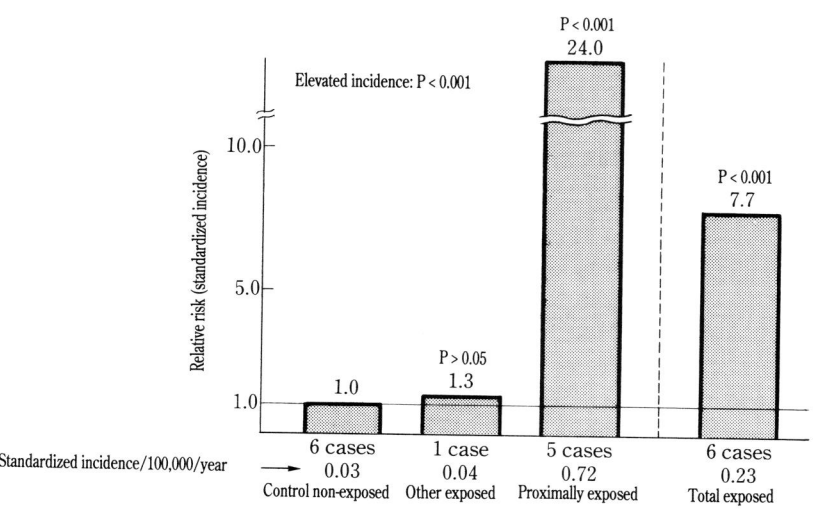

b

Figure 1   Relative risk (a) of parathyroid tumors and (b) parathyroid tumors with hyperparathyroidism among exposed survivors (Hiroshima Prefecture Tumor Registry, 1974–87)

pituitary gland tumors, these being respectively detected 21 and 22 years after exposure. Although a mere 2 cases were observed, an epidemiological study was performed comparing Marshall Islands residents with a non-exposed control population elsewhere in the United States which suggested a high incidence of this tumor among the exposed residents.

An investigation of atomic bomb survivors revealed 22 cases in the (NIC + 0 Gy) RERF autopsy population and 17 cases in the ≥ 0.01 Gy population, with no significant difference between the two populations. However, it is noteworthy that the 2 cases of malignant pituitary gland tumors were both observed in atomic bomb survivors, who were exposed to 2.08 Gy and 0.07 Gy respectively. Even at Hiroshima University, 16 pituitary gland tumor cases were found among atomic bomb survivors in 1960–85, and although only 1 case exhibited malignancy, this occurred in a survivor proximally exposed within 2.0 km of the hypocenter.

4. OTHER TUMORS

Recent improvements in diagnostic techniques have led to increased detection of carcinoid tumors. The Hiroshima prefectural tumor registry was established in 1973, and carcinoid tumor cases have been registered since 1978. Few cases were observed in the 1970s at either RERF or Hiroshima University, and it was not possible to establish a relationship with the atomic bomb. During the period 1978–87, 126 cases were registered in Hiroshima; excepting those born after the atomic explosion (17 cases), atomic bomb survivors accounted for 20 cases (18.3%) with the effect of exposure thus apparently small.

Thymic carcinoid tumors were comparatively rare, with only 3 cases observed; however, 2 of these occurred in atomic bomb survivors exposed at distances of 1.5 km and 5.0 km respectively, suggesting a need for future investigation.

With regard to the thymus, surgery was performed at Hiroshima University on only 6 atomic bomb survivors with thymomas between 1968 and 1984. During the same period, surgery was performed at Hiroshima University on malignant thymoma in 7 cases, of whom only 2 were atomic bomb survivors. Even in the 81 thymoma cases recorded in the Hiroshima tumor registry between 1978 and 1987, atomic bomb survivors accounted for only 7 cases (8.6%).

Table 2 shows the 10 cases of clinical endocrine tumors (including thyroid cancer) detected in prenatally exposed atomic bomb survivors by 1987. Thyroid cancer was the most common (5 cases), followed by adrenocortical tumors (4 cases) and pituitary gland tumors (1 case). Apart from 2 cases in the NIC population, the cases were in survivors directly exposed at 0.8–3.7 km, but for the 5 cases for whom doses were determined the T65D dose range was 0–0.73 Gy, which was not necessarily large; therefore at present it is not possible to say that a definite radiation effect exists. Care is thus necessary when considering thyroid cancer and adrenocortical tumors.

5. MULTIPLE ENDOCRINE AND GONADAL TUMORS

A study on the correlation between the organs affected and endocrine and gonadal tumors found 27 cases of multiple endocrine and gonadal tumors (MEGT) in autopsies performed at RERF[13]. All but one case involved the thyroid (i.e. 26 cases, 96.3%). Among them, the most frequent combination was tumors of the thyroid plus

Table 2   Clinical endocrine tumors in prenatally exposed atomic bomb survivors (up to 1989)

Case number	Sex	Details of exposure			Date of surgery		Endocrine tumors
		Gestational age (months)	Distance from hypocenter/day of entry into city	T65D kerma dose (Gy)	Year	Age (yrs)	Pathohistological diagnosis and accompanying symptoms
1	F	5	1.3 km	0.57	1972	26	Thyroid papillary carcinoma
2	M	7	2 days after bombing	NIC	1974	29	Adrenocortical adenoma; Cushing's syndrome
3	M	4	0.8 km	Unknown	1978	32	Thyroid papillary carcinoma
4	F	3	1.3 km	0.73	1980	34	Thyroid papillary carcinoma
5	F	2	1.7 km	0.10	1981	34	Adrenocortical adenoma; Cushing's syndrome
6	M	8	1.6 km	0.15	1981	35	Pituitary adenoma; acromegaly
7	F	6	2.5 km	Unknown	1983	37	Thyroid papillary carcinoma
8	F	7	3.6 km	0	1983	38	Adrenocortical adenoma; Cushing's syndrome
9	F	3	On day of bombing	NIC	1984	38	Thyroid papillary carcinoma
10	F	2	3.7 km	Unknown	1987	49	Adrenocortical adenoma; non-functioning

NIC = not in city at the time of bombing
F = female; M = male

ovaries (13 cases, 48.1%), which included 2 triple tumor cases, additionally involving a pituitary gland tumor. An increase in thyroid cancer and ovarian cancer hasalso been reported in atomic bomb survivors[14,15], with this being a likely combination. The second most frequent combination was tumors of the thyroid and pituitary glands (7 cases, 25.9%), which included 2 triple tumor cases involving an ovarian tumor. Two cases each occurred of tumors of the thyroid plus parathyroid, and thyroid plus carcinoid tumor. The MEGT incidence tended to increase with dose; in comparison to the 0 Gy population and those not in the city at the time of bombing, the relative risk rose gradually with dose, being 4.1 for those exposed to 0.01–0.09 Gy, 5.7 for those receiving 0.10–0.99 Gy, and 7.1 for those exposed to ≥ 1.00 Gy.

In order to investigate whether the same tendency exists clinically, clinical cases at Hiroshima University and RERF were studied together (Fig. 2). Five cases of tumors occurred in both the thyroid and ovaries, all of them in atomic bomb survivors. In contrast, the other cases—consisting of tumors in both the thyroid and suprarenal glands (4 cases), the pituitary gland and thyroid (2 cases), and pituitary gland and ovaries (1 case)—all occurred among non-exposed patients. Three of the four cases in which tumors developed in both the thyroid and adrenal glands suffered from a hereditary disease known as multiple endocrine neoplasia (MEN); all cases were observed in non-exposed patients, and no relationship to the atomic explosion appears to exist.

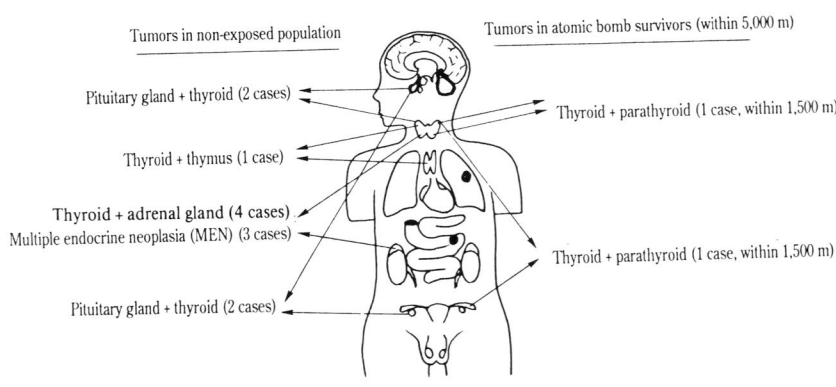

Tumors in non-exposed population

Tumors in atomic bomb survivors (within 5,000 m)

Pituitary gland + thyroid (2 cases)

Thyroid + parathyroid (1 case, within 1,500 m)

Thyroid + thymus (1 case)

Thyroid + adrenal gland (4 cases)
Multiple endocrine neoplasia (MEN) (3 cases)

Thyroid + parathyroid (1 case, within 1,500 m)

Pituitary gland + thyroid (2 cases)

1.   All cases were females.
2.   All 5 cases of thyroid + ovary cancers occurred in atomic bomb survivors.
3.   All 3 multiple endocrine neoplasia (MEN) cases (thyroid medullary carcinoma + adrenal pheochromocytoma) occurred in non-exposed populations.

MEGT = Multiple endocrine and gonadal tumors

Figure 2   Clinical MEGT cases at Hiroshima and RERF, 1971–82

CONCLUSION

Although reports have appeared concerning the relationship between radiation and endocrine and gonadal tumors in animals[16-18], the results cannot be easily applied to human beings.

The scarcity of data on non-thyroid endocrine tumors among atomic bomb survivors can be attributed to three factors: the long latency period, the low number of tumors, and the poor diagnostic techniques for identifying these tumors.

However, approximately half a century has now passed since the atomic bombs exploded. In recent years considerable advances have been made in diagnostic imaging techniques such as ultrasound and computed tomography (CT), in blood testing (e.g. for endocrine hormones and calcium etc.), in aspiration biopsy cytology, and in immunohistochemical techniques. In addition, the pathological processes involved in the development of carcinoid tumors have been clarified. All this has led to a significant improvement in the ability to diagnose endocrine tumors. Consequently, surgery on extremely small tumors and on non-functioning endocrine tumors is now possible, and an increasing number of reports is anticipated with relation to non-thyroid endocrine tumors in atomic bomb survivors.

To summarize, the non-thyroid endocrine tumors related to the atomic bomb are thought to be parathyroid tumors (including hyperparathyroidism), adrenocortical tumors accompanying Cushing's syndrome, MEGT, and in particular complications involving the thyroid and ovaries or thyroid and parathyroid (including thyroid and gonadal tumors). With respect to the endocrine glands and their tumors, however, numerous unresolved problems remain, including histopathological classifications, the relationship between secreted hormones and functions, radiosensitivity, oncogenes, tumor growth factors, the relationship between endocrine gland abnormalities and the development of other forms of cancer, and aging. It is hoped that further case data will be accumulated concerning atomic bomb survivors, including those from Nagasaki.

(*Nobuo Takeichi, Kiyohiko Dohi*)

REFERENCES

1. Iijima S, *et al.* Body injury in the initial stage - acute stage of atomic bomb injury. In: Committee for the compilation of materials on damage caused by the atomic bombs in Hiroshima and Nagasaki. Hiroshima and Nagasaki: the physical, medical, and social effects of the atomic bombings. Tokyo: Iwanami Shoten, 1981: 117–85.
2. Beebe GW, Usagawa M. The major ABCC samples. ABCC TR 12–68, 1968.
3. Milton RC, Shohoji T. Tentative 1965 radiation dose estimation for atomic bomb survivors, Hiroshima and Nagasaki. ABCC TR l-68, 1968.
4. Takeichi N, *et al.* Two cases of large functioning parathyroid adenoma in atomic bomb survivors. *Jap J Cancer Clin* 1983; **29**: 851–4. (*In Japanese*)
5. Takeichi N, Nishida T, Fujikura T, *et al.* Two cases of giant parathyroid adenoma in atomic bomb survivors. RERF TR l0–83, 1983.
6. Takeichi N, *et al.* Parathyroid gland tumors in A-bomb survivors, autopsy cases, Hiroshima, preliminary report. *J Hiroshima Med Ass* 1984; **37**: 439–41. (*In Japanese*)
7. Takeichi N, *et al.* Endocrine and gonadal tumors among A-bomb survivors. *J Hiroshima Med Ass* 1986; **39**: 334–9. (*In Japanese*)
8. Takeichi N, Dohi K, Ito H, *et al.* Parathyroid tumors in atomic bomb survivors in Hiroshima: first report of surgical cases, 1956–1988. *Hiroshima J Med Sci* 1991; **40**: 75–7.
9. Takeichi N, Dohi K, Yamamoto H, *et al.* Parathyroid tumors in atomic bomb survivors in Hiroshima: epidemiological study from registered cases at Hiroshima prefecture tumor tissue registry, 1974–1987. *Jpn J Cancer Res* 1991; **82**: 875–8.

10. Takeichi N, Dohi K, Ito H, *et al.* Parathyroid tumors in atomic bomb survivors in Hiroshima: a review. *J Radiat Res* 1991; (Suppl.): 189–92.

11. Takeichi N, Ito H, Okamoto H, *et al.* Analysis of 65 adrenocortical tumor cases (including A-bomb survivors in Hiroshima). Abstract of the first annual meeting of the Japan Association of Endocrine Surgeons 1989: 74.

12. Adams WH, Harper JA, Rittmaster RS, *et al.* Pituitary tumors following fallout radiation exposure. *JAMA* 1984; **252**: 664–6. 1984; **37**: 442–3.

13. Takeichi N, *et al.* Multiple endocrine tumors in A-bomb survivors, autopsy cases, Hiroshima, preliminary report. *J Hiroshima Med Ass* 198; **37**: 442–443. (*In Japanese*)

14. Takeichi N, Ezaki H, Dohi K. Thyroid cancer: Reports up to date and a review. *J Radiat Res* 1991; (Suppl): 180–8.

15. Tokuoka S. Ovarian neoplasms in atomic bomb survivors. In: Shigematsu I, Kagan A, editors. Cancer in atomic bomb survivors. *GANN Monograph on Cancer Res* 1986; **32**: 179–89.

16. Yokoro K. Radiation carcinogenesis. In: Sugawara T, editor. Radiation cellular biology. Tokyo: Asakura Shoten, 1986: 501–46. (*In Japanese*)

17. Yokoro K, *et al.* Endocrine experimental tumor. In: Imura S, Kato Y, *et al.* Endocrine experimental lecture 2, endocrine animal experimental method. Tokyo: Koudansha, 1982: 80–160. (*In Japanese*)

18. Berdjis CC. Pathogenesis of radiation-induced endocrine tumors. *Oncology* 1967; **21**: 49–60.

2

Benign Tumors

2. DIGESTIVE TRACT POLYPS, BENIGN GYNECOLOGIC TUMORS, AND OTHER BENIGN TUMORS

INTRODUCTION

Exposure to atomic bomb radiation is widely recognized as leading to an increased incidence of malignant tumors, and research is still continuing on various aspects of the topic. On the other hand, there has been a great scarcity of results concerning the relationship between radiation and benign tumors, with no explicit results determined at the present time. One reason for this is the lack of motivation, since benign tumors do not prove fatal. Furthermore, it is difficult to pursue determined research since major problems also surround the ascertainment rate in epidemiological studies.

However, certain disorders are recognized to play a significant role as precursors of malignant tumors e.g. polyps in the digestive system. Molecular biology techniques have in recent years clarified that one of these, polyps in the large intestine, is an important intermediary in the multi-stage process leading to the development of colorectal cancer[1]. It is also believed that genetic changes occur during the transition between normal epithelial cells of the intestine and polyp (adenoma) formation. Since genetic damage is thought to be an important mechanism involved in radiation-related carcinogenesis, it is extremely likely that radiation acts in a similar manner with benign tumors. It is therefore necessary to vigorously investigate the relationship between radiation and benign tumors. This chapter briefly reviews the research findings to date; however, it should be noted that certain benign tumors (tumors of the thyroid, parathyroid, salivary glands, and other endocrine glands) are dealt with in detail in other chapters and hence are not discussed here.

1. BENIGN TUMORS

Since the Radiation Effects Research Foundation (RERF) began the Adult Health Study in 1958, a fixed population of approximately 20,000 has undergone regular medical examinations once every two years, with follow-up examinations performed on the development of radiation-related diseases. The prevalence of benign tumors (including diseases 221–228 and 622 in the World Health Organization's International Classification of Diseases) was first analyzed in the 6th Adult Health Study report which covered the period 1968–80[2] (Fig. 1). The prevalence of benign tumors was found to increase significantly with dose, with the rate in the ≥ 2.0 Gy population being double that in the 0 Gy population and the tendency becoming more marked with the passage of time. As mentioned previously, it is extremely difficult to analyze epidemiological findings pertaining to benign tumors due to the large influence of the ascertainment rate, but since the diagnoses in the Adult Health Study are always performed according to standardized diagnostic criteria, the data is considered highly reliable.

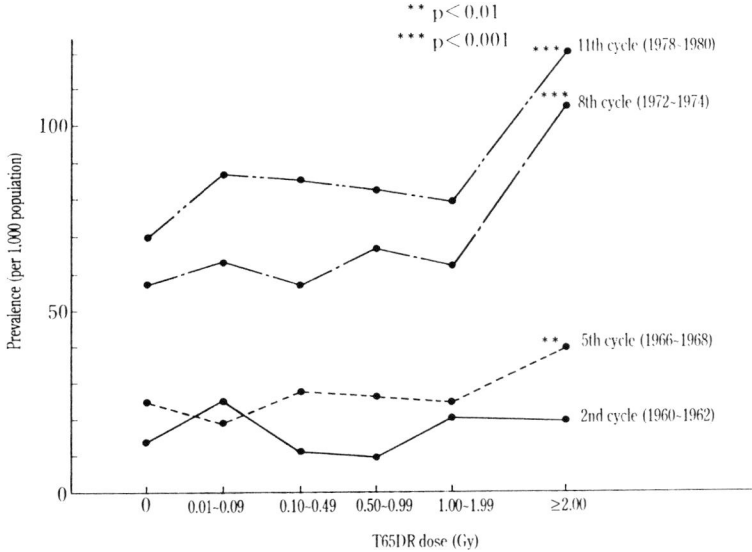

"Cycle" refers to the period of time (2 years) during which every subject in the Adult Health sample received one examination

Figure 1   Prevalence of benign tumors adjusted for city, sex and age, by radiation dose and observation period (adapted from Ref. 2)

Pathological epidemiology techniques are also valuable tools in benign tumor studies. Tumor registries in Hiroshima and Nagasaki, started in the 1950s, centered on the local medical associations and allowed compilation of data on tumor development in these areas. Although these data have primarily been utilized for studies on the relationship between radiation and malignant tumors, benign tumors have also been registered. A 1959 report revealed a significant difference in the frequency of benign tumors between atomic bomb survivors exposed within 1500 meters of the hypocenter and non-exposed individuals[3]. A later analysis of the tumor registry data for the RERF Life Span Study sample over the 10-year period 1973–82 also showed a high incidence of benign tumors in the ≥ 1.0 Gy population relative to the 0 Gy population, although the difference was not statistically significant[4].

Thus results also indicate that atomic bomb radiation caused an increased incidence of benign tumors, although variations are found in the organs in which the benign tumors are observed and the histologic types found. The following is a summary of the relationship between radiation and the organs with a relatively high frequency of benign tumors.

2. DIGESTIVE TRACT POLYPS

From the results of mass screening for gastric diseases, Ito et al[5] found that the frequency of gastric polyps in female atomic bomb survivors was slightly higher than in male survivors and that this was higher the national average, although no consideration was given to the conditions of exposure. An examination of the Adult Health Study data performed by Sawada et al[2] reveals that the gastric polyp prevalence in Hiroshima in the 1970s increased slightly with dose, although the tendency was not observed in Nagasaki. Also, this tendency was found among the youngest age group, but no difference was observed with regard to sex.

Yamamoto et al[6] investigated the frequency of benign digestive tract tumors based on autopsy data for the Life Span Study sample, and found 664 benign tumors among the 2,975 autopsy cases. Polyps were the most common form of benign tumor, with most occurring in elderly individuals. Almost all polyps had a maximum diameter of less than 5 mm and were well-defined solitary pendunculated adenomatous tumors. Polyps occurred most frequently in the large intestine, and in numerous cases of cancer of the large intestine (21%) benign polyps were also present. However, no relationship was found between development of benign tumors and exposure to the atomic bomb.

Therefore although some clinical and pathological epidemiology findings have suggested a relationship between gastric polyps and radiation, consistency is lacking and further studies are necessary.

3. GYNECOLOGICAL TUMORS

The most common benign gynecologic tumors are uterine myomas, but clinical reports commencing soon after the atomic explosion failed to demonstrate any effects due to atomic bomb radiation[7,8]. However, in the 6th report of the Adult Health Study, Sawada et al[2] showed that the incidence of uterine myoma increased significantly with an increase in dose, with the tendency particularly pronounced among young atomic bomb survivors. Even when the observation period of the Adult Health Study was extended to 1986, analyses showed a consistent relationship between radiation and uterine myoma[9]. Since there is no great difference in the gynecological examination rate in this population by radiation dose, the findings are believed to be extremely reliable; nevertheless, more detailed studies are required.

Ovarian tumors are another important type of benign gynecologic tumor. Experimental studies have shown that ionizing radiation produces atrophy of the ovarian follicles in mice ovaries, followed by over-secretion of gonadotropin, with the hormone imbalance causing a change in ovary cell reaction, facilitating the development of ovarian tumors[10]. Also, epidemiological studies have confirmed a relationship between atomic bomb radiation and the development of malignant ovarian tumors[11] although no association with radiation was found in several clinical studies on benign ovarian tumors in atomic bomb survivors[7,8,12]. However, in an analysis mainly utilizing tumor registry data for 70,030 females in the Life Span Study sample, Tokuoka et al[11] suggested an association between radiation dose and the development of benign ovarian tumors after observing 106 such tumors in the period 1950–80, with the frequency increasing with dose. However, an analysis of only the histologically confirmed cases did not reveal any statistical significance.

4. BENIGN TUMORS AT OTHER SITES

Reports have also appeared concerning benign tumors at other sites. Sanefuji et al[13] investigated the relationship between atomic bomb radiation dose and the development of urinary bladder tumors in the Life Span Study sample. Those cases diagnosed by cystoscopy alone were treated as papillary tumors of the bladder, but no relationship with radiation was demonstrated. Also, using bladder tissue sections from autopsies on atomic bomb survivors, Eto et al[14] performed a case-control study with regard to changes in the bladder transitional epithelium. Compared to the controls, the relative risk of papillary hyperplasia among heavily exposed ($\geqslant 1.0$ Gy) atomic bomb survivors was high (4.0 times), but the difference was not statistically significant.

Using autopsy data, Cirak et al[15] failed to find a relationship with radiation during studies on adenomatous hyperplasia of the pancreas duct epithelium.

Seyama et al[16] also used autopsy data to investigate primary intracranial tumors, but no association with radiation was found for the prevalence of latent adenomas in the pituitary gland.

CONCLUSION

As mentioned at the beginning, studies on benign tumors in atomic bomb survivors face various difficulties. However, studies performed in spite of these difficulties suggest a relationship with radiation exposure for certain benign tumors e.g. uterine myoma, and ovarian tumors, etc. Nevertheless, further studies are required in order to provide confirmation. Certain benign tumors are strongly related to malignant tumors, and it is important that further research into benign tumors in atomic bomb survivors be performed in order to investigate the mechanism by which radiation causes tumor development, since this may be involved in the process by which normal cells become malignant.

(Hideo Sasaki)

REFERENCES

1. Marx J. Many gene changes found in cancer. *Science* 1989; **246**: 1386–8.
2. Sawada H, Kodama K, Shimizu, *et al.* Adult Health Study report 6, results of six examination cycles (1968–80), Hiroshima and Nagasaki. RERF TR 3–86, 1983.
3. Harada T, Ishida M. Neoplasms among atomic bomb survivors, Hiroshima, tumor registry report 1. *J Nat Cancer Inst.* 1960; **25**: 1253–64. (ABCC TR 10–59, 1959).
4. Yamamoto T, Kajiwara H, Inai Y, *et al.* Benign and malignant tumors of A-bomb survivors among Hiroshima tissue registry. *Hiroshima J Med Sci* 1986; **39**: 406–8. (*In Japanese*)
5. Ito C, Matsusaka Y. Investigation of stomach diseases in atomic bomb survivors. Result of roentgenographic mass examination in past seven years. *Hiroshima J Med Sci* 1974; **27**: 633–40. (*In Japanese*)
6. Yamamoto T, Kato H, Smith GS. Benign tumors of the digestive tract among A-bomb survivors, 1961–70, Hiroshima. *Gann* 1975; **66**: 623–30. (ABCC TR 12–73, 1973).
7. Sawada H. Evaluation of gynecological tumors in the atomic bomb survivors. *Hiroshima J Med Sci* 1958; **7**: 187–97. (ABCC TR 6–59, 1959).

8. Ishibashi T, Sawazaki M, Shirasuna K. Reproductive organ tumor in the female survivors. *Hiroshima J Med Sci* 1962; **15**: 930–4. (*In Japanese*)

9. Wong FL, Yamada M, Sasaki H, *et al.* Non-cancer disease incidence in the atomic bomb survivors: 1958–1986. *Radiat Res* 1993; **135**: 418–30. (RERF TR 1–92, 1992).

10. Li MH, Gardner WU. Experimental studies on the pathogenesis and histogenesis of ovarian tumors in mice. *Cancer Res* 1947; **7**: 549–66.

11. Tokuoka S, Kawai K, Shimizu Y, *et al.* Malignant and benign ovarian neoplasms among atomic bomb survivors, Hiroshima and Nagasaki, 1950–80. *JNCI* 1987; **79**: 47–57. (RERF TR 8–86, 1986).

12. Yamabe T, Nakayama M, Suzuki K, *et al.* Study on malignant neoplasm of the atomic bomb survivors, investigation of ovarian pathology in the proximal survivors. *Nagasaki Med J* 1971; **47**: 399–401. (*In Japanese*)

13. Sanefuji H, Ishimaru T, Hara H, *et al.* Urinary bladder tumors among atomic bomb survivors, Hiroshima and Nagasaki, 1961–72. RERF TR 18–79.

14. Eto R, Ishimaru T, Tokunaga M. *Hiroshima J Med Sci* 1988; **37**: 11–15. (RERF TR 13–87, 1987).

15. Cirak RW, Yamakido R, Kawashima T, *et al.* Pancreatic ductal changes in atomic bomb survivors, Hiroshima and Nagasaki. ABCC TR 9–75, 1975.

16. Seyama S, Ishimaru T, Iijima S, *et al.* Primary intracranial tumors among atomic bomb survivors and controls, Hiroshima and Nagasaki, 1961–75. RERF TR 15–79, 1979.

3

Endocrine and Metabolic Diseases

3.1 THYROID DISEASES

INTRODUCTION

Interest in the relationship between radiation exposure and thyroid damage has risen since the accident at the nuclear power plant at Chernobyl in the former Soviet Union on April 26th 1986. It had been reported earlier that cervical irradiation in childhood caused an increased thyroid cancer incidence[1-4]; studies on atomic bomb survivors in Hiroshima and Nagasaki also found a high thyroid cancer incidence[5-11]. On the other hand, with regard to thyroid function, it is well-known that treatment of Graves' disease with [131]I (iodine-131) easily leads to delayed manifestation of hypothyroidism[12,13], and it has been reported that cervical irradiation also produces hypothyroidism[1-4]. Recently, reports have described increased incidence of nodular goiter and hypothyroidism among atomic bomb survivors[14-17] and residents of the Marshall Islands[18] exposed as a result of the atmospheric testing of nuclear weapons. This chapter summarizes the non-cancerous thyroid diseases produced by radiation exposure.

1. HISTOLOGIC CHANGES IN THE THYROID DUE TO EXTERNAL AND INTERNAL IRRADIATION

External thyroid irradiation occurs during the treatment of cervical lesions with X-rays and gamma rays, and occurred following the detonation of the atomic bombs in Hiroshima and Nagasaki. Internal thyroid irradiation occurs as a result of the administration of ^{131}I during treatment for hyperthyroidism and cancer, and occurred as the result of exposure to radioactive fallout during the hydrogen bomb tests in the Marshall Islands and in the Chernobyl nuclear accident. With regard to histologic changes produced by external irradiation, there is a slight contraction of follicles 3–6 weeks after irradiation[19], with fibrosis occurring in the thyroid after several months or years. A few of these cases exhibited hypothyroidism[20]. In general, exposure to 10–40 Gy of external irradiation is believed to lead to hypothyroidism, not immediately after exposure, but after a period of several months or years. Internal irradiation with ^{131}I produces virtually no morphological changes within the first week, but after 2–3 weeks there is the appearance of necrosis and inflammation of the follicles, edema, vasculitis accompanied by the development of thrombi, and hemorrhaging. Necrosis is still evident after 10 weeks, and after 3 years fibrosis with traces of the degenerated follicles can be observed. These phenomena are particularly marked in the central region rather than in the peripheral areas[21]. It has been reported that in general with regard to radiotherapy-produced carcinogenesis, the tissue damage produced by high doses is great, but induction of malignant neoplasms is rare[22]. That is, in the case of external irradiation, thyroid cancer rarely develops following exposure to $\geq$ 20 Gy[23]. Also, the absorption of several millicuries during the administration of ^{131}I as treatment for Graves' disease is equivalent to receiving a high dose of 10 Gy; the damage to thyroid tissue is great and the regenerative capacity is weak, leading to the supposition that there is no relationship to carcinogenesis. Large-scale studies in the United States[24] and Sweden[25] into the relationship between ^{131}I administration and the development of thyroid carcinoma have at the present time disproved the possibility of a causality relationship. However, a population receiving local external irradiation with a low X-ray dose (2.50–20 Gy) followed by ^{131}I therapy exhibited growth of small new follicles and fibrosis in the follicles, including a high incidence of atypical epithelium[26]. The radiation dose received by atomic bomb survivors was much less than during ^{131}I therapy, and the histologic changes following atomic bomb exposure were generally slight; however, it is postulated that during the process by which thyroid cancer develops there is degeneration of the follicle cells, fibrosis and regeneration of small follicles, and the appearance of atypical epithelium, and that the mechanism may involve proliferation of cells producing minute cancer, which then develops into clinical manifestations of carcinoma[26].

2. EXTERNAL IRRADIATION AND THYROID DAMAGE

An investigation of dose received during external irradiation in childhood for benign diseases (e.g. facial acne, enlargement of the tonsils, cervical adenopathy, and thymoma) showed that in almost all cases repeated fractional doses were administered with the cumulative total dose being 3.0–15 Gy[27]. The development of tumors in the thyroid and its vicinity would require fractional doses amounting to 10–60 Gy. Cases involving external therapeutic irradiation for hyperthyroidism received 10–20 Gy[28]. Several studies have already shown that X-ray irradiation of the head, neck and thorax during childhood leads to an increased risk of thyroid disease, and particularly thyroid cancer and hypothyroidism[1-4]. Fleming et al[1] performed observations on 298 cases over 5 years after receiving X-ray irradiation of the neck (dose range = 18–60 Gy) for malignant neoplasms such as Hodgkin's disease and leukemia etc. Thyroid abnormalities were observed in 36 cases (12.1%), and consisted of subclinical hypothyroidism with increases in only thyroid stimulating hormone (TSH) (17 cases), clinical hypothyroidism (9 cases), thyroid neoplasms (7 cases, consisting of thyroid cancer, 2 cases; adenoma, 2 cases; colloid nodule, 1 case; and undiagnosed nodules, 2 cases), thyroiditis (2 cases), and hyperthyroidism (1 case). The frequency of these diseases was significantly higher than among the non-exposed. DeGroot et al[2] studied a population of 416 patients irradiated with X-rays as treatment for enlargement of the tonsils or thymus etc., with an average irradiation dose of 10.52 Gy and an average absorbed thyroid dose of 4.51 Gy. Observations were carried out from 2 to 12 years, and revealed a high rate of thyroid cancer (41 cases). Also, positive results were obtained in 9% and 20% of cases respectively for the thyroglobin hemagglutination antibody test and the microsomal hemagglutination antibody test, rates higher than in healthy adults. Surgery was performed in 113 of the 416 cases, with the primary lesion in 14 cases (12.4%) being chronic thyroiditis. Spitalnik et al[3] performed a detailed investigation of the thyroid tissue in 68 cases who underwent surgery and had a history of external irradiation, and detected chronic thyroiditis in 46 cases (68%). It was reported that this did not occur in the control population, suggesting a relationship between radiation and the development of chronic thyroiditis. At an average of 19 years after irradiation, Kaplan et al[4] investigated thyroid function in 95 cases who received an average dose of 30 Gy during childhood external irradiation of the thyroid, and found hypothyroidism in 42 cases (44%). Making observations from 6 months to six and a half years after therapy, Oberfield et al[29] investigated 22 medulloblastoma cases who received an average thyroid dose of 24.0 Gy, and found increases in thyroid stimulating hormone (TSH) in 15 cases (68%).

3. INTERNAL IRRADIATION AND THYROID DAMAGE

Oral administration of ^{131}I is widely practised as a treatment for Graves' disease. The main action of this treatment is due to the release of beta radiation, with the maximum body penetration being of the order of 2 mm; gamma rays account for less than 1/10 of the radiation. There have been many reports on the late effects of ^{131}I therapy for Graves' disease[12,13]. Hypothyroidism in Graves' disease patients has been calculated to occur naturally at a rate of 0.7% in 1 year, and 7% in 10 years. On the other hand, administration of ^{131}I causes an extremely high incidence of dose-dependent hypothyroidism[13]. In other words, the incidence of hypothyroidism gradually increases over a period of years, with a reported annual increase of 2.3–3%; it is believed that at institutions where exposure is approximately 70 Gy this occurs at the high rate of 20–30%, with a rate of approximately 10% being unavoidable even if administration is conservative[30].

Reports on radiation thyroiditis are all concerned with the therapeutic use of ^{131}I, and none with external irradiation[31]. Many cases exhibit temporary symptoms, with slight throbbing pain and tenderness in the thyroid region 1–2 weeks after ^{131}I administration. It has been reported that occasionally large quantities of thyroid hormone released as a result of thyroid destruction produce a crisis, which occurs at a rate of 4–5% in Graves' disease patients treated with [131]I[32]. This does not occur when the thyroid dose is under 200 Gy; the frequency rises with increasing dose.

4. INTERNAL AND EXTERNAL IRRADIATION, AND THE RELATIONSHIP WITH BENIGN THYROID TUMORS

The nodular goiter risk from external thyroid irradiation is of the order of 50 times greater than from internal radiation[30], with external irradiation over 3 times more likely to cause benign thyroid tumors than carcinoma[33].

5. THE HIROSHIMA AND NAGASAKI ATOMIC BOMBS AND THYROID DAMAGE

The radiation emitted by the mid-air detonation of the atomic bombs can be broadly classified into two categories: the initial radiation that was emitted within one minute of the explosion, and the residual radiation which was observed later over a period of time at ground level. The initial radiation consisted mainly of gamma rays and neutron rays. The mid-air gamma ray and neutron doses within 1 km of the hypocenter of the Hiroshima explosion were respectively 2.55 and 1.91 Gy; the doses within 1 km of the Nagasaki explosion were 8.88 and 0.359 Gy respectively[34]. These doses would have been reduced in the case of shielding. Many of the substances that absorbed neutrons released in the atomic explosion as a result of the nuclear fission reactions involving uranium and plutonium were converted into radioactive isotopes. The materials which had become radioactive continued to emit beta rays over an extremely long period of time, frequently accompanied by the emission of gamma rays. Thus the materials in which radioactivity was induced by the neutron rays were an important source of residual radiation. The total gamma ray dose resulting from induced radio-activity at a point 1 meter above the ground at the hypocenter of the Hiroshima bomb and in the period up to 100 hours from the explosion was approximately 1.00 Gy, whereas in Nagasaki this total was approximately 0.40 Gy[35]. Besides radioactive fallout, residual radiation also originated from the products of nuclear fission derived from the uranium and plutonium, the uranium and plutonium that failed to undergo fission, and the radioactivity that was induced in the materials used to construct the atomic bomb which were subjected to bombardment from the neutrons. ^{89}Sr, ^{140}Br, ^{144}Pr, ^{95}Zr, ^{90}Sr, ^{137}Cs, ^{144}Ce, and ^{239}Pu that had failed to undergo fission were detected in the soil in the Nishiyama area of Nagasaki. The maximum total radiation dose due to radioactive fallout was 0.04–0.44 Gy in Hiroshima, and 0.30–1.49 Gy in the Nishiyama district of Nagasaki[35]. Thus, most of the radiation damage produced by the atomic bomb was that caused by the initial radiation, followed by the damage produced by exposure to induced radioactivity and radioactive fallout etc. On the other hand, residents exposed to radiation as a result of a nuclear power plant accident receive the radiation via two mechanisms: first, they are externally exposed to the gamma rays released from the radioactive gas flume; and second, internal exposure is suffered due to inhalation and transdermal absorption of radioactive iodine. The main nuclei produced by the nuclear fission are ^{137}Cs, ^{87}Sr, ^{90}Sr, ^{144}Ce and iodine, with the latter accounting for approximately one half of the total. The main form of radioactive iodine is ^{131}I. Immediately after the atomic explosion, ^{131}I is introduced into the body as a result of respiration and transdermal absorption, leading to internal irradiation of the thyroid. In addition ^{131}I falls to the earth and contaminates vegetables and pastures; by passing along the food chain, the ^{131}I causes contamination of milk, and is transferred to humans via the consumption of milk and vegetables[30].

A. Exposure to the Atomic Bomb and Benign Thyroid Tumors

Morimoto et al[10] compared 477 atomic bomb survivors who were exposed to ≥ 1 Gy and who were aged 20 or less at the time of bombing (ATB) with 501 atomic bomb survivors who were exposed to 0 Gy, and found 13 cases of nodular goiter among the atomic bomb survivors and 3 cases in the control population, with the high frequency in the atomic bomb survivor population being significant. Nagataki et al[15] investigated the effect of the Nagasaki explosion on the thyroid, and found that the frequency of thyroid nodules increased with increasing dose, and was significantly high among survivors aged ≤ 20 ATB. Radiation exposure in the

Nishiyama district of Nagasaki was due solely to radioactive fallout, with no direct exposure at the time of the explosion. Nagataki *et al*[15] studied thyroid effects among 180 residents of the same district 42 years after the atomic explosion and compared the results with a control population of 800 who were comparable in terms of sex and age. The nodular goiter frequency among the Nishiyama residents was 4.74%, significant in comparison to the 1.13% in the control population. These results show that the nodular goiter frequency increases even as a result of exposure to radioactive fallout.

B. Thyroid Disorders in Atomic Bomb Survivors

Many of the reports dealing with thyroid disease among atomic bomb survivors are concerned with thyroid cancer, with few reports on other thyroid disorders. Asano *et al*[11] confirmed the existence of 155 cases of Hashimoto's thyroiditis among the cases autopsied at the Radiation Effects Research Foundation (RERF) during the period 1954–74, but did not find a relationship with radiation exposure for either incidence or age ATB.

Studying atomic bomb survivors aged ≤ 20 ATB, Morimoto *et al*[10] found no difference in serum TSH or thyroglobulin between the ≥ 1 Gy and 0 Gy populations. On the other hand, when comparing the TSH levels in 6,112 survivors directly exposed within 1.5 km of the Hiroshima explosion with a population of 3,047 who were exposed at a distance greater than 3 km, Ito *et al*[14] found that the frequency of hypothyroidism among males in the 1.5 km population was 1.22%, compared to a value of 0.35% in the control population, with the corresponding figures for females being 7.08% and 1.18% (Fig. 1). An examination by dose shows that the frequency was 1.03% among males exposed to 0.01–0.99 Gy and 3.67% among males exposed to ≥ 2.0 Gy, with the respective figures for females being 6.23% and 7.26%, thus showing that the frequency of hypothyroidism increases with dose. Furthermore, it has been reported that the rate of positive results for the microsomal hemagglutination antibody test in the 1.5 km population was markedly lower than in the control population for both males and females. As shown in Fig. 2, investigations by Nagataki *et al*[16] and Inoue *et al*[17] into the thyroid effects of the Nagasaki atomic bomb showed that the rate of hypothyroidism was significantly high among the low-dose population, and was high among survivors aged between 10 and 39, particularly among women.

In the Nishiyama district of Nagasaki, which was contaminated by radioactive fallout from the atomic bomb, the level of radioactive ^{137}Cs in the soil was approximately double that of control areas 40 years after the atomic bomb was detonated, with the level in agricultural products showing an approximately tenfold increase. With regard to thyroid function, the level of free thyroxine (free T4) among Nishiyama residents was within the normal range but was significantly decreased relative to the control population, the difference being marked among the population aged ≤ 20 ATB[30].

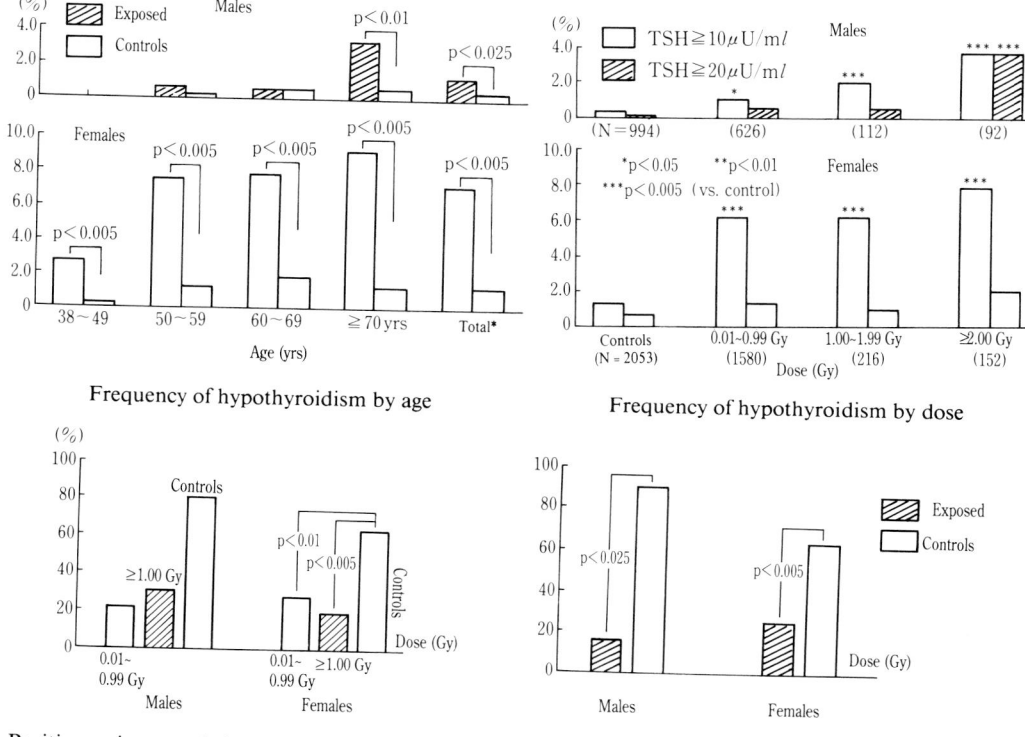

Frequency of hypothyroidism by age

Frequency of hypothyroidism by dose

Positive microsomal hemagglutination antibody tests among hypothyroidism cases by dose

Positive microsomal hemagglutination antibody tests among hypothyroidism cases by sex

Figure 1   Frequency of hypothyroidism among Hiroshima atomic bomb survivors[14]

6. THYROID DISEASE AMONG EXPOSED RESIDENTS OF THE MARSHALL ISLANDS

Subsequent to the atomic explosions at Hiroshima and Nagasaki, the residents of the Marshall Islands were exposed to strong radioactive fallout in the 1960's as a result of the hydrogen bomb tests. The incidence of thyroid cancer also increased among this exposed population, as did the incidence of hypothyroidism[18]. However, since this study was performed using old radiation dose standards, doubts surround the reliability of the dose estimates; because of this lack of accuracy, it is hoped that the study will be repeated.

CONCLUSION

Petroleum resources are finite, and in the future human beings will have to rely on atomic power as an energy source. Besides being an energy source, the use of radiation will become more widespread in medical treatment and in other industrial fields, and thus the risk of humans suffering radiation damage is rising. The thyroid

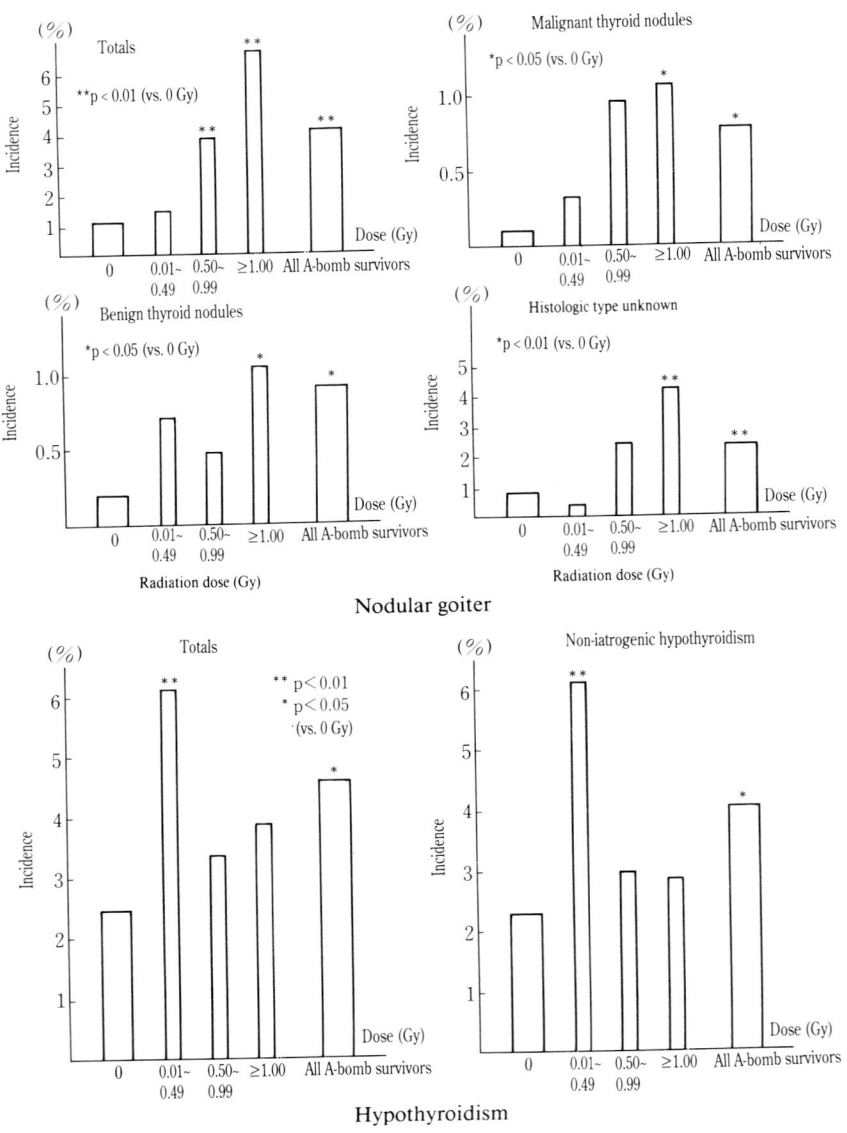

Figure 2   Thyroid disease among Nagasaki atomic bomb survivors[17]

is highly susceptible to radiation damage, and detailed long-term monitoring of the thyroid effects occurring among atomic bomb survivors from Hiroshima and Nagasaki is of great importance in the quest to clarify the damage that radiation inflicts on the thyroid.

(*Kouji Noma*)

REFERENCES

1. Fleming ID, Black TL, Thompson EI, *et al.* Thyroid dysfunction and neoplasia in children receiving neck irradiation for cancer. *Cancer* 1985; **55**: 1190–4.
2. DeGroot LJ, Reilly M, Pinnameneni K, *et al.* Retrospective and prospective study of radiation-induced thyroid disease. *Am J Med* 1983; **74**: 852–62.
3. Spitalnik PF, Straus II FH. Patterns of human thyroid parenchymal reaction following low-dose childhood irradiation. *Cancer* 1978; **41**: 1098–105.
4. Kaplan MM, Garnick MB, Gelber R, *et al.* Risk factors for thyroid abnormalities after neck irradiation for childhood cancer. *Am J Med* 1983; **74**: 272–80.
5. Socolow EL, Hashizume A, Neriishi S, *et al.* Thyroid carcinoma in man after exposure to ionizing radiation: a summary of findings in Hiroshima and Nagasaki. *N Engl J Med* 1963; **268**: 406–10.
6. Hollingsworth DR, Hamilton HB, Tamagaki H, *et al.* Thyroid disease: a study in Hiroshima, Japan. *Medicine* 1963; **42**: 47–71.
7. Wood JW, Tamagaki H, Neriishi S, *et al.* Thyroid carcinoma in atomic bomb survivors of Hiroshima and Nagasaki. *Am J Epidemiol* 1969; **89**: 4–14.
8. Jablon S, Tachikawa K, Belsky JL, *et al.* Cancer in Japanese exposed as children to atomic bombs. *Lancet* 1971; **1**: 927–32.
9. Parker LN, Belsky JL, Yamamoto T, *et al.* Thyroid carcinoma after exposure to atomic radiation: a continuing survey of a fixed population, Hiroshima and Nagasaki 1958–71. *Ann Intern Med* 1974; **80**: 600–4.
10. Morimoto I, Yoshimoto Y, Sato K, *et al.* Serum TSH, thyroglobulin and thyroid disorders in atomic bomb survivors exposed in youth: a study 30 years after exposure. RERF TR 20–85, 1986.
11. Asano M, Norman JE, Kato H, *et al.* Autopsy studies of Hashimoto's thyroiditis in Hiroshima and Nagasaki, 1954–74: relation to atomic bomb radiation. RERF TR 15–78, 1978.
12. Becker DV, McConahey WM, Dobyns BM, *et al.* The results of radioiodine treatment of hyperthyroidism: a preliminary report of the thyrotoxicosis therapy follow-up study. In: Fellinger K, Hofer R, editors. Further advances in thyroid research. *Verlag der Wiener Medizinischen Akademie* 1971; **1**: 603–09.
13. Maxson HR, Thomas ST, Seanger EL, *et al.* Ionizing irradiation and the induction of clinically significant disease in the human thyroid gland. *Am J Med* 1977; **63**: 967–78.
14. Ito C, Kato H, Mito K, *et al.* Study on the effect of atomic bomb radiation on thyroid function. *Hiroshima J Med Sciences* 1987; **36**: 13–24.
15. Nagataki S, Hirayu H, Izumi M, *et al.* Long-term effects of A-bomb radioactive fallout on the human body. *J Jap Soc Int Med* 1988; **77**: 229. (*In Japanese*)
16. Nagataki S, Hirayu H, Izumi M, *et al.* Long-term effects of A-bomb radiation on survivors. *J Jap Soc Int Med* 1989; **78**: 261. (*In Japanese*)
17. Inoue S, Toyama K, Shimaoka K, *et al.* Thyroid disease among atomic bomb survivors in Nagasaki (3rd report). *Nagasaki Med J* 1988; **63**: 587–92. (*In Japanese*)
18. Conard RA, Paglia DE, Larsen PR, *et al.* Review of medical findings in a Marshallese population twenty-six years after accidental exposure to radioactive fallout. New York: Brookhaven National Laboratory, Associated Universities. BNL 51261, 1981.
19. Liebow AA, Warren S, DeCoursey E. Pathology of atomic bomb casualties. *Am J Path* 1949; **25**: 853–1027.
20. McDougall IR, Costine LS, Donaldson SS, *et al.* Thyroid dysfunction after radiotherapy in children with Hodgkin's disease. *Clin Nucl Med* 1980; **5**: 22–3.
21. Feedberg AS, Kurland GS, Blumgart HL. The pathologic effects of ^{113}I on the normal thyroid gland of man. *J Clin Endocrinol Metab* 1952; **12**: 1315–48.
22. Clifton KH. Thyroid cancer: Reevaluation of an experimental model for radiogenic endocrine carcinogenesis. RERF TR 5–83, 1984.
23. Hiraoka T. Thyroid gland and radioactive rays. *Radiation Biology Research Communication* 1986; **21**: 259–72. (*In Japanese*)
24. Dobyns BM, Sheline GE, Workman JB, *et al.* Malignant and benign neoplasms of the thyroid in

patients treated for hyperthyroidism; a report of the cooperative thyrotoxicosis therapy follow-up study. *J Clin Endocrinol Metab* 1974; **38**: 976–98.

25. Holm LE, Dahlqvist I, Israelsson A, *et al.* Malignant thyroid tumors after iodine-131 therapy, a retrospective cohort study. *N Engl J Med* 1980; **303**: 188–91.

26. Takeichi N, Dohi K, Fujikura T, *et al.* Endocrine and gonadal tumors in atomic bomb survivors. *J Hiroshima Med Ass* 1986; **39**: 32–7. (*In Japanese*)

27. Refetoff S, Harrison JR, Karanfilski BT, *et al.* Continuing occurrence of thyroid carcinoma after irradiation to the neck in infancy and childhood. *N Engl J Med* 1975; **292**: 171–5.

28. Rubin PR, Casarett GW. Clinical radiation pathology. Philadelphia: WB Saunders, 1968; **11**: 721.

29. Oberfield SE, Allen JC, Pollack J, *et al.* Long-term endocrine sequelae after treatment of medulloblastoma: prospective study of growth and thyroid function. *J Pediatr* 1986; **108**: 219–23.

30. Yokoyama N, Nagataki S. Radiation and thyroid disease. *Clinic All-Round* 1986; **35**: 2264–8. (*In Japanese*)

31. Ishii J, Hara Y. Effects of radiation on the thyroid. *Japan Medical Journal* 1986; **3261**: 15–8. (*In Japanese*)

32. Beierwaltes WH, Johnson PC. Hyperthyroidism treated with radioiodine: a seven-year experience. *Arch Intern Med* 1956; **97**: 393.

33. DeGroot LJ, editor. The thyroid and its diseases. 5th ed. New York: John Wiley & Sons, 1984: 778.

34. Milton RC, Shohoji T. Tentative 1965 radiation dose (T65D) estimation for atomic bomb survivors. Hiroshima Radiation Effects Research Foundation. 1968; ABCC TR 1–68.

35. Takeshita K. Dose estimation from residual and fallout radioactivity — a real survey. *J Radiat Res* 1975; 16 (Suppl): 24.

3.2 PARATHYROID DISEASES

INTRODUCTION

The effects of radiation exposure on the parathyroid gland can be classified into acute damage and late effects. With regard to acute effects, hypoparathyroidism has been reported to occur between several months and one and a half years after ^{131}I treatment for hyperthyroidism. However, due to the extremely shallow tissue penetration of the beta rays from the ^{131}I, it is rare for hypoparathyroidism to actually be induced. No reports have appeared concerning acute effects of the atomic bombs on the parathyroid glands.

In Western countries X-rays were used until around 1960 to treat benign diseases such as thymal hypertrophy, tuberculous cervical lymphadenitis, and tinea capitis, etc. Thyroid tumors have been known to be induced by radiation exposure since around 1950, but the first report on the late effects on the neighboring parathyroid glands did not appear until the comparatively recent date of 1975.

This chapter considers hyperparathyroidism as a late effect of radiation exposure, focusing on data pertaining to the atomic bomb survivors.

1. HYPERPARATHYROIDISM DUE TO RADIOTHERAPY

Hyperparathyroidism is caused by tumors and hyperplasia of the parathyroid gland. Morbid excess hormonal excretion occurs, resulting in hypercalcemia, renal calculi, osteodynia, and bone fractures, etc.

The first report on the post-radiotherapy development of hyperparathyroidism described a case that developed approximately 40 years after therapeutic X-ray irradiation for a benign disease during the patient's childhood[1]. In the following year, Tisell et al[2] reported that out of 170 cases who underwent surgery for hyperparathyroidism, 14% had previously received 2.0–30 Gy of radiation during cervical radiotherapy, strongly suggesting an association with radiation exposure.

Several reports subsequently appeared concerning the post-radiotherapy development of hyperparathyroidism, stating that of the cases receiving surgery for the disease 11–30% had a history of radiotherapy, with the time period from radiotherapy to diagnosis of the disease indicating a long latency period of between 15 and 40 years[3-5]. On the other hand, the development of hyperparathyroidism was investigated in Sweden[6] and the U.S.A.[7] by performing long-term follow-up studies on patients who received radiotherapy. Tisell et al[6] found that of 444 patients who underwent cervical radiotherapy (parathyroid doses of 0.40–50.9 Gy), 14% developed hyperparathyroidism; by dose, 12% had received < 14 Gy and 29% ≥ 14 Gy, the latter high value indicating a significant relationship between dose and prevalence. Between 1974 and 1988, Cohen et al[7] monitored 4,297 patients who had received X-ray treatment of the tonsils while 16 years or under, and found that in comparison with the general population the medically irradiated population exhibited a high hyperparathyroidism incidence, the rate being approximately 2.9 times greater among those aged under 40, and approximately 2.5 times for those aged between 40 and 60.

Similarly to Western countries, X-ray treatment for benign diseases was performed in Japan until around 1960, but the development of hyperparathyroidism went virtually unnoticed, with the only report in 1991 referring to the fact that 8 out of 194 cases (4%) of hyperparathyroidism had a history of irradiation[8].

One further problem concerning cervical radiotherapy is the development of hyperparathyroidism following treatment with ^{131}I, but there is no agreement to date regarding this[9,10]. Since the age suitable for radioisotope treatment is relatively high, and as hyperparathyroidism is frequently accompanied by thyroid disease complications, it is difficult to judge whether hyperparathyroidism is actually induced by treatment with radioactive iodine, and further follow-up studies are awaited.

2. HYPERPARATHYROIDISM IN ATOMIC BOMB SURVIVORS

With regard to parathyroid disease among Nagasaki atomic bomb survivors, Matsumoto et al[11] reported in 1982 that of 13 cases that underwent surgery for primary hyperparathyroidism 3 cases were proximally exposed atomic bomb survivors, 1 case had entered the city within 1 week of the explosion, and 1 case had been exposed 4 km from the hypocenter and had previously received cervical radiotherapy. Takeichi et al[12] surveyed the incidence of parathyroid tumors among 4,136 autopsy cases in the period 1961–77. The crude incidence per 1,000 autopsy cases among early entrants and survivors exposed to a T65 dose[13] of 0 Gy was 1.8, with the figures being 4.12 and 13.4 respectively for the populations exposed to 0.01–0.49 Gy and $\geqslant 0.50$ Gy, thus demonstrating a high incidence among the heavily exposed populations.

Furthermore, Takeichi et al[14] used tumor registries compiled from data at medical facilities throughout Hiroshima prefecture during 1978–87 to study the parathyroid tumor incidence, and found 23 cases. The standardized annual incidence per 100,000 was 0.05 among the non-exposed population, and 0.81 among proximally exposed atomic bomb survivors (i.e. those within 2 km of the hypocenter), with the proximally exposed population thus exhibiting a high incidence, approximately 16.2 times greater than the non-exposed population. However, almost all parathyroid tumor cases developed hyperfunction and exhibited hypercalcemia, with many cases detected by chance following blood tests. Consequently, data must be treated on the assumption that there is no difference between the contrasted populations with regard to the proportion of subjects undergoing serum calcium tests.

Accordingly, during the period 1986–88 Fujiwara et al[15-17] determined the serum calcium levels in all the approximately 6,000 subjects in the Adult Health Study conducted by the Radiation Effects Research Foundation (RERF), which consisted of Hiroshima and Nagasaki atomic bomb survivors and controls. People with high calcium levels were subjected to detailed tests for parathyroid hormone etc., and the relationship between hyperparathyroidism diagnoses and exposure to the atomic bomb was investigated. Out of the approximately 4,000 subjects studied in

Hiroshima, 19 cases of hyperparathyroidism were diagnosed. The prevalence among women in the 0 Gy population (DS86 calculations,[18]) was 0.3%, but was 1.9% in the ≥ 1 Gy population, demonstrating a clearly increased prevalence as a result of exposure to the atomic bomb (Fig. 1).

The prevalence increased with decreasing age at the time of bombing (ATB), with the incidence in the 1 Gy population being 2.8 times greater than in the non-exposed (0 Gy) population among those aged ≥ 20 ATB, and 11.1 times greater for survivors aged 0–9 ATB (Fig. 2).

The hyperparathyroidism prevalence among females was approximately 3 times greater than amongst males, but there was no difference between the sexes with regard to the effect of radiation exposure.

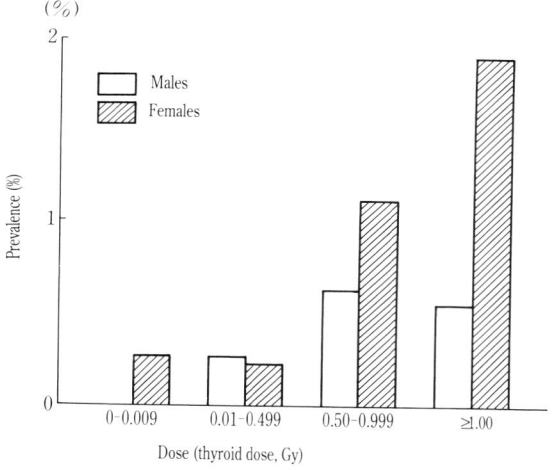

Figure 1   Prevalence of hyperparathyroidism, Hiroshima, Aug. 1986–July 1988 (*adapted from Ref. 16*)

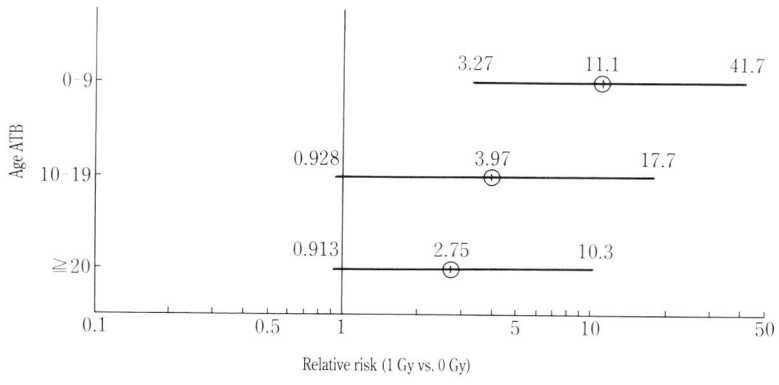

Figure 2   Relative risk of hyperparathyroidism by age ATB

3. HISTOLOGIC TYPE

Approximately 80–85% of primary hyperparathyroidism is due to parathyroid adenoma, about 10% due to hyperplasia, and only rarely due to cancer. With respect to the development of hyperparathyroidism following therapeutic irradiation, some reports state that the percentages are unchanged[19,20], whereas another report claims that the percentage due to carcinoma is higher[21]; however, the number of cases considered by each of these studies is small, and it is not possible to arrive at a conclusion.

In a study on atomic bomb survivors, Fujiwara et al[15] stated that 7 out of 9 surgical cases had adenoma and 2 cases exhibited hyperplasia, but due to the small number of cases no conclusion was reached concerning radiation dose and histologic type.

4. COMPLICATIONS OF HYPERPARATHYROIDISM AND THYROID DISEASE

Hyperparathyroidism is known to be a frequent complication of thyroid disease, but the frequency is even higher following radiation exposure, and when it accompanies thyroid cancer the rate among medically irradiated patients is approximately 9 times greater than among those not receiving such treatment[5]. Cohen et al[7] reported that approximately 84% of post-radiotherapy hyperparathyroidism occurred with the development of thyroid tumors, and 31% with thyroid cancer.

Studying atomic bomb survivors, Fujiwara et al[15] found that of 16 hyperparathyroidism cases among survivors exposed to $\geqslant 0.01$ Gy, the disease was a complication of thyroid disease in 6 cases, with 2 of these having thyroid cancer.

CONCLUSION

Of the tumors induced by exposure to the atomic bomb, most attention has been paid to malignant tumors. However, a study of hyperparathyroidism revealed that benign tumors also increased after a long latency period, raising a new problem for research concerning exposure to atomic bomb radiation in that even after the passage of approximately half a century since exposure to the atomic bomb, it is necessary to pursue further studies on the atomic bomb survivors.

(Saeko Fujiwara)

REFERENCES

1. Rosen IB, Strawbridge GH, Bain J. A case of hyperparathyroidism associated with radiation to the head and neck area. *Cancer* 1975; **36**: 1111–4.
2. Tisell LE, Carlsson S, Lindberg S, *et al.* Autonomous hyperparathyroidism: a possible late complication of neck radiotherapy. *Acta Chir Scand* 1976; **142**: 367–73.
3. Prinz RA, Paloyan E, Lawrence AM, *et al.* Radiation-associated hyperparathyroidism. A new syndrome? *Surgery* 1977; **82**: 296–302.
4. Palmer JA, Mustard RA, Simpson WJ. Irradiation as an etiologic factor in tumours of the thyroid, parathyroid and salivary glands. *Canadian J Surg* 1980; **23**: 39–42.

5. Hedman I, Tisell LE. Associated hyperparathyroidism and nonmedullary thyroid carcinoma: the etiologic role of radiation. *Surgery* 1984; **95**: 392–7.
6. Tisell LE, Carlsson S, Fjälling M, *et al.* Hyperparathyroidism subsequent to neck irradiation. Risk factors. *Cancer* 1985; **56**: 1529–33.
7. Cohen J, Gierlowski TC, Schneider AB. A prospective study of hyperparathyroidism in individuals exposed to radiation in childhood. *JAMA* 1990; **264**: 581–4.
8. Kanbe M, Kurita T, Fujimoto Y, *et al.* Eight cases of primary hyperparathyroidism following external neck radiation. *Folia Endocrinologia Japonica* 1991; **67**: 352. (*In Japanese*)
9. Bondeson AG, Bondeson L, Thompson NW. Hyperparathyroidism after treatment with radioactive iodine. Not only a coincidence? *Surgery* 1989; **106**: 1025–7.
10. Fjälling M, Dackenberg A, Hedman I, *et al.* An evaluation of the risk of developing hyperparathyroidism after ^{131}I treatment for thyrotoxicosis. *Acta Chir Scand* 1983; **149**: 681–6.
11. Matsumoto T, Sakai H, Tokunaga S, *et al.* Radiation-induced hyperparathyroidism. *Geka* (Surgery) 1982; 44 (Suppl): 831–6. (*In Japanese*)
12. Takeichi N, Fujikura T, Nishida T, *et al.* Parathyroid gland tumors in A-bomb survivors, autopsy cases, Hiroshima, preliminary report. *J Hiroshima Med Ass* 1984; **37**: 439–41. (*In Japanese*)
13. Milton RC, Shohoji T. Tentative 1965 radiation dose estimation for atomic bomb survivors, Hiroshima and Nagasaki. ABCC TR 1–68.
14. Takeichi N, Dohi H, Ito H, *et al.* Parathyroid tumors in atomic bomb survivors in Hiroshima. A review. *J Radiat Res* 1991; 32 (Suppl): 189–192.
15. Fujiwara S, Sposto R, Ezaki H, *et al.* Hyperparathyroidism among atomic bomb survivors in Hiroshima. *Radiat Res* 1992; **130**: 327–8.
16. Fujiwara S. Radiation-induced hyperparathyroidism. *Igaku no ayumi* (Advances in Medicine) 1990; 153: 363. (*In Japanese*)
17. Fujiwara S. Hyperparathyroidism. *J Radiat Res* 1991; 32 (Suppl): 245–8.
18. Roesh WC, editor. US-Japan joint reassessment of atomic bomb radiation dosimetry in Hiroshima and Nagasaki, final report, DS86. Vol. 1 and 2. Hiroshima: Radiation Effects Research Foundation, 1987.
19. Katz A, Braunstein GD. Clinical, biochemical, and pathologic features of radiation-associated hyperparathyroidism. *Arch Intern Med* 1983; **143**: 79–82.
20. Hedman I, Hansson G, Lundberg LM, *et al.* A clinical evaluation of radiation-induced hyperparathyroidism based on 148 surgically treated patients. *World J Surg* 1984; **8**: 96–105.
21. Christman TJ, Chapple CR, Noble JG, *et al.* Hyperparathyroidism after neck irradiation. *Br J Surg* 1988; **75**: 873–4.

3.3 DIABETES MELLITUS

INTRODUCTION

The frequency of diabetes mellitus in Japan is known to be steadily increasing; the rate in the atomic bomb survivor population is 10%, extremely high in comparison with populations in other areas of the country[1]. An interesting problem concerning the mechanism by which diabetes mellitus develops is whether the high incidence among atomic bomb survivors is due to aging of the population or whether it is somehow related to atomic bomb radiation. This chapter discusses the effect of radiation on the pancreas, and the relationship between radiation exposure and the prevalence and incidence of diabetes mellitus. For certain types of data it is difficult to make comparisons with respect to time since diagnostic techniques and criteria have varied with time. This chapter reviews the current state of knowledge regarding diabetes mellitus.

1. THE EFFECT OF RADIATION ON THE PANCREAS

A. Effect of X-Ray Irradiation

The pancreas is believed to have a comparatively low sensitivity to radiation[2]. Although few reports have dealt with the effect of radiation exposure on pancreatic tissue, Oughterson et al[3] reported the absence of evidence concerning morphological abnormalities in the pancreatic islets of Langerhans among victims who died in Japan due to the atomic bomb during the initial period following the atomic bombing.

   With regard to experimental studies on the effect of radiation on pancreatic tissue, Rauch and Stentrom[4] performed localized irradiation of rat pancreas, either with a single X-ray dose of 6.0 Gy or a series of 2.0 Gy doses over a period of several days resulting in a cumulative dose of 8.0–16.0 Gy. Observations were performed at 1 day, 2 days, and 2 months after exposure, to determine whether histologic changes had occurred in the pancreas, but no clear changes were detected. In 1981 Tsubouchi et al[5] performed whole-body irradiation of hamsters with 350 Gy and 100 Gy, and reported secretory cell lesions and the disappearance of secretory granules 4 hours after irradiation. However, in the case of 100 Gy irradiation, although the beta cell count decreased until 1 day after irradiation, it then tended to increase thereafter until the 4th or 5th day.

   Barkalaya[6,7] and Tsubota et al[8] performed animal experiments in order to determine whether incomplete insulin secretion from the pancreas occurred as an acute effect of radiation. Both authors irradiated rats with what was believed to be a dose that would cause death in 50% of the irradiated subjects, and studied the effect on pancreatic endocrine function. Tsubota et al performed a single whole-body irradiation of the rats with 8.0 Gy of 25MV X-rays. As shown in Table 1, a temporary excess blood glucose level was apparent at 5 hours and 2 days after irradiation, with the blood insulin level relatively low and the blood glucagon level high in comparison with the blood glucose level; however, the insulin secretion itself

Table 1   Changes in blood glucose, insulin, glucagon and cortisol levels after X-ray irradiaton (8 Gy)

	Controls (n = 5)	Time after irradiation		
		5 hrs (n = 3)	2 days (n = 3)	7 days (n = 3)
Blood glucose (mg/dl)	125.2 ± 5.5	*1 180.3 ± 9.4	*2 180.3 ± 3.1	148.5 ± 20.9
Blood insulin (μU/ml)	20.2 ± 4.3	*3 37.0 ± 3.6	24.0 ± 5.7	21.7 ± 3.3
Blood glucagon (pg/ml)	396.4 ± 35.7	494.3 ± 60.1	592.3 ± 123.6	443.3 ± 29.6
Blood cortisol (μg/dl)	7.1 ± 0.7	5.6 ± 1.3	6.7 ± 0.2	7.3 ± 0.3

*significantly different from control. (*1 : $P < 0.01$, *2 : $P < 0.001$, *3 : $P < 0.05$) Mean ± S.E.

did not decrease. Also, pancreatic perfusion experiments showed reappearance of the hyperglycemic state, and no difference in hypersecretion between the irradiated population and a control population with respect to insulin and glucagon secretion at 5 hours and between 1 and 7 days after irradiation. In the previously mentioned experiment by Tsubouchi et al[5] involving whole-body irradiation with 350 and 100 Gy, blood insulin levels decreased 12 hours after irradiation with 350 Gy, but following irradiation with 100 Gy the level returned to normal 2–4 days after irradiation, and tended to register an increase on the 5th day (Fig. 1).

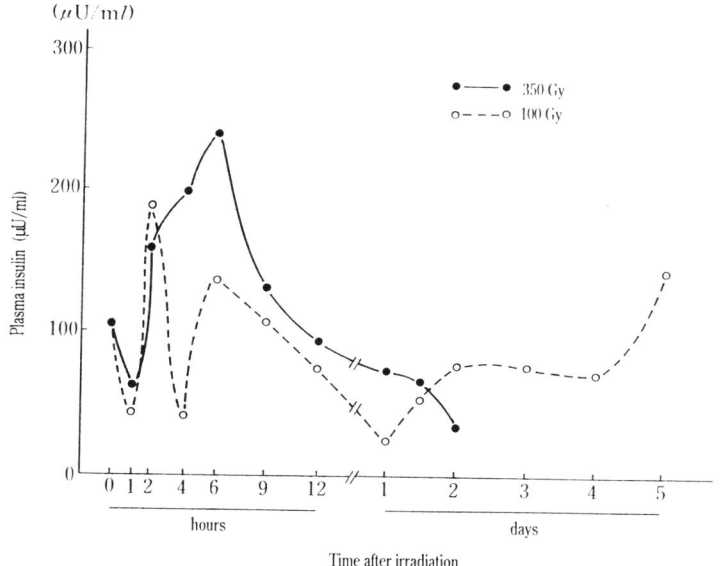

Figure 1   Plasma insulin levels following whole-body irradiation (adapted from Ref. 5)

B. Effect on Atomic Bomb Survivors

With respect to results concerning the atomic bomb survivors, Ito[9] studied the insulin reaction of Hiroshima survivors 26–28 years after exposure during the 50 g glucose tolerance test (GTT). The estimated doses received[10] were believed to be ≥ 0.316 Gy for survivors directly exposed within 1.5 km of the hypocenter, and 0 Gy for survivors directly exposed at distances greater than 3.0 km. Since the blood insulin level varies greatly with the blood glucose level and age, a comparative study was performed by age and the diabetes type based on the criteria defined by the Japan Diabetes Association. An examination of blood glucose and blood insulin (immunoreaction insulin, IRI) levels in the 40–59 year old population with normal type GTT levels revealed that the proximally exposed (≤ 1.5 km) exhibited a slightly higher insulin reaction than the distally exposed (≥ 3.0 km) (Fig. 2). For other age groups and diabetes types the proximally exposed population did not exhibit a lower insulin reaction, and no reduction in insulin secretion was seen among the proximally and heavily exposed population.

Epidemiological data has also been used to investigate the relationships between radiation exposure and prevalence of diabetes mellitus, and between diabetes mellitus incidence and diabetic complications.

Rundnick et al[12] investigated the relationship between radiation exposure and prevalence of diabetes mellitus for 3,851 atomic bomb survivors resident in Hiroshima and included in the first examinations of atomic bomb survivors in the Adult Health Study sample of the Atomic Bomb Casualty Commission (ABCC) detection program and clinical survey between 1958 and 1960. The diagnostic criteria used for determination of diabetes mellitus were either a blood glucose level when the stomach was empty of ≥ 125 mg/dl, or a glucose tolerance when the

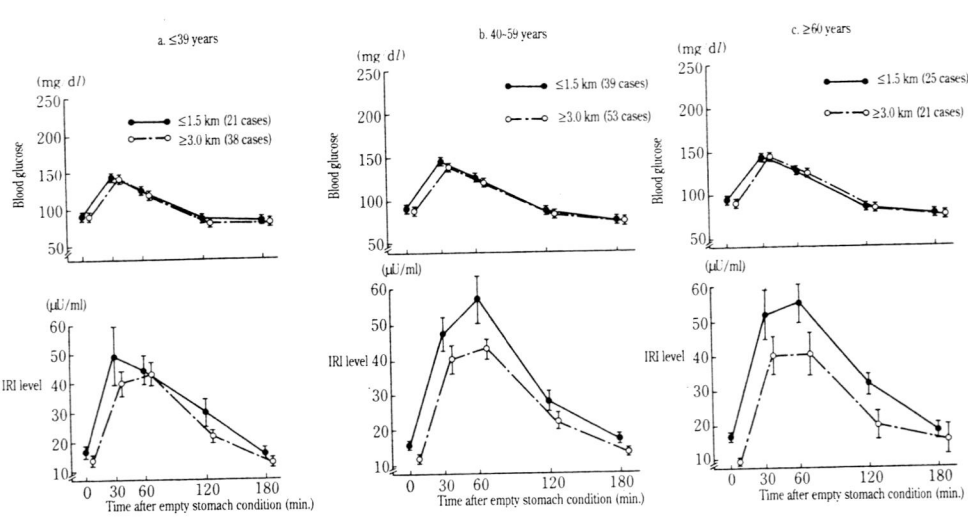

Figure 2   Normal type blood glucose and immunoreaction insulin (IRI) levels by distance from hypocenter

stomach was empty equal to 1.75 g per 1 kg of body weight followed 2 hours later by a blood glucose level of ≥ 140 mg/dl. Although these values are lower than the current diagnostic criteria, no statistically significant relationship was observed between radiation exposure and diabetes mellitus prevalence. Furthermore, similar results were reported at the same facility by Freedman et al[13] and Belsky et al[14]. Later epidemiological studies on diabetes mellitus have assumed no relationship between radiation exposure and diabetes mellitus.

Wada et al[15-17] compared atomic bomb survivors with non-exposed diabetes mellitus patients with regard to age at the onset of the disease and clinical observations. No difference was observed between the two populations, suggesting that radiation exposure has no effect on the development of diabetes mellitus. In 1971 Kawate et al[18] investigated the frequency of diabetes mellitus in atomic bomb survivors tested at the Hiroshima Atomic Bomb Survivors Health Clinic based on the 50 g glucose tolerance test (GTT), and compared directly and proximally exposed survivors (≤ 2.0 km) with a distally exposed population consisting of individuals who were either exposed directly at distances greater than 3.0 km or who entered the city after August 10th 1945. As shown in Table 2, no difference in diabetes mellitus frequency was observed between the proximally and distally exposed populations.

Further, Ito et al[19] measured GTT in some of the patients undergoing examination at the Hiroshima Atomic Bomb Survivors Health Clinic over the 21-year period 1963–83, and, in 2,843 cases in which follow-up studies were possible, compared diabetes mellitus incidence between atomic bomb survivors exposed within 1.9 km of the hypocenter with those receiving exposure at distances greater than 3.0 km. As can be seen from Table 3, the percentage of non-obese individuals who initially exhibited normal type GTT results but who within 1 year developed results indicative of diabetes mellitus type amounted to 0.89% for the proximally exposed (≤ 1.9 km) population and 0.65% for the distally exposed population, with the figures for those initially with borderline type being 5.73% and 5.49% respectively; thus there was no difference observed between the two populations[20]. Even among the obese patients, although the percentage who developed diabetes mellitus was

Table 2   Frequency of diabetes mellitus by age and distance from hypocenter

	(A) 20 ~ 39 years			(B) 40 ~ 59 years			(C) ≤ 60 years		
	No. of examinees	No. of diabetes cases	%	No. of examinees	No. of diabetes cases	%	No. of examinees	No. of diabetes cases	%
(1) Proximally exposed survivors	175	5	2.9	198	23	11.6	169	39	23.1
(II) Distally exposed survivors	94	4	4.1	93	13	13.9	76	26	34.2
(1)–(II)x^2	0.06			0.14			3.70		

Table 3   Annual rate of diabetes mellitus development in the ≤ 1.9 km and ≥ 3.0 km populations (cumulative data over 1~19 year period)

(a) Non-obese population

Initial GTT test		Distance from hypocenter ≤ 1.9 km (n = 754) (%)	≥ 3.0 km (n = 685) (%)	Significance
Normal type		0.89	0.65	None
Borderline type	B – 1 (2 hr P.G. < 140)	2.91	2.72	None
	B – 2 (140 ~ 169)	6.93	6.31	None
	B – 3 (≥ 170 mg/dl)	12.36	11.69	None
	Total	5.73	5.49	None

(b) Obese population

Initial GTT test		Distance from hypocenter ≤ 1.9 km (n = 72) (%)	≥ 3.0 km (n = 73) (%)	Significance
Normal type		4.51	3.08	None
Borderline type	B – 1 (2 hr P.G. < 140)	7.62	6.82	None
	B – 2 (140 ~ 169)	13.26	15.11	None
	B – 3 (≥ 170 mg/dl)	28.07	15.38	None
	Total	14.25	12.09	None

n = no. of subjects

GTT = glucose tolerance test
2 hr P.G. = plasma glucose level 2 hours after 75 g glucose tolerance test

over double that observed amongst non-obese individuals, no difference was found with respect to exposure status. Studies on the frequency of diabetes mellitus complications (proteinuria, diabetic retinopathy, hyperlipidema, and ischemic heart disease) again showed no difference with respect to exposure status[19].

CONCLUSION

The pancreas is believed to have low radiosensitivity, and no histologic or endocrinological effects have been reported after irradiation with several Grays even in the immediate post-irradiation period. With regard to the relationship between radiation exposure and development of diabetes mellitus, reports have appeared concerning decreased insulin secretion, diabetes mellitus prevalence and incidence, and accompanying complications, but all findings have been negative.

(Jun-ichiro Ogawa, Chikako Ito)

REFERENCES

1. Ito C. Prevalence and incidence of diabetes mellitus in atomic bomb survivors in Hiroshima. In: Kosaka K, Kuzuya K, editors. *Tonyobyogaku* (Diabetes mellitus) Tokyo: Shindan-to-chiryo, 1991: 11–26. (*In Japanese*)
2. Mossman KL. Radiation effects in nuclear medicine. In: Herbet J, da Rocha AFG, editors. Textbook of nuclear medicine. Vol. 1: Basic science. Philadelphia: Lea & Febiger, 1984: 282–302.
3. Oughterson AW, Warren S. Pathology of atomic bomb in Japan. New York: McGraw Hill, 1956: 296–316.
4. Rauch GF, Stentrom KW. Effects of X-ray radiation on pancreatic function. *Gastroenterology* 1952; **20**: 595–603.
5. Tsubouchi S, Suzuki H, Ariyoshi H, *et al.* Radiation-induced acute necrosis of the pancreatic islet and the diabetic syndrome in the golden hamster (Mesocricetus auratus). *Int J Radiat Biol* 1981; **40**: 95–106.
6. Barkalaya AI. Radioimmunologic analysis of insulin secretion during acute radiation sickness. *Radiologia* 1975; **15**: 127–9. (*English abstract; article in Russian*)
7. Barkalaya AI. Radioimmunologic study of insulin secretion during acute radiation sickness. *Radiologia* 1977; **17**: 596–9. (*English abstract; article in Russian*)
8. Tsubota M, Dalimunthe D, Kawate R, *et al.* Effects of 25 MV whole-body X-ray irradiation on endocrinous function of pancreas of rats. *J Hiroshima Med Ass* 1980; **33**: 1112–8. (*In Japanese*)
9. Ito C. Plasma insulin response in atomic bomb survivors. Proceedings of the 15th Atomic Casualty Council Meeting; 1975 June 16; Nagasaki. Nagasaki: Nagasaki Atomic Bomb Casualty Council 1975: 42–9. (*In Japanese*)
10. Milton CC, Shohoji T. Tentative 1965 radiation dose estimation for atomic bomb survivors. ABCC TR 1–68, 1968.
11. Kuzuya S. Standardization of oral glucose tolerance test. *J Japan Diab Soc* 1970; **13**: 1–7. (*In Japanese*)
12. Rundnick PA, Anderson PS, Jr. Diabetes mellitus in Hiroshima, Japan. A detection program and clinical survey. *Diabetes* 1962; **11**: 533–43. (ABCC TR 16–61, 1961).
13. Freedman LR, Blackard WG, Sagan LA, et al. The epidemiology of diabetes mellitus in Hiroshima and Nagasaki. *Yale J Biol Med* 1965; **37**: 283–99. (ABCC TR 18–64, 1964).
14. Belsky JL, Tachikawa K, Jablon S. The health of atomic bomb survivors: a decade of examination in a fixed population. *Yale J Biol Med* 1973; **46**: 284–96. (ABCC TR 9–71, 1971).
15. Wada, S, Yamakido M. Studies for onset age of diabetes mellitus in relation to atomic bomb. *Japan J of Clin & Exp Med* 1958; **40**: 584–8. (*In Japanese*)

16. Wada S, Matsuura J, Yamakido M. Studies for diabetes mellitus in relation to atomic bomb. *J Hiroshima Med Ass* 1963; **16**: 229–34. (*In Japanese*)
17. Wada S, Yamakido M, Amano H, *et al.* Studies for diabetes mellitus in relation to atomic bomb. *J Hiroshima Med Ass* 1967; **20**: 237–50. (*In Japanese*)
18. Kawate R, Naito Y, Noma K, *et al.* Metabolic changes with age in Hiroshima atomic bomb survivors. *J Hiroshima Med Ass* 1971; **24**: 1196–204. (*In Japanese*)
19. Ito C, Hasegawa K, Kato M, *et al.* Clinical investigation proximate exposed group. Report 1. A study for prevalence rate of diabetes mellitus. *J Nagasaki Med Ass* 1984; **59**: 349–55. (*In Japanese*)
20. Kosaka K, *et al.* Criteria for diabetes mellitus. *J Japan Diab Soc* 1982; **25**: 857–66. (*In Japanese*)

4

Hematologic and Hematopoeitic Organ Disease

4 HEMATOLOGIC AND HEMATOPOEITIC ORGAN DISEASE

INTRODUCTION

Numerous people perished in the immediate aftermath of the massive explosion as a result of trauma and burns, of whom many died after 1 week to 10 days with high temperatures and hemorrhaging despite suffering only slight trauma or burns. Also, numerous cases exhibited marked post-exposure fatigue, general malaise, appetite loss, nausea, vomiting, and thirst, after which the symptoms became milder and general body condition temporarily recovered; but this was followed by the occurrence of epilation, subcutaneous bleeding and general malaise etc., and then death due to inexplicable symptoms. Due to the sense of anxiety caused by the fact that even apparently healthy individuals might at any time become ill and die, these symptoms were termed atomic bomb illness. This atomic bomb illness was essentially caused by radiation-produced damage to the bone marrow. This chapter reviews the literature based on studies conducted immediately after the bombing with regard to the most important topics of anemia and leukopenia, with particular emphasis on analyses of the changes occurring during the initial period.

1. LEUKOPENIA

Hiroshima atomic bomb survivors exhibited leukopenia, initially lymphopenia, followed by a rapid disappearance of granulocytes. A minimum level was observed approximately 1 month later, after which recovery occurred, in some cases rapidly and in others gradually. Naturally many bone marrow aplasia cases died without exhibiting any recovery. The severity and pattern of illness were strongly dose-dependent, although to a small extent individual differences were also observed. The changes occurring between the 1st week and 1st month of the initial period following exposure were dramatic. The atomic bombing was unprecedented in human experience, and with the extreme incineration in Hiroshima there are extremely few records of leukocyte counts. The Army Medical School[1] described conditions in the following way: "On the day of the bombing, the medical facilities were swamped dealing with a deluge of patients, and it was absolutely impossible to make detailed observations. Every person with burns received equal treatment without any consideration given to the extent of the injuries, including people who died in the initial period with slight burns, and thus it was difficult to perform observations on the early symptoms of radiation damage." It is quite surprising that even under these difficult circumstances the Army Medical School and the Kure Naval Station[2] monitored some leukocyte counts until August 13th. This section reviews the data concerning the bewildering changes in the numbers and types of leukocytes from the acute period through the subacute period, and then to the recovery period.

A. Acute Period

The leukocyte counts from 1 week to at most 10 days after the bombing were less than 4,000 in 32 out of 118 cases (27%) (Table 1)[1,2]. A study performed by Kikuchi (Kyoto University) in 1942 on healthy people in the Hiroshima area found an average leukocyte count of 7,424, and in 42 cases found none with less than 4,000. All the 11 cases in Table 1 with less than 1,000 leukocytes were exposed within 200 meters of the hypocenter. Even so, there were some cases exposed within 200 meters with leukocyte counts over 6,000 in the 1st week, and other cases exposed at 1,500–2,000 m with leukocyte counts of less than 3,000 (Table 2). At the present time details concerning the relationship between dose and exposure status for these cases are not clear. Despite the fact that some proximally exposed cases exhibited normal leukocyte counts in the 1st week, and that some relatively distally exposed cases exhibited marked leukopenia, this was probably due primarily to exposure conditions such as shielding, although it also necessary to give consideration to individual differences. The question of shielding is important, and in cases where parts of the body were completely shielded much of the hematopoietic function is believed to have been preserved. Table 3 shows the classifications of leukocytes in cases exhibiting marked leukopenia. The study, which comprises the only data available from this period, was performed at Iwakuni Naval Hospital. Lymphopenia was marked, but granulocytes also exhibited a marked decrease relative to the absolute granulocyte count[3]. The greatest interest during this period of marked leukopenia focuses on what happened in the bone marrow, but data are extremely scarce. Referring to 2 of the cases shown in Table 3 for whom bone marrow examinations were performed, it was stated that "Bone marrow tests in 2 cases revealed a greatly decreased nucleated cell component, and especially myeloid cells had at this time already almost vanished from the bone marrow; the two or three mature granulocytes that were detected with difficulty exhibited marked toxic degeneration. Bone marrow megakaryocytes also greatly decreased, and those detected showed marked degenerative changes. On the other hand, small lymphocytes were relatively abundant (20–40%). Reticular cells increased, and the observed increase in plasma cells merits particular attention."

Table 1   Leukocyte counts at 1 week after bombing in cases exposed within 1 km (at the Army Medical School, Kure Naval Station, and Iwakuni Naval Hospital)

Leukocyte count	0 ~ 1,000	1,000 ~ 2,000	2,000 ~ 3,000	3,000 ~ 4,000	4,000 ~ 5,000	5,000 ~ 6,000	6,000 ~ 7,000	7,000 ~ 8,000	8,000 ~ 9,000	9,000 ~ 10,000	Total
Individuals with varying degrees of injury	11	2	8	5	18	9	13	4	6		76
Healthy workers			3	3	2	6	15	5	7	1	42
Total	11	2	11	8	20	15	28	9	13	1	118
			32 (27%)			86 (73%)					

Table 2   Leukocyte counts by distance from the hypocenter at 1 week after bombing[2]

Leukocyte count Distance from hypocenter (m)	0 ~ 500	500 ~ 1,000	1,000 ~ 2,000	2,000 ~ 3,000	3,000 ~ 4,000	4,000 ~ 5,000	5,000 ~ 6,000	6,000 ~ 7,000	7,000 ~ 8,000	8,000 ~	Total
> 200 m	6 (26)	5 (22)		1 (4)	2 (9)	4 (17)		5 (22)			23
1,500 ~ 2,000 m			1 (5)	7 (35)	2 (10)	3 (15)	2 (10)	4 (20)	1 (5)		20

(Percentages indicated in parentheses)

Table 3   Leukocyte data for 9 leukopenia cases at 1 week after bombing[2]

Subject	1	2	3	4	5	6	7	8	9
Date of examination	Aug. 12	Aug. 12	Aug. 12	Aug. 12	Aug. 12	Aug. 12	Aug. 13	Aug. 12	Aug. 13
Erythrocyte count	410	420	420	265	328	375	413	282	326
Leukocyte count	400	150	400	400	150	250	400	300	300
Estimated no. of leukocytes	50[*1]	50	50	20	13	100	30	20	50
Lymphocytes	28	30	14	(1)[*2]	0	8	(5)[*2]	(1)[*2]	16
Monocytes	6[*1]	4	10	0	0	4	(2)[*2]	(1)[*2]	16
Myelocytes	0	0	0	0	0	0	0	0	2
Metamyelocytes	0	0	0	0	0	4	0	0	0
Stabs	20	8	16	0	(2)[*2]	26	(1)[*2]	0	10
Segs	40	50	60	(12)[*2]	(11)[*2]	56	(22)[*2]	(18)[*2]	70
Eosinophils	0	4	0	0	0	2	0	0	0
Basopils	0	0	0	0	0	2	0	0	0
Plasma cells	2	0	0	0	0	0	0	0	0
Erythroblasts	0	4	0	(7)[*2]	0	0	0	0	2

[*1]The number of cells for case #1 was 96, i.e. less than 100, and the values are shown unchanged.
[*2]Due to the low calculated number of cells, only the actual number of cells is shown.

Tables 4 and 5 show autopsy findings for cases who died at this time. Table 4 shows the autopsies performed at Ninoshima and the later detailed comments by Amano[4]. Each case was proximally exposed within 400–650 meters of the hypocenter, with death occurring on the 4th or 5th day. In every case whole organs were diagnosed as agranulocytosis, with the phrasing used by Amano in the autopsy reports suggesting a complete absence of granulocytes. Major Yamashina[5] of the army left records on 12 autopsies performed during the period August 10th–15th. References to the hematopoietic organs that were gleaned from the documents are presented in Table 5. The leukocyte counts in the 4 cases examined were all normal.

Table 4   Acute period autopsy data (at Ninoshima)[4]

Subject	Distance from hypocenter (m)	Date of autopsy	Spleen	Lymph nodes	Bone marrow	Autopsy diagnosis
1. Male, 40 yrs.	400	Aug. 10th	Marked atrophy	Absent	Absent	Agranulocytosis (granulocytopenia exhibited throughout body)
2. Male, 15 yrs.	650	Aug. 11th	Marked atrophy	Absent	Absent	Agranulocytosis
3. Male, 32 yrs.	650	Aug. 11th	Marked atrophy	Absent	Absent	Agronulocytosis

Table 5   Hematopoietic data from autopsy records for subjects who died soon after atomic bombing[15]

Subject	Distance from hypocenter (m)	Date of autopsy	WBC	Spleen	Lymph nodes	Bone marrow
3. Female, 15 yrs.	1000	Aug. 11	9500	—	—	—
5. Male, 39 yrs.	1000	Aug. 12	9500	—	—	*1 Adequate cell counts. Reticular cells, macrophages, and plasma cells observed. Granulocytes, primarily eosinophils.
6. Female, 13 yrs.	1500	Aug. 13	—	—	—	*2 Predominantly plasma cells and eosinophils; no hematopoietic function
9. Male, 25 yrs.	1500	Aug. 14	7500	—	—	Cellular marrow.
10. Female, 25 yrs.	2000	Aug. 14	9500	Marked atrophy	—	*3 Considerable number of cells, primarily eosinophils, reticular cells and plasma cells.
11. Male, 25 yrs.	1200	Aug. 14	5500	—	—	No plasma cells.
12. Male, 33 yrs.	700	Aug. 15	—	—	Marked leukopenia	*6 At first glance, an apparently normal bone marrow. Plentiful granulocytes, shift to the left, slight increase in plasma cells. Difficult to conceive that this bone marrow was exposed to radiation.

Bone marrow specimens were available in 6 cases, with all but 2 showing an increase in plasma cells. Increases were also observed in reticular cells and eosinophils, and are similar to the bone marrow studies on leukopenia cases at the afore-mentioned Iwakuni Naval Hospital. However, the cell counts in Yamashina's cases were particularly high. On the other hand, the spleen exhibited marked atrophy in the 12th case. At first glance the patient appeared to have had a normal bone marrow, but actually exhibited a marked decrease in lymphocytes in the lymph nodes; the extreme destruction of the lymph system was the same as in the marked splenic atrophy evident in Amano's 3 cases. Lymphopenia in the peripheral blood was the phenomenon most apparent in the initial period, thus adding pathological support to this.

B. Subacute Period

Immediately after the atomic explosion there were complaints of fatigue, general malaise, loss of appetite, nausea, vomiting, and thirst, but several days later these symptoms became milder, with the so-called midterm recovery period lasting from the end of the 1st week to the 4th week. After this a number of people exhibited epilation and a variety of symptoms leading to an increased bleeding tendency (e.g. subcutaneous bleeding, leukopenia and thrombopenia), followed by death. These are referred to as both subacute and midterm death patterns, but in many cases leukocyte counts which were initially normal decreased, registering a minimum from late August to early September. Time sequential monitoring of leukocyte counts was performed in extremely few cases, but 1 case reported by Nakao et al.[3] was thought to be typical of these in terms of the clinical course (Table 6). The case was a 14-year-old boy, exposed at an unknown distance from the hypocenter, who exhibited nausea, vomiting, and loss of appetite for 3 days after exposure. It can be surmised that he received a considerable dose of radiation (vomiting is a good indicator of radiation dose, with the time between exposure and onset of vomiting decreasing with increasing dose). The leukocyte count was in the normal range on August 11th, but the absolute total of lymphocytes was only 840, already indicating mild lymphopenia. Leukopenia progressed rapidly after August 20th, agranulocytosis developed, and the patient died on the 27th. The number of deaths following such a pattern reached a maximum in late August, after which they decreased. Of the 13 deaths at the Hiroshima No.1 Army Hospital (Ujina) in late August and early September, only 2 had leukocyte counts over 1,000 (2,200 and 1,100 respectively). Leukopenia during this period was granulocytopenia, and indicated relative lymphocytosis. Of 22 cases observed at Hiroshima No.1 Army Hospital (Ujina), Iwakuni Naval Hospital and Hiroshima Ryouyousho, lymphocytes accounted for ≥ 70% of leukocytes in 11 cases[3]. However, in these cases also, the absolute total of leukocytes had decreased. Data obtained at Hiroshima Ryouyousho clearly show the period during which the leukocyte count reached a minimum and the number of days after the bombing at which it occurred (Table 7). That is, the time until appearance of leukopenia decreased with increasing severity of the patient's illness, with the minimum leukocyte count being observed late in mild cases. For those subjects who died, there is approximate agreement between minimum leukocyte count and the period in which death occurred. However, in some cases death occurred as the leukocyte count was beginning to recover[3]. This was due to progressive pneumonia which developed during the agranulocytic period.

Table 6   Case initially exhibiting normal leukocyte counts but later exhibiting marked leukopenia[3]

Date of examination	Aug. 11	Aug. 20	Aug. 21	Aug. 23	Aug. 25	Aug. 27
Erythrocyte count	406	337	391	205	169	268
Hemoglobin	70	60	65	51	48	70
Leukocyte count	4,200	1,100	1,000	350	170	120
Estimated cell count	50	20		6		2
Lymphocytes	20 (840)*	70 (770)		5 (292)		1 (60)
Monocytes	4 (162)	5 (55)		0		0
Myelocytes	0	0		0		0
Metamyelocytes	2 (84)	10 (110)		0		1 (60)
Stabs	30 (1,260)	10 (110)		0		0
Segs	44 (1,848)	0		0		0
Eosinophils	0	0		1 (58)		0
Basophils	0	0		0		0
Plasma cells	0	0		0		0
Nucleated erythrocytes	0	5 (55)		0		0

( ) Parentheses indicate actual numbers observed.

Almost all autopsies on cases who died during the subacute period revealed agranulocytosis or aplastic anemia[4]. These observations were essentially the same as those seen in the acute period deaths, with the differences believed to have been due to differences in radiation dose. Most of the cases in this population were exposed at between 700 m and 1,800 m from the hypocenter[3,4], slightly further than those who died in the acute period.

Many individuals recovered despite exhibiting leukopenia during the subacute period. Normal hematopoiesis suddenly became evident in the bone marrow, and leukocyte counts rose, although some patients recovered at an extremely slow rate. In severe cases bone marrow recovery began in the 6th week, returning to approximately normal levels in the 9th week. During this period myelocytes and metamyelocytes in some instances temporarily appeared in peripheral blood; marked eosinophilia was also observed in some individuals. In the recovery of leukocyte counts, first there was an increase in lymphatic cells, followed by an increase in

Table 7   Relationship between physical condition and number of days after the bombing at which leukocyte counts were at a minimum[6]

Physical condition	No. of days after bombing 20	22	24	26	28	30	32	34	36	38	40	42	44	Total	Average no. of days
Death		4	3	3	4	4	3							21	27
Serious condition			5	3	2	1	8	1						20	29
Moderate symptoms				2	1		4	4		1				12	32
Mild symptoms						1		1	2	2			1	7	37
Extremely mild symptoms	1							1		1	1			4	36
Total	1	4	8											64	

granulocytes. Fujii *et al*[6] reported that in 75% of cases, restoration of hematopoietic function began with a recovery of lymphocytes.

C. Leukocyte Counts at 3–4 Months

In this period 16 out of 44 cases had counts of $\leq 4,000$, with 1 case of 600[7]. Granulocyte counts of $\leq 2,000$ were observed in 6 out of 43 cases. However, all of the others were believed to exhibit normal values.

D. Leukocyte Counts at 1 Year and 2 Years

A study of leukocyte counts at 1 year after the bombing[8] revealed that counts of under 4,000 were observed in 78 out of 523 cases (14.9%), showing a clearly greater number of leukopenia cases than in the control population (6 out of 173 cases, 3.5%). However, there was no constant relationship between the cases exhibiting leukopenia and either distance from the hypocenter or appearance of symptoms at the time of bombing. No difference with the controls was observed in neutrophil, eosinophil or lymphocyte counts.

A study at 2 years 2 months after the bombing[9] found leukocyte counts under 4,000 in 9 out of 243 cases (3.7%), approximately the same as in the control population (6 out of 173 cases, 3.5%) and showing a decrease from the level at 1 year after the bombing. No difference with the controls was observed in neutrophils or lymphocytes, and the bone marrow data was virtually normal.

E. Leukocyte Counts at 10 Years

The average leukocyte count in 1947 was approximately 9,000, but this had fallen to 5,500 by 1956[10]. No significant difference was observed between the exposed and control populations. The reduction in the average leukocyte count observed in 1956 was probably due to factors such as improvements in the environment, food, and use of antibiotics etc.

F. Studies on Individuals Proceeding Close to the Hypocenter

At the Army Medical School, apart from 1 case with a leukocyte count of 3,200 all individuals had counts of at least 5,000 and exhibited no abnormalities.

Furthermore, examinations of atomic bomb survivors resident in the Otake area were performed by Yamamoto[11] in 1952, Hirose[12] in 1953, Yokoro[13] in 1954, and Yamada et al[14] in 1955. Recovery of leukopoietic function was slow, with the examination of 15,510 individuals between 1954 and 1957 by the Hiroshima Atomic Bomb Casualty Council revealing 3.1% to have a leukocyte count of under 4,000. Therefore, by 1957 complete recovery of hematopoietic function was observed.

Conclusion

It should be stated that the identification of the reduced leukocyte count in the initial period following the bombing was without doubt due to the astuteness of the medical researchers at the time who collected the limited number of instruments and examined the people who exhibited post-bombing vomiting, bloody stool and high fever, and who then died for no apparent reason. It was extremely strange that the people who immediately after the bombing complained of fatigue, general malaise, loss of appetite, nausea, vomiting and thirst demonstrated an improvement within days, but after a recovery period of 1–4 weeks exhibited a wide range of symptoms such as epilation, subcutaneous bleeding, and infections resulting from leukopenia, which was then followed by death. The condition was termed atomic bomb illness, and it is easy to imagine the fear generated. In actual fact many of these symptoms were a result of leukopenia, and after approximately 10 years the leukopenia had virtually disappeared, with recovery of normal hematopoietic function. From that time not only testing for leukopenia but also immunological techniques became widely available, and it is ironic that this was the period in which leukocyte abnormalities had almost vanished. However, the fact that hematopoietic function had returned to normal after 10 years and did not again display abnormalities testifies to the resilience of the human body.

2. ANEMIA

A. Acute Period

No detailed data are available until approximately 7–10 days after the bombing. However, many early deaths occurred in individuals who despite a leukocyte count of 150 had an erythrocyte count of 4.2 million. Only 2 out of the 9 leukopenia cases shown in Table 3 with a leukocyte count of under 1,000 had an erythrocyte count below 3 million. However, 8 out of the 9 exhibited a marked decrease in hemoglobin to less than 45% of normal, and displayed hypochromic anemia. According to blood data for healthy individuals in the Hiroshima area in 1942, a healthy male erythrocyte count was 4.54 million with 95% hemoglobin, and a healthy female erythrocyte count was 4.35 million with 94% hemoglobin, making it difficult to believe that Hiroshima residents suffered from iron deficiency before the atomic bombing. The reason for hypochromic anemia in this period is uncertain.

B. Subacute Period

Numerous anemia patients were observed between 2 and 4 weeks after the bombing. In many cases erythrocyte counts and hemoglobin levels decreased after early September, marking a minimum around September 20th[3]. All anemia cases at this time had a color index of > 1.0. There is the fear that the test values were greatly affected by hemorrhaging (including bleeding due to trauma and gastrointestinal tract bleeding) and dehydration symptoms (due to burns etc.), but almost all the anemia exhibited in this period was normochromic or hyperchromic. Compared to leukopenia, anemia appeared late, and since recovery was very slow, the subacute period lasted until around October. Katsube[15] of Hiroshima Teishin Hospital reported on atomic bomb survivors exposed within 2 km. In October signs of recovery appeared, with 41% of cases having an erythrocyte count of over 4 million; however, although in November the number with leukocyte counts of under 4,000 had fallen to 4.9%, a full 19.9% had erythrocyte counts of under 3.5 million (Table 8).

Table 8   Erythrocyte counts between August and November for survivors exposed within 2 km[15]

Erythrocyte count/m^3 \ Month	Aug.	Sep.	Oct.	Nov.
0–100	1 (1.6)	0 (0)	0 (0)	0 (0)
100–150	0 (0)	0 (0)	0 (0)	0 (0)
150–200	2 (3.3)	1 (0.8)	1 (1.5)	0 (0)
200–250	4 (6.7)	11 (7.2)	6 (3.1)	2 (1.2)
250–300	12 (20.0)	21 (15.8)	11 (5.1)	5 (3.00)
300–350	16 (26.7)	41 (30.8)	25 (12.6)	26 (15.7)
350–400	9 (15.0)	26 (20.0)	74 (37.1)	79 (47.6)
400–450	7 (11.7)	26 (20.0)	71 (35.6)	47 (23.3)
450–500	4 (6.7)	5 (3.8)	9 (4.5)	6 (3.6)
500–550	2 (3.3)	2 (1.6)	2 (1.0)	1 (0.6)
550–	3 (5.0)	0 (0)	0 (0)	0 (0)
Total	60	133	199	166
			Total	558

(   ) Parentheses indicate percentages.

C. Morphological Abnormalities in Erythrocytes

Of 34 individuals examined at Ono Army Hospital between September 6th and 17th, only 3 exhibited morphological abnormalities in erythrocytes, with 2 cases of anisocytosis and 1 case with both polychromatic erythrocytes and basophilic stippling. On the other hand, Katsube[15] observed a high frequency of abnormality at Hiroshima Teishin Hospital, particularly among cases who died. Morphological abnormalities were observed in the erythrocytes of 5 out of 8 patients hospitalized in the Osaka University Medical School[16]. Table 9 shows data concerning an interesting case for whom erythrocytic morphological abnormalities were absent in early September, but which became apparent in late September when marked anemia was observed; from early October improvements in the anemia were accompanied by disappearance of the erythrocytic morphological abnormalities.

Out of the 34 cases hospitalized at Ono Army Hospital between early and mid-September, 16 underwent bone marrow aspiration. In 5 of these erythroblasts accounted for less than 10%, with 3 others under 20%. Erythrocyte counts ranged from 2.42 million to 4.41 million (mean = 3.56 million) and a hemoglobin range of 55% to 86% (mean = 66.4%). The granulocytes indicated normal bone marrow in 6 of the 10 cases. Although 3 of the other cases showed slightly delayed recovery, 1 case exhibited marked eosinophilia though neutrophil recovery was delayed. With regard to erythroblasts in the same population, 1 case displayed mild recovery but 9 exhibited decreased erythroblast formation, with the G/E (granuloid/erythroid) values being respectively 9.0, 5.3, 500, 8.6, 3.7, 8.6, 3.8, 8.3, and 15.0; even when the granulocytes were in the recovery period the erythroblast recovery was delayed.

Table 9   Changes in peripheral blood and morphological abnormalities in patients hospitalized at Osaka University Hospital[16]

Date of examination	1/9	9/9	11/9	14/9	20/9	26/9	1/10	8/10	26/10	6/11
Erythrocyte count	443	325	342	332	231	192	150	328	289	399
Hemoglobin (%)	78	60	63	85	49	44	41	53	71	81
Leukocyte count	2100	2000	1900	1300	1600	1500	800	2800	4700	7900
Basophils	0	0[*1]	0	0	1.5	0[*2]	0	1	0	0[*3]
Eosinophils	0	1	0	0	0	0	1	0	3	0
Monocytes	4	5	4	3	0	13.3	30	8	6	32
Metamyelocytes	2	0	2	0	0	2	1	0	0	
Stabs	24	34	33	15	13.5	20	30	20	15	26
Segs	43	27	27	23	4.5	18	7	50	49	34.5
Lymphocytes	27	32	34	58	80.5	46.7	31	21	27	7.5
Erythroblasts	(1)	0	0	0	1	0	0	0	0	
Polychromasia	—	—	—	—	+	+	+	—	—	—
Basophilic stippling	—	—	—	—	+	+	+	—	—	—
Anisocytosis	—	—	—	—	+ +	+ +	+ +	+	+	—
Poikilocytosis	—	—	—	—	+ +	+ +	+ +	+	+	—

[*1]Total of leukocyte classification was only 99, so actual figures are given.
[*2]Total was 150, so figures were adjusted proportionally
[*3]Total was 140.5, so figures were adjusted proportionally

Erythrocyte counts and hemoglobin levels 3–4 months after the bombing were examined in 43 cases at the Ujina Army Hospital between October 15th and November 20th. Hemoglobin levels were 80% or more in 17 cases, but were 60–79% in 11 cases, 40–59% in 9 cases, and less than 40% in 6 cases. Although 11 cases had erythrocyte counts above 4 million, counts were 3–4 million in 13 cases, 2–3 million in 1 case, and under 2 million in 4 cases. In 21 of these 28 cases the color index was ≥ 1.0, indicating continued normochromic anemia. Reticulocytes were 10% or more in 12 out of 25 cases. Anemia was still present in November.

D. Observations at 1 Year after Bombing

Kikuchi et al[8] reported that 90 out of 523 atomic bomb survivors (17.2%) had erythrocyte counts of less than 3 million. In a non-exposed control population of 173 individuals examined at the same time, erythrocyte counts of under 3 million were found in 2.8% of the cases. Many anemia cases were observed at 1 year after the bombing. Bone marrow examinations were conducted at this time on 17 cases. Even though almost complete reconstitution of the granulocytes was observed, the erythroblast findings indicated 2 hypoplastic cases, with 1 of these exhibiting extreme hyperplasia with erythroblasts at 3.2%.

E. Observations at 2 Years 2 Months after Bombing

Kikichi et al[9] reported that erythrocyte counts of less than 3 million were observed in 11.8% of cases at 2 years 2 months after the bombing, a decrease from 17.2% at 1 year.

F. Observations at 10 Years after Bombing

Anemia gradually decreased thereafter, and the 1956 Radiation Effects Research Foundation (RERF) study on 4,196 individuals revealed no significant difference between exposed and non-exposed populations in hemoglobin levels, erythrocyte counts, hematocrit values, mean cell volumes, and mean cell hemoglobin levels etc.

G. Studies by the Atomic Bomb Casualty Council

The Atomic Bomb Casualty Council started to conduct additional analyses on medium severity anemia (hemoglobin levels of 9 g/dl or less)[17,18]. Almost all cases were iron deficiency anemia, but some cases were observed due to renal failure or rheumatism-related anemia etc. In addition to these, the existence of normochromic anemia of no apparent cause was observed with no abnormalities in the leukocytes and platelets, and this was termed atomic bomb refractory anemia[19,20]. However, this population included cases who were proximally exposed survivors and city entrants (i.e. individuals who entered the city shortly after the bombing), and as expected it is unclear whether there is a close relationship with exposure.

Today no type of anemia is believed to be closely related to exposure, and the anemia observed in atomic bomb survivors should probably be treated as being the same as anemia in non-exposed patients.

(Hiroo Dohy)

REFERENCES

1. Japanese Army Medical School. Report on Hiroshima disaster by the atomic bomb. *Genshibakudan saigai chousa Houkokushu* [Collection of the reports on the investigation of the atomic bomb casualties] Vol. 1. Tokyo: Japan Society for the Promotion of Science, 1953: 285–412. (*In Japanese*)
2. Kure C. Report on the atomic bomb in Hiroshima city (From a medical point of view). *Genshibakudan saigai chousa Houkokushu* [Collection of the reports on the investigation of the atomic bomb casualties] Vol. 1. Tokyo: Japan Society for the Promotion of Science, 1953: 423–436. (*In Japanese*)
3. Nakao K, Kobayashi G, Kato S, *et al.* Hematological studies on the effect of atomic bomb radiation. *Genshibakudan saigai chousa Houkokushu* [Collection of the reports on the investigation of the atomic bomb casualties] Vol. 1. Tokyo: Japan Society for the Promotion of Science, 1953: 649–62. (*In Japanese*)
4. Amano S, editor. Report of the diseases of atomic bomb (Report 1–4). *Genshibakudan saigai chousa Houkokushu* [Collection of the reports on the investigation of the atomic bomb casualties] Vol. 1. Tokyo: Japan Society for the Promotion of Science, 1953:285–412. (*In Japanese*)
5. Yamashina S. Report on the scientific records of the atomic bomb disaster, preliminary report of the returned materials from AFIP, Research Institute for Nuclear Medicine and Biology. Hiroshima: Hiroshima University, 1973. (*In Japanese*)
6. Fujii M, Shirai H, Sawasaki H, *et al.* Effect on human beings of the attack of atomic bomb in Hiroshima city. *Genshibakudansaigai chousa Houkokushu* [Collection of the reports on the investigation of the atomic bomb casualties] Vol. 2. Tokyo: Japan Society for the Promotion of Science, 1953: 1282–99. (*In Japanese*)
7. Nakao K, Kekei H, Kato S, *et al.* Statistical observations of peripheral blood picture of the atomic bomb survivors in Hiroshima prefecture 3–4 months after the exposure. *Genshibakudansaigai chousa Houkokushu* [Collection of the reports on the investigation of the atomic bomb casualties] Vol. 1. Tokyo: Japan Society for the Promotion of Science, 1953: 663–6. (*In Japanese*)
8. Kikuchi T, Wakisaka K, Setsuda T, *et al.* The results of the health examination one year after the atomic bomb exposure in Hiroshima city - with special reference to the hematological findings. *Genshibakudan saigai chousa Houkokushu* [Collection of the reports on the investigation of the atomic bomb casualties] Vol. 2. Tokyo: Japan Society for the Promotion of Science, 1953: 834–9. (*In Japanese*)
9. Kikuchi T, Wakisaka K, Setsuda T, *et al.* The results of the health examination two years and two months after the atomic bomb exposure in Hiroshima city - with special reference to the hematological findings. *Genshibakudan saigai chousa Houkokushu* [Collection of the reports on the investigation of the atomic bomb casualties] Vol. 2. Tokyo: Japan Society for the Promotion of Science, 1953: 859–71. (*In Japanese*)
10. Wald N, Truax WE, Sears ME, *et al.* Hematological findings in Hiroshima and Nagasaki atomic bomb survivors: a 10 year review. *J Hiroshima Med Ass* 1963; **16**: 1082–91.
11. Yamamoto T, Hirose F, Himeno T, *et al.* Hematological studies of the inhabitants of Otake exposed to atomic bomb in Hiroshima 7 years ago, especially of the member of volunteer labor units at the time of exposure. *Acta Hematologica Japonica* 1953; **16**: 253. (*In Japanese*)
12. Hirose F, Yamamoto T, Himeno T, *et al.* Blood picture of the persons in Otake town exposed to the atomic bomb at Hiroshima 8 years ago. *Acta Hematologica Japonica* 1954; **17**: 307–8. (*In Japanese*)
13. Yokoro K, Hirose F, Yamamoto T, *et al.* Blood pictures of the inhabitants of Otake town exposed to the atomic bomb at Hiroshima before 9 years. *Acta Hematologica Japonica* 1955; **18**: 254–55. (*In Japanese*)

14. Yamada A, Yokoro K, Wada N, *et al.* Blood pictures of the inhabitants of Otake town exposed to the atomic bomb at Hiroshima before 10 years. *Acta Hematologica Japonica* 1956; **19**: 248–9. (*In Japanese*)

15. Katsube G. Studies on the atomic bomb I, Hiroshima type. *Genshibakudan saigai chousa Houko-kushu* [Collection of the reports on the investigation of the atomic bomb casualties] Vol. 2.Tokyo: Japan Society for the Promotion of Science, 1953: 1306–13. (*In Japanese*)

16. Fukushima K, Kitani T, Nishifuji S, *et al.* Peripheral blood pictures and bone marrow findings of the atomic bomb survivors. *Genshibakudan saigai chousa Houkokushu* [Collection of the reports on the investigation of the atomic bomb casualties] Vol. 2. Tokyo: Japan Society for the Promotion of Science, 1953: 1140–54. (*In Japanese*)

17. Taketomi Y, Abe T, Okita H, *et al.* Clinical survey of blood dyscrasias among Hiroshima A-bomb survivors by the periodical health examination (Report 5). *J Hiroshima Med Ass* 1980; **33** (3): 316–9. (*In Japanese*)

18. Abe T, Dohy H, Okita H, *et al.* Clinical survey of blood dyscrasias among Hiroshima A-bomb survivors by the periodical health examination. Report 6. *Nagasaki Med J* 1981; **55**: 802–808. (*In Japanese*)

19. Dohy H, Abe T, Okita H, *et al.* Clinical survey of blood dyscrasias among Hiroshima A-bomb survivors by the periodical health examination. Report 7. *J Hiroshima Med Ass* 1983; **35**: 455–8. (*In Japanese*)

20. Dohy H, Abe T, Okita H, *et al.* Clinical survey of blood dyscrasias among Hiroshima A-bomb survivors by the periodical health examination. Report 8. *J Hiroshima Med Ass* 1983; **35**: 212–6. (*In Japanese*)

5

Psychoneurological and Psychological Effects

5 PSYCHONEUROLOGICAL AND PSYCHOLOGICAL EFFECTS

This chapter reviews what is known about the psychoneurological and psychological effects of exposure to the atomic explosion, although the position regarding such effects has not been clarified.

1. PSYCHONEUROLOGICAL STUDIES

Little research has been performed on the psychoneurological effects of the atomic bomb and very few reports have covered the period from immediately after the atomic explosion up to the present day. Konuma[1] supposes that "since the events surrounding the atomic bombing so greatly exceeded the usual conditions involved in the development of psychiatric and neurotic symptoms, it was not possible to observe the formation of symptomatic mental disorders and neuroses," and in reference to the period in which late effects appeared stated that "it can be considered that autonomic ataxia or psychosomatic diseases accompanied the various after-effects, but these were treated as usual after-effects; few cases received examination and treatment in psychoneurological departments, and thus the opportunity for diagnosis was missed."

The first report concerning the psychoneurological effects of the atomic bomb was by Okumura and Hikida[2], who randomly selected 50 survivors out of 192 who were hospitalized at the Omura National Hospital and survived for 3 months after the bombing. While referring to past histories of illness, they studied the damage to the psychoneurological system caused by the bombing by separating observations into three time frames: the 2–3 week period until the end of August (initial stage), the one month period from early September to early October (intermediate stage), and from mid-October to early November (late stage). The subjects studied did not include severe cases who died within 3 months, and it was difficult to ascertain accurate facts relating to mental disorders immediately after the bombing. Following a detailed examination of their histories to determine initial stage psychogenic reactions, the only mental disorders found in the 50 cases were 3 cases of affective stupor and 1 case who was unable to walk. In the intermediate stage patients were still suffering from thermal burns and trauma, and exhibited neurasthenia-like symptoms. In the late stage patients with specific diatheses tended to display neuroses, and it was concluded that the development of psychoneurological disorders was a result of a deterioration of the environment and physical condition caused by exposure.

Tsuiki et al[3] conducted a study in 1951 after noting that although no atomic bomb survivors exhibited clear illness, quite a few were not healthy and complained of various neurotic disorders. It was found that the psychoneurological symptoms became more pronounced with increasing severity of acute radiation illness symptoms, with the complaints (in decreasing order of frequency) being weariness, lack of spirit, introversion, and poor memory.

Tsuiki et al[4] and Nishikawa and Tsuiki[5] studied patients who exhibited neurosis-like symptoms during general examinations of atomic bomb survivors at Nagasaki University in February and December 1956. Out of a total of 7,297 patients, 73 were found to have psychiatric disorders. Neurosis-like symptoms were discovered in 533 patients, with the vast majority exhibiting neurasthenia. Among the patients with neurosis-like symptoms, the number who exhibited symptoms of acute radiation illness was significant in comparison with the population who did not[4]. Electroencephalography was performed on 30 of the patients with neurosis-like symptoms who were selected from the population that displayed symptoms of acute radiation illness, with abnormalities clearly evident in 3 cases. Autocorrelation curves were obtained for these 30 cases, with the power spectrum showing a clear difference from normal individuals. From this it was concluded that although some of the atomic bomb survivor neurosis cases could without doubt be considered to have developed pure neurosis due to psychogenic factors, it would generally be appropriate to regard others as a form of encephalopathy or somatopathy caused by organic or functional disorders produced by radiation[5].

In August 1953 Konuma et al[6] studied 132 survivors living in the city of Otake who had been exposed while working as volunteers in Hiroshima. The subjects were exposed at 1.5 to 2 km from the hypocenter, and despite quickly fleeing from the area suffered thermal burns, with many exposed to the "black rain" that fell immediately afterwards. To a certain degree they displayed symptoms of acute radiation illness, and later complained of after-effects. The range of complaints of those subjects whose symptoms continued for 8 years after exposure implies autonomic ataxia, suggesting a population exhibiting diencephalic syndrome. Konuma et al[6-10] noted that these symptoms or complaints resemble those of cephalic trauma after-effects. As a result, atomic bomb radiation illness is indirectly reflected in organic and functional disorders of the central nervous system centering on the diencephalon, and it was estimated that there was a high likelihood that accompanying psychogenic reactions based on these disorders would be the appearance of neurotic and psychosomatic symptoms.

Izumi et al[11] obtained encephalograms for 27 of the above-mentioned Otake residents studied by Konuma et al, and found 8 cases with severe abnormal waves which could be interpreted as originating in the subcortical brain stem. However, they considered it would be dangerous to attribute all of these abnormalities to the atomic bombing without considering diseases such as cerebral arteriosclerosis etc. In 1956 they obtained encephalograms for 39 atomic bomb survivors who were resident in the city of Kure and who either complained of many symptoms at that time or possessed hematologic abnormalities, but no relationship was observed between exposure to the bomb and encephalographic abnormalities[12].

2. PSYCHOLOGICAL STUDIES

In 1949–50 Kubo[13] studied the immediate post-bombing behavior of some Hiroshima atomic bomb survivors by conducting individual interviews with 54 survivors selected from the academic staff of Hiroshima University. The stimuli which the survivors received were classified in order of time, and the behavior of survivors during each cluster of stimuli was analyzed. The first cluster of stimuli were flash, blast and destruction. The second cluster of stimuli consisted of injuries, cries and fires. The third cluster were fires, sounds, black rain, rumors, and streams of sufferers; the latter had leaders. The fourth cluster of stimuli were the terrible sights of death, injury and burns, direct views of the collapse and obliteration of buildings throughout the city, and exposure to numerous rumors and tragic tales from other people. The fifth cluster were assaults by later sights and sounds. The sixth cluster was Japan's surrender on August 15th. After exposure to the 1st and 2nd clusters of stimuli, some respondents (i.e. the survivors who were the subjects of this study) were stupefied and at a complete loss (blankness). The 1st and 2nd cluster of stimuli were situations unlike anything the survivors had ever experienced before. The situation was one of terrifying panic, since people felt that another unexpected catastrophe might befall them. Some reported at this stage observing psychologically abnormal individuals. Following the period of blankness, the survivors acted in a blind manner which could be termed post-catastrophe behavior. The 3rd cluster of stimuli performed the role of reinforcing the catastrophic situation, and survivors displayed fragmentary actions which are similar to post-catastrophe behavior, and as time passed they became oriented toward life-saving, and proceeded to seek refuge. Although the 1st, 2nd and 3rd clusters of stimuli were experienced on the 1st day, the psychological effects at that time could not be judged according to any previously known criteria for any individual. The survivors were conscious of the destruction of their personalities. At the same time anxieties were greatly enhanced by worries of a predicted repeat catastrophe. Persons experiencing the 4th, 5th and 6th clusters of stimuli exhibited various behavioral patterns, but the contents of their observations were vague, with virtually all behavioral experiences wiped from their memory.

In August 1954 Kondo et al[14] studied the memory, fatigue, and emotional and diencephalon excitation of 90 survivors living in Otake. Recall of memory among survivors was below average, but there was no significant difference between the populations with severe and mild complaints. No difference between the exposed and controls was observed in the study of emotional excitation and fatigue tests using Flicker values, or in studies on diencephalon excitation using a psychogalvanometer.

Lifton[15] described the conditions in the initial period after the bombing in "Death in Life," stating that "The most striking psychological feature of this immediate experience was the sense of a sudden and absolute shift from normal existence to an overwhelming encounter with death... Beyond death imagery *per se*, there was a widespread sense that life and death were out of phase with one another, no longer properly distinguishable... Related to the sense of death in life was a total disruption of individual and social order [i.e. the loss of both human relationships and a physical environment]... Such disruption reaches deeply into psychic experience."

The following introduces some of Lifton's comments pertaining to the psychological effects of the bombing. "*Hibakusha* [atomic bomb survivors] began to undergo a process of 'psychic closing-off'; that is, they simply ceased to feel... The survivors who were exposed to intense stimuli tried to protect themselves by 'psychic closing-off' from the threatening stimuli from without or within. The latter took the form of guilt and shame." The first step towards psychological recovery was a vacuous state: "The vacuum state could, paradoxically, be a prelude to symbolic rebirth." Through reunions with old friends who could revive memories of times before the bombing and by talking over experiences of the bombing with other survivors, human relationships were gradually restored.

"On the other hand, the manifestations of toxic radiation effects aroused in the minds of the people a special terror, and survivors again lapsed into anxiety. Rumors concerning the horror of the atomic bombing such as 'all who had been exposed to the bomb in the city would be dead' and 'trees, grass and flowers would never again grow in Hiroshima' provided a further severe shock to the survivors."

After 1950 "the fear of late effects became greatly magnified by the increased incidence of leukemia and cancer among the atomic bomb survivors. The threat of late effects became an indefinite extension of earlier 'invisible contamination'."

"The term 'A-bomb disease' was applied not only to earlier invisible contamination and later leukemia and cancer, but also to such innocuous conditions as fatigue, sensitivity to hot weather, borderline anemia, and susceptibility to cold."

"The psychosomatic bind is self-perpetuating, part of a vicious circle." Thus physical symptoms produced psychological anxiety, and psychological anxiety led to physical symptoms.

"As compared to usual hypochondriac and phobic patterns encountered in psychiatric work, those in *hibakusha* are much more directly related to actual bodily assaults that can result from atomic bomb exposure."

Lifton concludes with his impression of psychological studies on the atomic bomb survivors by saying, "The special difficulty in Hiroshima is that no one is ever certain where radiation effects and psychological manifestations begin."

Information concerning the atomic bombing and late radiation effects were usually treated as important news in Hiroshima, and the survivors were greatly affected by such reports. Topics which frequently cropped up in newspapers included "atomic bomb illness," "atomic bomb neurosis," "marriages of atomic bomb survivors," "suicides of atomic bomb survivors," "atomic bomb orphans," and "orphaned elderly." Studies on the marital status and suicides among the survivors were conducted by the Atomic Bomb Casualty Commission (ABCC), but the rates of non-marriage and suicide among the survivors were not found to be high[16].

In 1990 Yamada *et al*[17] examined the relationship between exposure and complaints by comparing the frequencies of various symptoms among 11,876 subjects of the 1962–65 ABCC Adult Health Study. The analysis excluded subjects who were suffering from organic diseases. The subjects were classified into 4 populations: those who were exposed within 2 km of the hypocenter and exhibited symptoms of acute radiation illness; those exposed within 2 km of the hypocenter but who did not exhibit symptoms of acute radiation illness; those exposed at distances of 3 km or more; and those not in the city at the time of bombing. The proximally exposed population who exhibited symptoms of acute radiation illness showed the highest frequency for each of the following categories: physical symptom rates pertaining to heart disease and disorders of the peripheral vascular system, nervous system and sense organs; degree of fatigue; frequency of illness; habits such as excess smoking and alcohol consumption etc.; and emotional disorders such as dread and anxiety. The frequency of complaints among the population with acute radiation symptoms was greater than among the population not exhibiting such symptoms, with the tendency still evident after adjustment for DS86 doses. The above suggests that the survivors tended to complain of various physical and mental symptoms, and that this tendency can be considered to be a psychological effect of exposure.

3. EXPOSED CHILDREN AND CHILDREN EXPOSED PRENATALLY

With respect to the effect of the bombing on the mental development of children, Sutow et al[18] conducted a neurological and psychological study in 1952 comparing prenatally exposed children in Nagasaki with a group of controls, and found that the prenatally exposed children displayed a significantly high frequency of both neurological abnormalities such as nystagmus and behavioral problems such as sleep disorders. However, psychometric tests such as the Bender score and Goodenough score etc. failed to show a difference between the two populations. In a 1953 study on intelligence and physical ability, Ando[19] found no significant difference between exposed children and the control population.

CONCLUSION

In a discussion on the psychological effects on the atomic bomb survivors in Hiroshima and Nagasaki, it is important to comprehend the complexity of the damage inflicted by the atomic explosions. The calamity was produced as a result of the combined effects of thermal rays, blast and radiation, with many of the people in Hiroshima and Nagasaki (and particularly those exposed within 2 km of the hypocenter) suffering serious physical injury. Large numbers of buildings were destroyed and socioeconomic damage was great. Many of the survivors not only suffered personal injury immediately after the bombing, but also witnessed radical changes in their environment due to family bereavement and the breakdown of daily life etc. Furthermore, even in the years that followed they suffered from late effects and anxiety regarding late effects, with the result that the bombing had long-term psychological effects. The fact that numerous survivors complained of a diverse range of symptoms can be viewed as one of the psychological manifestations of the effect of exposure. However, many points concerning the psychiatric and psychological effects remain unresolved, and further studies are necessary.

(*Michiko Yamada, Hideo Sasaki*)

REFERENCES

1. Konuma M. Neuropsychiatric consideration of the atomic bomb sickness and its sequelae. In: Hiroshima University A-bomb Dead Memorial Functions Committee (*Hiroshima Daigaku Genbaku Shibotsusha Irei Gyoji Iinkai*), The atomic bombing and Hiroshima University - "Light of fate" (*Genbaku to Hiroshima Daigaku - "Seishi no Hi"*). 1977: 96–105. (*In Japanese*)

2. Okumura N, Hikida H. Results of pyschoneurological studies on atomic bomb survivors. *Kyushu Neuropsychiatry* 1949; **I**: 50–2. (*In Japanese*)

3. Tsuiki S, Ueno K, Segawa K, *et al.* Clinical experiences in the Department of Psychiatry, Nagasaki University for five years after the end of the Second World War. *Psychiatrica Neurologica Japonica* 1951; **53**: 229. (*In Japanese*)

4. Tsuiki S, Yuzuriha T, Anzo E, *et al.* Psychiatric investigations on people exposed to the atomic bomb. *Nagasaki Med J* 1958; **33**: 637–9. (*In Japanese*)

5. Nishikawa T, Tsuiki S. Psychiatric investigations of atomic bomb survivors. *Nagasaki Med J* 1961; **36**: 717–22. (*In Japanese*)

6. Konuma M, Furutani M, Kubo S. Diencephalic syndrome as a delayed A-bomb effect. *Japanese Medical Journal* 1953; **1547**: 4853–60. (*In Japanese*)

7. Konuma M. Psychiatric and psychosomatic case studies on the after-effects on A-bomb survivors. Report of the Cooperative Research, Ministry of Education. Medicine and Pharmacy 1953. Tokyo: *Nihon Gakujutsu Shinkokai* 1954: 375. (*In Japanese*)

8. Konuma M. Interpretation of the complaints and symptoms assuming diencephalon syndrome as a late effect of the atomic bomb. *Nagasaki Med J* 1961; **36**: 706–16. (*In Japanese*)

9. Konuma M. Psychosomatic problems as the late effects of atomic bomb exposure. In: Koyama T, Tabuchi A, Watanabe S, editors. Nuclear medicine. Tokyo: Kanehara Shuppan, 1963: 338–400. (*In Japanese*)

10. Konuma M, Miyake M, Furutani M, *et al.* Psychoneurological study concerning A-bomb after-effects. *Naika no Ryoiki* (Journal of Medicine, Radiatrics, and Dermatology). 1954; **2**: 261–6. (*In Japanese*)

11. Izumi C, Hayakawa T, Izumi K. Electroencephalographic researches of Hiroshima atomic bomb casualty. *J Hiroshima Med Ass* 1955; **8**: 671–7. (*In Japanese*)

12. Izumi C, Hayakawa T, Amano T. Electroencephalographic further researches of Hiroshima atomic bomb casualty on after-effects 10 years later. *Hiroshima Med J* 1967; **5**: 20–5. (*In Japanese*)

13. Kubo Y. A study of A-bomb sufferers' behavior in Hiroshima. A socio-psychological research on A-bomb and A-energy (I). *Japan J of Psychol* 1952; **22**: 103–10. (*In Japanese*)

14. Kondo T, Yoshioka I, Kida S, *et al.* Psychological researches on the cases accompanied 8 years with after-effects of atomic bombs casualty at Hiroshima. *J Hiroshima Med Ass* 1966; **9**: 95–101. (*In Japanese*)

15. Lifton RJ. Death in life - survivors of Hiroshima. New York: Random House, 1967.

16. Matsumoto YS. Social impact on atomic bomb survivors, Hiroshima and Nagasaki. ABCC TR 12–19, 1969.

17. Yamada M, Kodama K, Wang FL. The long-term psychological sequelae of atomic bomb survivors in Hiroshima and Nagasaki. Proceedings of the Medical Basis for Radiation - Accident Preparedness III: The Psychological Perceptive; 1990 Dec 5–7; Oak Ridge.

18. Sutow WW, Hamada M, Kawamoto S. Neurological and psychometric examination of children exposed *in utero* to the atomic bomb in Nagasaki. USAEC NYO-4472, 1953.

19. Ando T. The effect of the atomic bomb at Hiroshima on the physical and mental development of children. *Hiroshima Med J* 1958; **6**: 951–1016. (*In Japanese*)

6

Ocular Lesions

6.1   ATOMIC BOMB CATARACTS

INTRODUCTION

Ocular damage due to the atomic bomb can be classified into the following three categories[1]:

A. Direct Injury Immediately after Exposure

The ocular injuries observed immediately following exposure included eyelid burns due to thermal radiation, mechanical ocular injuries caused by the bomb blast, ocular trauma produced by foreign bodies such as glass fragments, and retinal damage due to looking directly at the flash from the bomb.

B. Lesions due to Radiation Illness

Ocular damage accompanying atomic bomb radiation illness consisted of retinopathy produced as a result of severe anemia, tendencies to hemorrhage, and infection.

C. Late Effects

Besides atomic bomb cataracts, a late effect observed after healing of eyelid burns was eyelid deformity due to scars, with subsequent changes in the cornea and conjunctiva etc. In order to investigate whether atomic bomb exposure accelerated ocular aging, the decreased amplitude of ocular accommodation was studied, but no definite conclusion was forthcoming. Also, studies were performed to determine whether the incidence of age-related cataracts (an aging phenomenon of the lens) was higher among atomic bomb survivors, but this has not yet been clarified.

Atomic bomb cataracts were the first late radiation effects detected among Hiroshima and Nagasaki atomic bomb survivors, and were also the lesions most frequently observed as late effects due to the lens being the most radiosensitive part of the eye[2].

The first recognized case of atomic bomb cataract in Hiroshima was reported by Ikui[3] to be in 1948, and the first in Nagasaki detected by Hirose and Fujino[4] in June 1949. The next was reported in December 1949 by Cogan et al[5], which was then followed by numerous other studies.

1. RADIATION CATARACTS

Cataracts are a disease in which the transparent lens becomes opaque, leading to reduced vision. Irradiation is one of the many causes of this condition.

A. Development of Radiation Cataracts

There is one epithelial layer in the anterior subcapsular region of the lens, with cells proliferating in the most peripheral region of the equator. The cells divide normally with the mature cell losing its nucleus, which migrates towards the posterior pole, forming transparent lenticular fibers. When the lens is exposed to radiation and the cells in the equatorial cell proliferation zone become damaged, the pseudo-epithelial cells swell, and with their nuclei intact migrate more slowly than normal cells along the inner side of the posterior capsule towards the posterior pole, where they accumulate and produce lenticular opacity (Fig. 1).

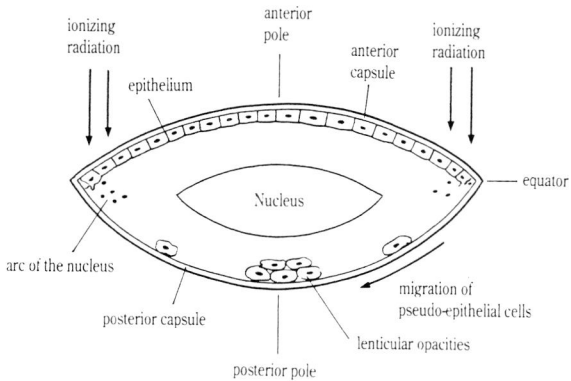

Figure 1   Development of radiation-induced posterior subcapsular opacity

B. Characteristics of Radiation Cataracts

1) The lens undergoes the same type of morphological changes when exposed to radiation, irrespective of the particular form of ionizing radiation[6].

2) For a given absorbed dose of radiation, the severity of the lens damage produced is dependent on the form of radiation, as indicated by the relative biological effectiveness (RBE). With respect to cataract development, fast neutrons have a greater RBE than X-rays and gamma rays. For radiation with a high RBE, cataracts are produced by a sub-lethal dose of whole-body irradiation.

3) With increasing radiation dose, the latency period before cataract development is shortened and the cataract severity increases.

4) The change is greater with decreasing age, but there are also individual differences with regard to radiosensitivity.

5) The initial observations characteristic of radiation cataracts are as follows[6]. Opacity initially develops on the inner surface of the posterior polar capsule of the lens. Punctate or disciform opacity forms, and part expands into a doughnut-shaped configuration. Examination by slit-lamp biomicroscope reveals the surface of the opacity to be granular with a polychromatic sheen. The opacity is separated between a position on the inner surface of the posterior capsule and a location slightly anterior to that, forming an opacity with a bivalve configuration.

6) Opacity on the inner surface of the posterior polar capsule which resembles that of radiation cataracts is also produced by cataracts with complications of pigmentary degeneration of the retina or uveitis, steroid-induced cataracts, and age-related

cataracts which originate from the inner surface of the posterior capsule, and it is therefore necessary to distinguish between these.

2. ATOMIC BOMB CATARACTS

A. Clinical Aspects

The clinical aspects of atomic bomb cataracts are extremely similar to those of cataracts induced by radiation from sources other than the atomic bomb. Even if lens opacity is observed on the inner surface of the posterior polar capsule, there is hesitation about attributing it to the atomic bomb, since mild changes are also observed among non-exposed individuals.

Sinskey[7] stated that for a diagnosis of atomic bomb cataract it is not sufficient to detect the presence of granules in only the posterior subcapsular axial region, and that the minimum positive findings should be a definite minute subcapsular axial plaque observed with a slit-lamp biomicroscope.

Studying Nagasaki atomic bomb survivors, Tokunaga[8] suggests lenticular evidence required for diagnosis as an atomic bomb cataract to be (1) punctate opacities in the disjunction zones, and (2) tuff-like opacities in the cortex of the posterior pole.

Studying Hiroshima atomic bomb survivors, Dodo and Toda[9] suggest the following two morphological characteristics as diagnostic standards for atomic bomb cataracts: (1) localized lenticular opacity on the inner surface of the posterior polar capsule presenting a polychromatic sheen, and (2) punctate or massive opacity anterior to the posterior capsule.

It was stated that a diagnosis of atomic bomb cataract is possible providing four conditions are met, i.e. observation of the above-mentioned lenticular opacity, a history of direct proximal exposure to the atomic bomb, the absence of ocular disease that could lead to complicated cataracts, and non-exposure to considerable doses of ionizing radiation other than the atomic bomb.

B. Histopathological Characteristics of Atomic Bomb Cataracts

In agreement with the clinical findings, marked changes occur in the cortex on the inner side of the lenticular posterior capsule. Granular disintegration and amorphous changes are observed in the lenticular fibers, but there are no characteristic histopathological findings due to the form of radiation[1].

C. Classification of Atomic Bomb Cataracts by Severity

During the 4-year period following October 1957, 128 people were examined at Hiroshima University, with atomic bomb cataracts observed in 58 of the 248 eyes examined (23.4%); these were then classified into the four categories of severity described below (Table 1, Fig. 2)[9].

1) Minute degree. Cataracts with a minute degree of severity have localized lenticular opacity with a polychromatic sheen on the inner surface of the posterior

Table 1   Classification of atomic bomb cataracts by severity[9]

Observations	Degree of severity			
	Minute	Slight	Moderate	Severe
Localized opacity on inner surface of posterior polar capsule	+	+	+	+
Opacities located in subcapsular cortical layer of posterior polar region	−	punctate	small clumps	large
Shadows upon transillumination Photographic reproduciton by transillumination	− impossible	± impossible	+ possible	+ + possible
Subjective visual disorders	−	−	−	+
Incidence among 58 eyes with atomic bomb cataract (%)	33 (56.9)	15 (25.9)	4 (6.9)	6 (10.3)

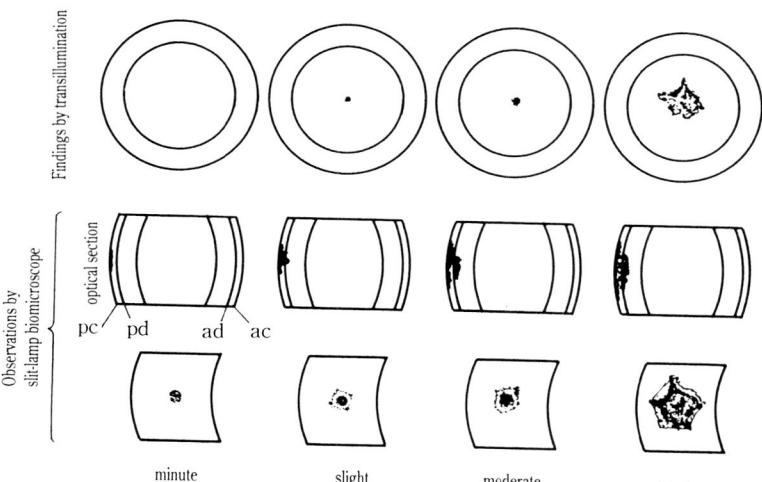

Figure 2   Classification of atomic bomb cataracts by severity[9]
ac = anterior capsule
ad = anterior disjunction
pc = posterior capsule
pd = posterior disjunction

polar capsule, but the opacity is not observable even with transillumination using a direct ophthalmoscope with a + 8D lens. Detection is only possible by slit-lamp biomicroscopy following dilatation of the pupil.

2) A slight degree of severity indicates minute punctate opacity anterior to the posterior capsule (the posterior disjunction zone), with faint opaque shadows observed by transillumination.

3) A moderate degree of severity indicates observation during transillumination of round opaque shadows with a diameter of 1 mm or less in the central axial region of the lens. Slit-lamp biomicroscopy also reveals small clump-like (or tuff-like) opacities anterior to the plaque on the posterior capsule.

4) A severe degree means that transillumination reveals a rather large, round, opaque shadow in the posterior polar region which is several millimeters in diameter and frequently protrudes in several directions.

When lenticular opacities become moderate or great in severity, it is possible to detect confirmatory opaque shadows even by transillumination, but these may not produce visual disturbance. Subjective visual disorders only exist when cataracts are severe; and such cases later underwent cataract surgery. The atomic bomb cataracts observed today are minute or slight, while moderate ones are rare[9].

D. Incidence of Atomic Bomb Cataracts

As with radiation dose, there is a correlation between the incidence and degree of severity of atomic bomb cataracts and the age at the time of exposure. Consequently, a correlation also exists between distance from the hypocenter, shielding conditions (which are related to radiation dose), the presence and degree of epilation, and other symptoms of acute radiation illness[1].

1. *Distance from the Hypocenter*

Studies performed in the Ophthalmology Clinic of the Hiroshima Red Cross Hospital from June 1953 to October 1954 showed that the incidence of atomic bomb cataracts among atomic bomb survivors within 2.0 km of the hypocenter was 54.7%, whereas it was 10.8% among those exposed at distances greater than 2.0 km.

Studies in the Department of Ophthalmology of Hiroshima University between October 1957 and September 1961 found the atomic bomb cataract incidence among survivors exposed within 1.0 km of the hypocenter to be 70%, and 30% among those exposed at 1.0–2.0 km, with the incidence decreasing rapidly among survivors exposed at distances greater than 1.6 km[2].

In order to exclude errors and obstructions to diagnoses due to the intervention of age-related changes in the lens, a study was performed at Hiroshima University between February 1958 and September 1959 on survivors exposed during infancy. The study aimed at accurately comprehending the lenticular changes caused by atomic bomb radiation[11].

The incidence of atomic bomb cataracts among those aged 1–4 years at the time of bombing was 13.5%. As in the case of survivors exposed as adults, the incidence showed a marked decrease at distances greater than 1.6 km (Table 2).

A study performed in the Ophthalmology Department of Nagasaki University between July 1953 and December 1956 found the incidences to be 57.4% among survivors exposed within 1.8 km of the hypocenter, and 45.8% among those exposed

Table 2   Frequency of atomic bomb cataracts among survivors prenatally exposed in Hiroshima[11]

Distance from hypocenter (km)	Number of eyes examined	Number of eyes with atomic bomb cataracts (%)	
		Definite	Suspected
0 ~ 1.0	18	10 (55.6)	2 (11.1)
1.0 ~ 1.2	20	10 (50.0)	0
1.2 ~ 1.4	18	4 (22.2)	2 (11.1)
1.4 ~ 1.6	50	6 (12.0)	1 (2.0)
1.6 ~ 1.8	30	0	0
1.8 ~ 2.0	38	1 (2.6)	2 (5.3)
2.0 ~ 3.0	56	0	1 (1.8)
Total	230	31 (13.5)	8 (3.5)

within 2.4 km, with the statistical limit for atomic bomb cataract development believed to be 1.8 km.

2. Epilation and Shielding Conditions

A study on Hiroshima and Nagasaki atomic bomb survivors[7] found a high correlation between the severity of scalp epilation and lenticular opacity on the inner surface of the posterior capsule (Fig. 3). The Nagasaki study showed that for individuals displaying no epilation the incidence of such opacity decreased with greater shielding and increasing distance from the hypocenter (Figs. 4 and 5).

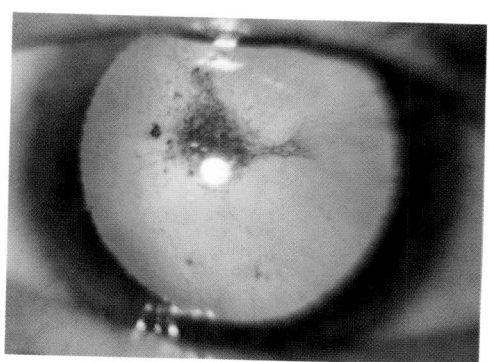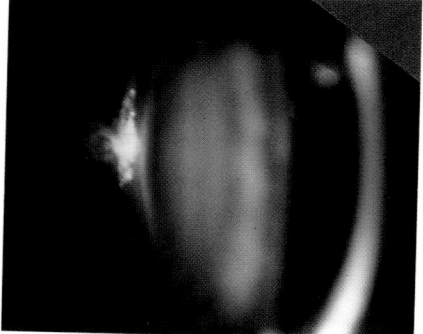

Figure 3   Atomic bomb cataract (right eye)

Male, 61 years (photograph taken in April 1966). Aged 40 years at time of bombing. Exposed under eaves of wooden house 820 meters from hypocenter. Exhibited gingival bleeding and total cranial epilation. At 55 years, underwent surgery for atomic bomb cataract in left eye, with visual acuity improved from 0.2 to 0.8. At the time of the photograph, right visual acuity was 0.2, corresponding to severe cataract.
Left: disciform opacity lens with partial radial extension
Right: opacity in lenticular posterior polar region separated into 2 layers, on the inner surface of the polar capsule and in the subcapsular cortical layer

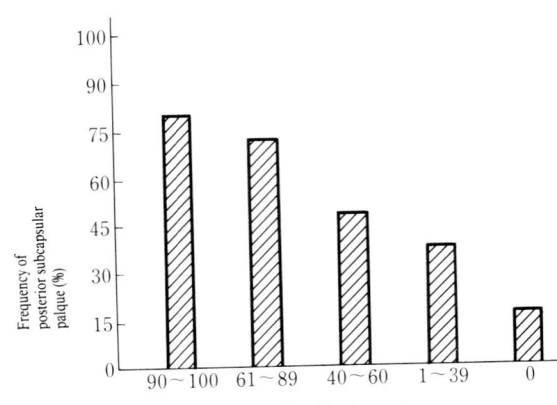

Figure 4   Correlation between epilation and frequency of posterior subcapsular plaque

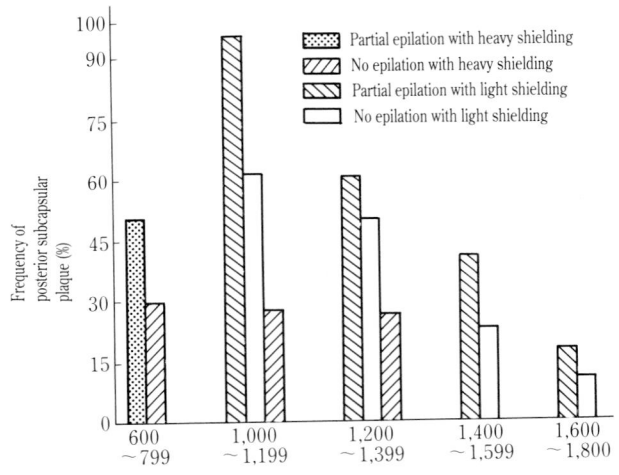

Figure 5   The effects of epilation, shielding, and distance from the hypocenter on the frequency of posterior subcapsular plaque[7]

3. *Acute Radiation Illness*

A study was performed at the Nagasaki Atomic Bomb Casualty Commission between November 1959 and August 1960 on atomic bomb survivors for whom an estimated radiation dose was available[12]. The subjects were divided into two groups according to whether or not they had exhibited symptoms of acute radiation illness. The frequency of lenticular opacity in the posterior polar region (shown in Table 3) was generally higher among the survivors who had displayed symptoms of acute radiation illness.

Table 3   Frequency of lens opacity of posterior polar region by dose and exposure status (Nagasaki)[12]

Estimated dose (Gy)	With acute radiation symptoms (+) (%)	Without acute radiation symptoms (–) (%)	Number of opacities per number of people examined	(%)
0 ~ 0.49	(17.4)	(5.3)	5/42	(11.9)
0.50 ~ 0.99	(22.2)	(31.3)	9/34	(26.5)
1.00 ~ 1.99	(56.5)	(41.9)	26/54	(48.1)
2.00 ~ 4.99	(58.1)	(42.9)	21.38	(55.3)
≥ 5.00	(90.0)	—	9/10	(90.0)
Total	48/105 (45.7)	22/73 (30.1)	70/178	(39.3)

E. Atomic Bomb Cataracts with Respect to Time

Atomic bomb cataracts developed within several months to several years following exposure. Severe cases developed quickly, with an extended latency period for mild cases. Lenticular opacity develops with a severity varying from minute to severe depending on the received dose of radiation, after which progression ceases. In a small number of cases the opacity progresses, and there are cases in which opacity decreases.

As in the case of age-related cataracts, cataract surgery is performed when opacity increases and visual acuity worsens to the point at which it constitutes a hindrance to daily life. No postoperative abnormalities were observed[1].

(Kanji Choshi)

REFERENCES

1. Committee for the Compilation of Materials on Damage Caused by the Atomic Bombs in Hiroshima and Nagasaki. *Hiroshima-Nagasaki no Genbaku Saigai.* (Hiroshima and Nagasaki: the physical, medical and social effects of the atomic bombings.) Tokyo: Iwanami Shoten, 1979: 127–32. (*In Japanese*)
2. Hiroshima University A-bomb Dead Memorial Functions Committee (*Hiroshima Daigaku Shibotsusha Irei Gyoji Iinkai*). Genbaku to Hiroshima Daigaku - *"Seishi no Hi"* (The atomic bombing and Hiroshima University — "Light of fate"). 1977: 105–12. (*In Japanese*)
3. Ikui H. Ocular lesions caused by the atomic bombing of Nagasaki and Hiroshima: early disorders. *J Hiroshima Med Ass* 1967; **20** (Suppl): 160. (*In Japanese*)
4. Hirose K, Fujino S. Cataracts due to atomic bomb exposure. *Acta Soc Ophthalmol Jpn* 1950; **54**: 449–54. (*In Japanese*)
5. Cogan DG, Martin SF, Kimura SJ. Atomic bomb cataracts. *Science* 1949; **110**: 654–5.
6. Cogan DG, Donaldson DD, Reese AB. Clinical and pathological characteristics of radiation cataracts. *Arch Ophthalmol* 1952; **47**: 55–70.
7. Sinskey RM. The status of lenticular opacities caused by atomic radiation, Hiroshima and Nagasaki, Japan 1951–1953. *Am J Ophthalmol* 1955; **39**: 285–93.
8. Tokunaga T. Atomic bomb radiation cataract in Nagasaki. *Acta Soc Ophthalmol Jpn* 1959; **63**: 1211–30. (*In Japanese*)
9. Dodo T, Toda S. Ophthalmological late effects among A-bomb survivors, especially A-bomb cataracts. In: Koyama T, Tabuchi A, Watanabe S, editors. *Genshi Igaku* (Nuclear Medicine). Tokyo: Kanehara Shuppan, 1963: 400–8. (*In Japanese*)

10. Kandori F, Masuda Y. Statistical observations of atomic bomb cataracts. *Am J Ophthalmol* 1956; **42**: 212–4.

11. Toda S, Hosokawa Y, Choshi K, *et al.* Ocular changes in A-bomb survivors exposed during infancy. *Folia Ophthalmol Jpn* 1964; **15**: 96–103. (*In Japanese*)

12. Hirose I, Okamoto A. Interrelationship between lenticular opacity of the posterior pole and estimated exposure doses of the atomic bomb survivors in Nagasaki (preliminary report). *Nagasaki Med J* 1961; **36**: 781–2. (*In Japanese*)

7

Circulatory Diseases

7 CIRCULATORY DISEASES

INTRODUCTION

The question of whether circulatory diseases are a late effect of exposure to atomic bomb radiation attracted attention quickly since in Japan these diseases have, along with cancer, been of importance due to their high prevalence and mortality rates. However, many circulatory diseases have their origin in arteriosclerosis, and since various factors are involved in their development, such as the long period before manifestation, comparatively few reports have dealt with the late effects of atomic bomb exposure.

This chapter reviews the literature pertaining to the circulatory diseases that occur following radiotherapy for malignant tumors, and also to animal experiments involving irradiation; in addition, there is a discussion of reports related to whether circulatory diseases are a late effect of atomic bomb radiation.

1. RADIATION AND CIRCULATORY DISEASE

A chronological examination of the literature concerning radiation and circulatory disease shows that until the 1960s the circulatory system was believed to be comparatively resistant to ionizing radiation[1,2]. Subsequently, however, many reports appeared describing the development of pericarditis, myocarditis, and conduction abnormalities following irradiation of the mediastinum as treatment for malignant tumors, and the effect of ionizing radiation on the heart is today widely recognized[3,4].

However, confirmation has not yet been forthcoming for either the relationship between ionizing radiation and ischemic heart disease and cerebrovascular diseases (which have their origin in arteriosclerosis), or concerning the pathogenesis involved[3,5].

Nevertheless, as described below, an association between ionizing radiation and vascular lesions has been confirmed in animal experiments[6-10]. Also, several case studies have detailed the development of ischemic heart disease following radiotherapy for Hodgkin's disease and breast cancer[11-17]. Furthermore, some reports have recently appeared concerning post-radiotherapy follow-up studies[18-26]. Other case studies have described the development of cerebral infarction following cervical irradiation and the occurrence of obstructive peripheral artery disease in the lower extremities following irradiation of the pelvis[28-39].

A. Ionizing Radiation and Vascular Lesions: Animal Experiments

Stewart et al[6] noted chronic development of fibrosis in the pericardium and myocardium following experimental irradiation of rabbit hearts. In rabbits, Fajardo et al[7] observed swelling of the capillary endothelium and occlusion of the intima by means of an electron microscope. Vascular lumen lesions and thrombus formation were observed simultaneously, and it was suggested that irradiation caused microvasculopathy, leading to fibrosis accompanied by ischemia[6,7].

Amronim and Solomon[8] compared the effects in rabbits of irradiation alone and in conjunction with a high cholesterol diet, and observed a marked occurrence of coronary sclerosis in the irradiated high cholesterol diet population. Coronary sclerosis was significantly advanced in comparison to the sum of the degree of coronary artery lesions in the radiation-only population plus the changes in the high-cholesterol only population, and it was speculated that there is an additive effect between irradiation and the high-cholesterol diet[8].

Similar conclusions were obtained in rat and pigeon experiments[9,10], i.e. that the presence of both radiation and hypercholesterolemia is necessary for development of coronary sclerosis.

B. Post-Radiotherapy Ischemic Heart Disease

A case study of myocardial infarction following radiotherapy was reported by Pearson[11] in 1958. There have since been several clinical and pathological autopsy case studies concerning death due to myocardial infarction and ischemic heart disease after therapeutic irradiation of the mediastinum for Hodgkin's disease, breast cancer, or seminoma etc[11-17]. However, these case studies have failed to confirm a causal relationship between ionizing radiation and ischemic heart disease.

On the other hand, occasional recent reports have described long-term follow-up studies on irradiated patient populations. For example, Host and Loeb[18] performed a randomized trial involving over 1,000 patients who had undergone surgery for breast cancer, and after 5 years found an excess mortality from myocardial infarction in the population irradiated with cobalt-60 (^{60}Co). Also, in a retrospective study on 957 Hodgkin's disease patients, Bovin and Hutchinson[19] found indications of an increased ischemic heart disease mortality risk after 1 year. However, since the patient populations in these studies underwent mediastinal irradiation in an obsolete procedure, it is believed that, instead of being adequately shielded, the heart received an immense dose of radiation, strongly suggesting that a large radiation dose to the heart leads to ischemic heart disease.

With regard to patients treated by recent radiotherapy techniques which give due consideration to cardiac shielding, studies on Hodgkin's disease patients were performed by Hancock et al[20], Mauch et al[21] and Brusius et al[22], the latter using autopsy data. However, no significant difference in the ischemic heart disease mortality rate was observed between the irradiated and control populations. Follow-up studies on seminoma patients also showed no increased ischemic heart disease mortality risk[23-26]; however, few of these studies covered a period exceeding 20 years, and it is possible that extension of the period might lead to a significant difference in the rates[27]. Also, the follow-up studies so far performed have mainly dealt with mortality rates, but in order to confirm a relationship between radiation exposure and ischemic heart disease it is necessary to perform long-term follow-up studies, incorporating known risk factors concerning ischemic heart disease, on the incidence in a large population[3,5].

C. Post-Radiotherapy Cervical and Cerebrovascular Disease

As with ischemic heart disease, case studies have appeared concerning the post-radiotherapy development of cervical and cerebrovascular disease[28-33]. For example, reports have appeared on the subsequent development of stenosis and occlusion of the carotid artery following radiotherapy for pharyngeal cancer[28-30], thyroid cancer[30], Hodgkin's disease[30,31], breast cancer[30], and parotid gland tumors[29] etc.; on rare occasions there have been reports concerning development of the diseases following radiotherapy for hyperthyroidism[29,32] and tonsillitis[33].

Furthermore, Elerding et al[34] performed a 9-year follow-up study on 910 cervically irradiated patients, and observed cerebrovascular disease in 6.3% of the patient population, a significantly high rate relative to the control population which suggested a causal relationship between radiation and cerebrovascular disease. However, in order to confirm this, it is necessary to perform a study on the incidence of cerebrovascular disease in a larger population.

Moreover, it has also been reported that, as found in animal experiments, hypercholesterolemia acts as a promoter in radiation-induced arteriosclerosis[30].

There have also been reports on the subsequent development of intracranial cerebrovascular disease following radiotherapy of the head[35-37].

D. Peripheral Vascular Disease and Radiotherapy

Although reports on radiotherapy and peripheral vascular disease have not been as numerous as with the carotid artery, some reports have described the post-irradiation development of occlusive vascular disease[38,39].

Occlusive vascular disease has been reported to frequently develop in smokers who undergo irradiation of bones in the leg[38] or pelvic cavity[39].

Findings pertaining to the post-radiotherapy development of occlusive vascular disease in the coronary artery, carotid artery, intracerebral artery, and peripheral artery, as well as in irradiation experiments involving animals, strongly suggest that arteriosclerotic disease may frequently occur following radiotherapy. No significant difference in ischemic heart disease mortality rates has been observed with recent radiotherapy techniques, but follow-up studies on patients have been comparatively short, and in order to observe the effects of relatively low-dose exposure it is necessary to further extend the follow-up periods. Furthermore, it is believed that the risk increases for patients who both smoke and exhibit hypercholesterolemia, and it is necessary to carefully design studies that incorporate known confounding risk factors.

2. CIRCULATORY DISEASE AND ATOMIC BOMB RADIATION

Approximately half a century has already passed since atomic bombs were dropped on Hiroshima and Nagasaki, and there has been an abundance of reports during this period on the late effects of atomic bomb radiation. However, the reports have focused on leukemia and cancer, the effects which received early recognition, and relatively few reports have appeared concerning circulatory disease. This section examines reports in the literature dealing with the mortality rates, prevalence, incidence, electrocardiographic abnormalities, and blood pressure abnormalities etc. pertaining to circulatory disease.

A. Circulatory Disease Mortality Rates

With the aim of conducting research on the late effects of atomic bomb radiation, the Atomic Bomb Casualty Commission (ABCC; the present-day Radiation Effects Research Foundation, RERF) in 1950 established various study populations. One of these, the Life Span Study sample, consisted of approximately 120,000 subjects; continuous surveys on the mortality rates from various diseases in this population have been performed[40], and the results of the analyses periodically published. Until the 5th Life Span Study report, which covered the period 1950–66, no relationship was suggested between atomic bomb radiation and mortality rates from cerebro-vascular disease and other circulatory disorders[41]. However, the 6th report, which analyzed data for the period 1950–70, became the first to recognize the effect of radiation on mortality due to circulatory disorders other than cerebrovascular disease in females[42]. That is, the circulatory disease mortality rate during this follow-up period increased in females in all populations exposed to a T65D dose of ≥ 0.10 Gy, with the increase particularly marked in the ≥ 0.50 Gy population. Although the same tendency was not confirmed in the second part of the 9th report (Kato et al.,[43]), which covered the years 1950–78, an increased mortality rate from non-malignant diseases was observed in the ≥ 2.0 Gy population.

Recently Shimizu et al[44] employed the DS86 dose estimates when summarizing mortality from non-malignant disease among the Life Span Study sample for 1950–85, and found a more distinct increase in the circulatory disease mortality rate among the heavily exposed populations. That is, an increase in the mortality rate from non-malignant disease was observed in the ≥ 2 Gy populations, and particu-larly after 1965 among the population aged under 40 at the time of bombing. Among the non-malignant diseases, high mortality rates were observed for circulatory and digestive tract diseases; cerebrovascular and heart diseases were each circulatory disorders for which the mortality rates increased in the heavily exposed populations (Fig. 1). However, in comparison with cancer, the increase in relative risk for the heavily exposed populations was small. Moreover, a large percentage of the heart disease mortalities were accounted for by ischemic heart disease[44].

The above outlined the results obtained from long-term studies on a fixed population. Kurihara et al[45] analyzed mortality statistics for atomic bomb survivors throughout Hiroshima prefecture over the period 1968–72, and found a significantly high relative mortality risk from hypertensive disease. In contrast, significantly low mortality rates were found for heart disease and stroke[45–47]. These findings agreed with those by Munaka et al[48] for Hiroshima and Mine et al[49,50] for Nagasaki. Hayakawa et al[51] further extended the observation period and analyzed the causes of death among atomic bomb survivors in Hiroshima prefecture between 1973 and 1977. The findings were similar to those of Kurihara et al,. i.e. among atomic bomb survivors, the hypertensive disease mortality rate was high, but the mortality rates

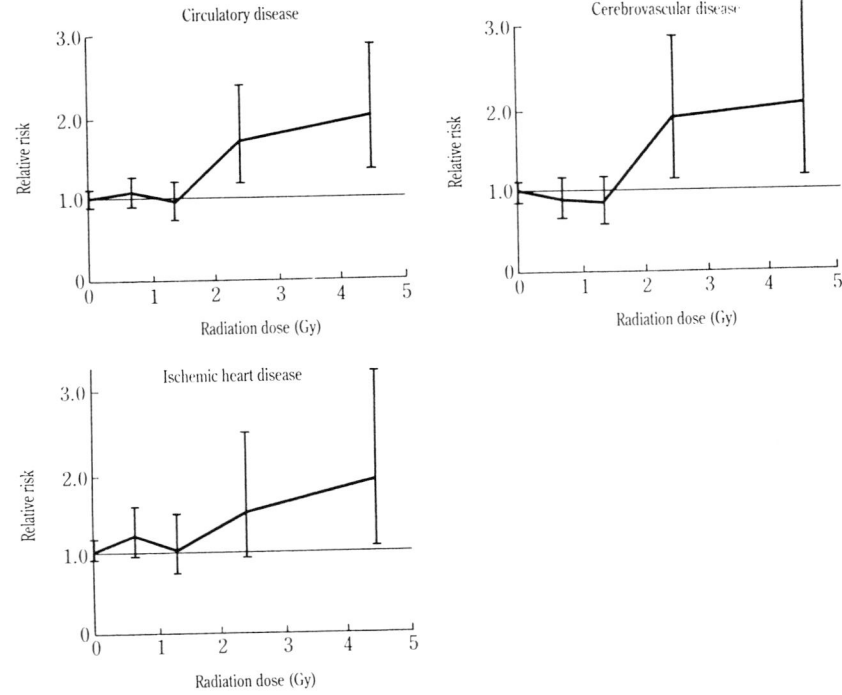

Figure 1   The relative mortality risks by DS86 dose of circulatory disease, cerebrovascular disease, and ischemic heart disease among the Life Span Study sample aged under 40 years ATB, 1966–85[44]
ATB = at the time of bombing

for cardiac and cerebrovascular disease were low; the latter could also be attributed to thorough health management procedures, but since it is well known that these mortality rates vary greatly with location, it might be due to the atomic bomb survivors tending to be in the city of Hiroshima[45–47,51].

B. Prevalence of Circulatory Disease

Since 1958 the ABCC-RERF has conducted surveys at regular 2-year intervals on an Adult Health Study sample consisting of approximately 20,000 subjects. The large majority of circulatory disease studies on this population found no relationship between exposure to atomic bomb radiation and the prevalence of ischemic heart disease, cerebrovascular disorders, and hypertensive heart disease[52–60]. However, according to the report by Yano and Ueda[61] covering the period 1958–60, only among females in Hiroshima was a significantly high prevalence of ischemic heart disease found in the proximally exposed population.

Shimizu et al[62] also performed a study on circulatory disease prevalence among a specific (legally determined) population of atomic bomb survivors in Hiroshima city, but found no significant difference in the prevalences of hypertensive heart disease or ischemic heart disease with respect to either distance from the hypocenter or exposure conditions.

C. Incidence of Circulatory Disease

Little research has been performed on the relationship between circulatory disease incidence and exposure to atomic bomb radiation, with the diseases under study limited to ischemic heart disease and cerebrovascular disorders[57,58,63,64].

Circulatory disease studies on the Adult Health Study sample have been performed since the outset, but Johnson et al[57,58] reported no relationship between atomic bomb radiation and the incidences of ischemic heart disease and cerebrovascular disorders for the period 1958–1964. However, in a study on the 16-year period from 1958 to 1974, Robertson et al[63] became the first to observe a possible increase (0.05 < p < 0.10) in cerebrovascular disorders and ischemic heart disease among heavily exposed Hiroshima females, with the tendency being particularly marked among women aged under 50 at the time of bombing (ATB).

Kodama et al[64] later extended the study to cover the 20-year period 1958–1978, and reported that the incidence of cerebrovascular disease among Hiroshima females increased significantly with dose, and that a high incidence was observed among Nagasaki males exposed to T65D doses of 1.00–1.99 Gy. The ischemic heart disease incidence was found to show a significant radiation-related increase only among Hiroshima females. An examination of this increase in circulatory disease incidence among Hiroshima females with respect to observation period reveals that the incidence became significant after 1969, and that it was especially marked among survivors aged under 30 ATB (Fig. 2). Since these diseases develop from arteriosclerosis it is possible to understand the long latency period, and also the observed effect of radiation on young atomic bomb survivors, who are believed to have a higher sensitivity to radiation. However, it is difficult to explain the effects being primarily seen among females, and is necessary to confirm the results by extending the observation period and revising data collection methods etc.

D. Pathological Studies

There have been few pathological autopsy studies pertaining to the relationship between circulatory disease and atomic bomb radiation[65–68].

According to ABCC pathology reports, neither the 1950–62 study[65] nor the 1950–65 study[66] discovered a relationship between radiation exposure and cerebrovascular disorders or ischemic heart disease in either Hiroshima or Nagasaki. Similarly, Yamamoto et al[67] found no relationship with radiation exposure in a study covering the period 1961–75.

On the other hand, investigating autopsy cases at the Hiroshima Atomic Bomb Hospital, Matsushita et al[68] found that the frequency of myocardial infarction among survivors exposed within 2 km of the bomb was 2.4 times greater than among the non-exposed population; similarly, they reported a high frequency of pericarditis, cardiomegaly and cor pulmonale among the exposed population.

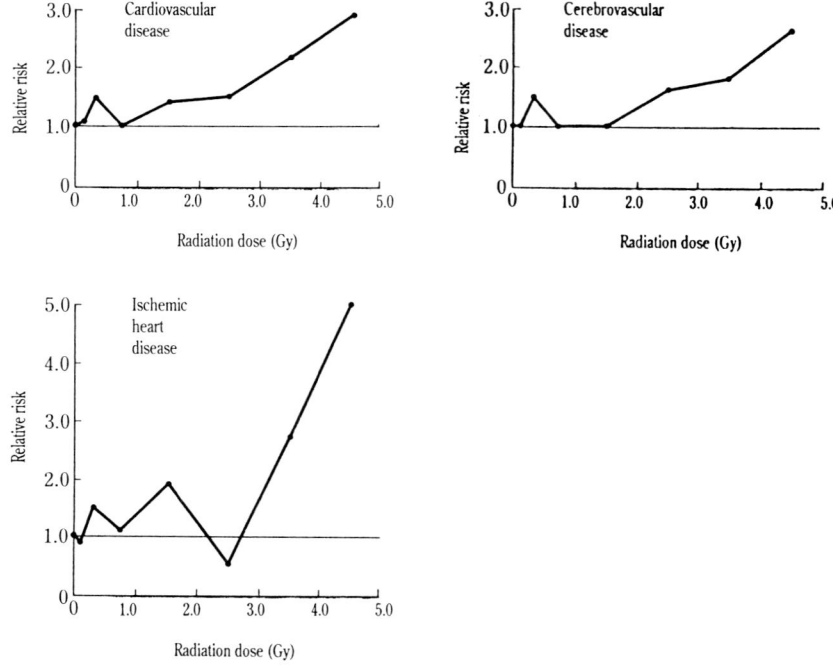

Figure 2   The relative risks by DS86 of cardiovascular disease, cerebrovascular disease, and ischemic heart disease among Hiroshima females in the Adult Health Study sample, 1958–78[64]

E. Other Clinical Observations Related to Arteriosclerosis

Cerebrovascular disorders and ischemic heart disease, typical diseases which develop from arteriosclerosis, have already been discussed. This section therefore considers research on roentgenologically detected aortic arch calcification[69,70] and pulse wave velocity[71].

In the 6th report of the RERF Adult Health Study, Sawada et al[69] stated that the prevalence of arterial disease (mostly calcification of the aortic arch diagnosed by chest X-ray) tended to increase with dose, a phenomenon observed in both Hiroshima and Nagasaki, and also in both males and females. For every age group, the prevalence was higher in the heavily exposed population[69]. (Fig. 3).

Takayama et al[70] investigated the relationship between radiation exposure and calcification and tortuosity of the thoracic aorta by performing computed radiography observations on both exposed and non-exposed subjects examined at the Hiroshima Atomic Bomb Survivors Health Clinic. High rates of calcification and tortuosity of the thoracic aorta were found among the exposed population, particularly among those aged over 70.

Pulse wave velocity was investigated by Mito et al[71] and Takayama et al[72], but on each occasion no difference was observed between the exposed and non-exposed populations.

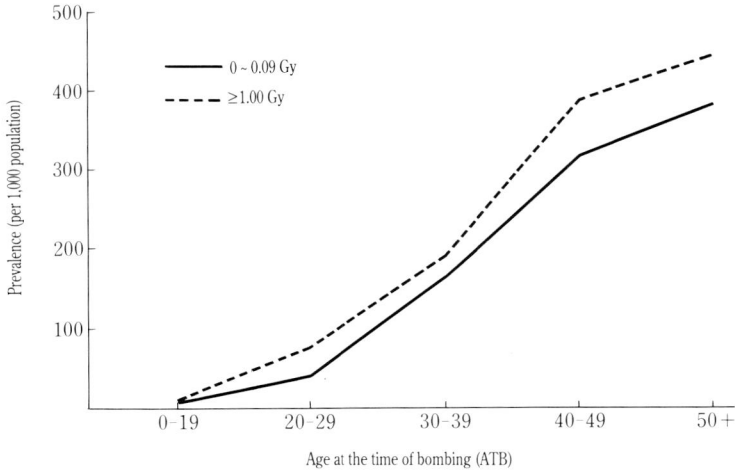

Prevalence (per 1,000 population)

0 ~ 0.09 Gy

≥1.00 Gy

0–19   20–29   30–39   40–49   50 +

Age at the time of bombing (ATB)

"Cycle" refers to the period of time (2 years) during which every subject
in the Adult Health Study sample received one examination

Figure 3   Prevalence of arterial disease by radiation dose and age ATB in the 9th examination cycle[69]

F. Electrocardiographic Abnormalities

In the ABCC Adult Health Study, the reports by Hollingworth & Anderson[53] and Ueda & Yano[73] did not find an increased frequency of electrocardiographic (ECG) abnormalities among the proximally exposed atomic bomb survivor population. However, in a later report covering the period 1958–60, Yano & Ueda[74] found an increased frequency of ECG abnormalities among the proximally exposed population, and in particular noted a significant increase in ST-T wave abnormalities among proximally exposed males aged 50–69.

With regard to studies on subjects outside this fixed population, Uraki et al[75,76] many years ago reported an unexpectedly high rate of right bundle-branch block among atomic bomb survivors. Miyanishi et al[77] studied atomic bomb survivors who underwent ECG examination at the Hiroshima Atomic Bomb Survivors Health Clinic in 1970, but found no significant difference between the proximally and distally exposed populations with respect to frequency of ECG abnormalities. Also, Hasegawa et al[78] studied atomic bomb survivors who between 1970 and 1982 simultaneously underwent glucose tolerance tests and electrocardiographic examination at the same institute. A comparison of the frequency of ECG abnormalities between the population directly exposed within 1.9 km of the hypocenter and the population directly exposed at distances greater than 3.0 km revealed a significantly high rate of Q/QS abnormality and ST depression among males in the directly and proximally exposed population. Similarly, Tadehara et al[79] studied atomic bomb survivors who received ECG examinations at the same institute during a one-year period beginning in 1988, and also found that elderly males showed a significantly high rate of ischemic electrocardiographic changes.

G. Blood Pressure Abnormalities

For both Hiroshima and Nagasaki, the ABCC Adult Health Study initially found no relationship between radiation exposure and the prevalence of hypertension[53,54]. However, in the 3rd report, Finch and Anderson[55] noted that among Hiroshima males the average systolic and diastolic pressures were lower among the population who were exposed within 2 km of the hypocenter and who suffered from acute radiation illness; among the population exposed within 2 km of the hypocenter but not suffering from acute radiation illness, the pressures were higher and statistically significant. However, in the 5th and 6th reports of the Adult Health Study[59,69], which employed T65D dose estimates, no significant association was found between blood pressure and dose. Studying the same Adult Health Study sample, Sasaki et al[80] found no definite variation with radiation dose for systolic, diastolic and pulse pressures.

Kamada et al[81] found no difference in blood pressure abnormalities between the population exposed within 500 meters and those exposed at distances greater than 2 km. In a report on the cold pressor test for blood pressure, Sasaki[82] studied the Nagasaki Adult Health Study sample in 1960 but found no difference in hyperreactor rate among the various atomic bomb survivor populations.

It can therefore be concluded that the majority of studies found that exposure to the atomic bomb had no effect on blood pressure.

H. Cardiac Function

There have been extremely few reports on atomic bomb exposure and abnormal ventricular function. Using systolic time intervals for the Hiroshima RERF Adult Health Study population, it was only among males aged 40–44 at the time of study that the exposed population exhibited a prolonged pre-ejection period (PEP) index, increased PEP/LVET (LVET = left ventricular ejection time), and abnormal ventricular function. However, echocardiograms showed no relationship between exposure and abnormal ventricular function[84-86].

I. Other Disorders

Besides the studies described above, ABCC/RERF has also published reports on the relationship between atomic bomb exposure and both rheumatic and congenital heart disease, but in each case no relationship to atomic bomb radiation was found[87,88].

To summarize, radiation exposure had an effect on the incidences and mortality rates of ischemic heart disease and cerebrovascular disorders, and also affected the prevalence of calcification of the aortic arch. In addition, some electrocardiographic studies also indicated that exposure caused electrocardiographic changes consistent with ischemic heart disease. However, in all studies problems remain regarding the accuracy of data and the number of cases etc., and further research is necessary in order to establish whether a relationship does exist between radiation exposure and circulatory disease.

CONCLUSION

A consideration of the literature pertaining to the post-radiotherapy development of occlusive vascular disease in the coronary, carotid, intracranial and peripheral arteries, together with the published results of animal irradiation experiments, suggests a strong likelihood that arteriosclerotic disease is frequently induced by radiotherapy. However, the epidemiological studies performed thus far have not been adequate, and it is necessary to further extend the follow-up period, particularly with respect to the effect of comparatively low-dose exposure. Also, although it is believed that the risk is further increased among patients who both smoke and exhibit hypercholestemia, further carefully designed studies are required that take into consideration known confounding risk factors.

The literature pertaining to circulatory disease and exposure to atomic bomb radiation suggests that exposure exerts an effect on the incidence and mortality rates of ischemic heart disease and cerebrovascular disorders, and also on the prevalence of calcification of the aortic arch; ischemic electrocardiographic changes also indicate an effect. However, the effects are small in comparison with the carcinogenic effects of the atomic bomb radiation. Various problems remain with all the reports regarding the accuracy of data (including the accuracy of death certificate entries) and the number of cases etc., and further research is necessary in order to establish whether a relationship does exist between circulatory disease and the previous exposure to atomic bomb radiation.

(*Kazunori Kodama*)

REFERENCES

1. Warren S. Effects of radiation on the cardiovascular system. *Arch Path* 1942; **34**: 1070–9.
2. Desjardins AV. Action of roentgen rays and radium on the heart and lungs. *Am J Roentgenol* 1932; 27: 153–76.
3. Stewart JR, Fajardo LF. Radiation induced heart disease: an update. *Prog Cardiovas Dis* 1984; **28**: 173–94.
4. Tominaga K, Shinkai T. Radiation-induced heart disease. *The Saishin Igaku* 1982; **37**: 2095–102.
5. Corn BW, Trock BJ, Goodman RL. Irradiation-related heart disease. *J Clin Oncol* 1990; **8**: 741–50.
6. Stewart JR, Fajardo LF, Cohn KE, *et al.* Experimental radiation-induced heart disease in rabbits. *Radiology* 1968; **91**: 814–7.
7. Fajardo LF, Stewart JR. Pathogenesis of radiation-induced myocardial fibrosis. *Lab Invest* 1973; **29**: 244–57.
8. Amronim GD, Gildenhorn HL, Solomon RD, *et al.* The synergism of X-irradiation and cholesterol-fat feeding on the development of coronary artery lesions. *J Atheroscler Res* 1964; **4**: 325–34.
9. Gold H. Production of arteriosclerosis in the rat. Effect of X-ray and high fat diet. *Arch Pathol* 1961; **71**: 268–72.
10. Artom C, Lofton HB, Clarkson TB. Ionizing radiation atherosclerosis and lipid metabolism in pigeons. *Radiat Res* 1965; **26**: 165–77.
11. Pearson H. Incidental dangers of X-ray therapy. *Lancet* 1958; **1**: 222.
12. Prentice RTW. Myocardial infarction following radiation. *Lancet* 1965; **2**: 388.
13. Feher J. Myocardial infarction following radiation. *Lancet* 1965; **2**: 643–4.
14. Stewart JW, Cohn EK, Fajardo LF, *et al.* Radiation-induced heart disease. *Radiology* 1967; **89**: 302–10.

15. Tracy GP, Brown DE, Johnson LW, *et al.* Radiation-induced coronary artery disease. *JAMA* 1974; **228**: 1660–2.
16. McReynolds RA, Gold GL, Roberts WC. Coronary heart disease after mediastinal irradiation for Hodgkin's disease. *Am J Med* 1976; **60**: 39–45.
17. Horimoto M, Igarashi T, Masaki Y, *et al.* A case of coronary artery disease probably elicited by mediastinal radiation. *J Jap Soc Int Med* 1988; **77**: 873–9.
18. Host H, Loeb M. Post-operative radiotherapy in breast cancer: long-term results from the Oslo study. *Int J Radiat Oncol Biol Phys* 1986; **12**: 727–32.
19. Bovin JF, Hutchinson GB. Coronary heart disease mortality after irradiation for Hodgkin's disease. *Cancer* 1982; **49**: 2470–5.
20. Hancock SL, Hoppe RT, Horning SJ, *et al.* Intercurrent death after Hodgkin's disease therapy in radiotherapy and adjuvant MOPP trials. *Ann Intern Med* 1988; **109**: 183–9.
21. Mauch P, Tarbell N, Weinstein H, *et al.* Stage IA and IIA supradiaphragmatic Hodgkin's disease: prognostic factors in surgically staged patients treated with mantle and para-aortic irradiation. *J Clin Oncol* 1988; **6**: 1576–83.
22. Brusius FC, Waller BF, Roberts WC. Radiation heart disease. Analysis of 16 young necropsy patients who received over 3,500 rads to the heart. *Am J Med* 1981; **70**: 519–30.
23. Lederman GS, Sheldon TA, Chaffey JT, *et al.* Cardiac disease after mediastinal irradiation for seminoma. *Cancer* 1987; **60**: 772–6.
24. Peckham J, McElwain TJ. Radiotherapy of testicular tumors. *Proc Roy Soc Med* 1974; **67**: 14–7.
25. Willan BD, McGowan DG. Seminoma of the testis: experience with radiotherapy. *Int J Radiat Oncol Bio Phys* 1985; **11**: 1769–75.
26. Hunter M, Peschel RE. Testicular seminoma. Results of the Yale University experience, 1964–1984. *Cancer* 1989; **64**: 1608.
27. Silberberg JM. Myocardial infarction in patients treated with mantle radiotherapy. *J Clinic Oncol* 1989; **7**: 541.
28. Glick B. Bilateral carotid occlusive disease. *Arch Pathol Lab Med* 1972; **93**: 352–5.
29. Levinson SA, Close MB, Ehrenfeld WK, *et al.* Carotid artery occlusive disease following external cervical irradiation. *Arch Surg* 1973; **107**: 395–7.
30. Silverberg GD, Britt RH, Goffinet DR. Radiation-induced carotid artery disease. *Cancer* 1978; **41**: 130–7.
31. Marty AT, Logan JA. Radiation-induced amaurosis fugax. *Indiana Med* 1984; **77**: 90–1.
32. Hayward RH. Arteriosclerosis induced by radiation. *Surg Clin North Am* 1972; **52**: 359–66.
33. Rotman M, Seidenberg B, Rubin I, *et al.* Aortic arch syndrome secondary to radiation in childhood. *Arch Intern Med* 1969; **124**: 87–90.
34. Elerding SC, Fernandez RN, Grotta JC, *et al.* Carotid artery disease following external cervical irradiation. *Ann Surg* 1981; **194**: 609–15.
35. Werner MH, Burger PC, Heinz ER, *et al.* Intracranial atherosclerosis following radiotherapy. *Neurology* 1988; **38**: 1158–60.
36. Montanera W, Chui M, Hudson A. Meningioma and occlusive vasculopathy: coexisting complications of past extra-cranial radiation. *Surg Neurol* 1985; **24**: 35–9.
37. Kyoi K, Kurino Y, Sakaki T, *et al.* Therapeutic irradiation for brain tumor and cerebrovasculopathy. *Neurol Surg* 1989; **17** (2): 163–70.
38. Amemiya A, Yamaguchi A, Sakurai K. Radiation-induced occlusion of the artery in the distal lower extremity. *Jpn J Surg* 1987; **17**: 178–81.
39. Pettersson F, Swedenborg J. Atherosclerotic occlusive disease after radiation for pelvic malignancies. *Acta Chir Scand* 1990; **156**: 367–71.
40. Beebe GW, Usagawa M. The major ABCC samples. ABCC TR 1968; 12–68.
41. Beebe GW, Kato H, Land C. JNIH-ABCC Life Span Study report 5: mortality and radiation dose, October 1950–September 1966. ABCC TR 11–70, 1970.
42. Jablon S, Kato H. JNIH-ABCC Life Span Study report 6: mortality among A-bomb survivors, 1950–70. ABCC TR 10–71, 1971.
43. Kato H, Brown CC, Hoel DG, *et al.* Life Span Study report 9, part 2: mortality from causes other than cancer among atomic bomb survivors, 1950–78. RERF TR 5–81, 1981.

44. Shimizu Y, Kato H, Schull WJ, *et al.* Life Span Study report II, part III: Non-cancer mortality in the years 1950–1985 based on the recently revised doses (DS86). *Radiat Res* 1992; **130**: 249–66. (RERF TR 2–91, 1991).

45. Kurihara M, Munaka M, Hayakawa N, *et al.* Mortality statistics among atomic bomb survivors in Hiroshima prefecture, 1968–1972. *J Radiat Res* 1981; **22**: 451–71.

46. Kurihara M, Munaka M, Hayakawa N, *et al.* Mortality statistics among A-bomb survivors in Hiroshima prefecture, 1968–1972. Annual Report of Research Institute for Nuclear Medicine and Biology. *Hiroshima University* 1981; **22**: 235–55.

47. Kurihara M, Munaka M, Hayakawa N, *et al.* Mortality statistics among A-bomb survivors in Hiroshima prefecture - other causes of death than malignant neoplasms in 1968–1972. *J Hiroshima Med Ass* 1982; **35**: 359–62.

48. Munaka M, Watanabe T, Sumida H, *et al.* A study on the demographics of atomic bomb survivors. Proceedings of the 15th Meeting of the Late Atomic Bomb Effects Research Meeting. Hiroshima: Hiroshima Atomic Bomb Casualty Council, 1975: 8–13.

49. Mine M, Nakamura T, Mori H, *et al.* Statistical studies on cause of death among A-bomb survivors from 1970 to 1976 in Nagasaki city. *J Hiroshima Med Ass* 1980; **33**: 401–3.

50. Mine M, Nakamura T, Mori H, *et al.* The current mortality rates of A-bomb survivors in Nagasaki city. Report 2. *J Hiroshima Med Ass* 1982; **35**: 363–5.

51. Hayakawa N, Munaka M, Kurihara M, *et al.* Mortality statistics by cause of death among A-bomb survivors in Hiroshima Prefecture, 1973–1977. Annual Report of Research Institute for Nuclear Medicine and Biology. *Hiroshima University* 1981; **22**: 235–55.

52. Switzer S. ABCC-JNIH Adult Health Study Hiroshima 1958–59. Hypertension and ischemic heart disease. ABCC TR 01–61, 1961.

53. Hollingworth JW, Anderson PS. Adult Health Study Hiroshima. Preliminary report 1958–59. ABCC TR 11–61, 1961.

54. Sagan L, Seigel D. ABCC-JNIH Adult Health Study report 2: 1958–60 cycle of examinations Nagasaki. ABCC TR 12–63, 1963.

55. Finch SC, Anderson PS. ABCC-JNIH Adult Health Study report 3: 1958–60 cycle of examinations Hiroshima. ABCC TR 19–63, 1963.

56. Freedman LR, Fukushima K, Seigel DG. ABCC-JNIH Adult Health Study report 4: 1960–62 cycle of examinations Hiroshima and Nagasaki. ABCC TR 20–63, 1963.

57. Johnson KG, Yano K, Kato H. Cerebral vascular disease in Hiroshima. Report of a six-year period of surveillance, 1958–64. ABCC TR 23–66, 1966.

58. Johnson KG, Yano K, Kato H. Coronary heart disease in Hiroshima. Report of a six-year period of surveillance, 1958–64. ABCC TR 24–66, 1966.

59. Belsky JL, Tachikawa K, Jablon S. ABCC-JNIH Adult Health Study report 5: results of the first five examination cycles, 1958–68 Hiroshima and Nagasaki. ABCC TR 9–71, 1971.

60. Hamilton HB, Brody JA. Review of the thirty years study on Hiroshima and Nagasaki atomic bomb survivors. III. Future research and health surveillance, health surveillance studies. *J Radiat Res* 1975; 16 (Suppl.): 138–48.

61. Yano K, Ueda S. ABCC-JNIH Adult Health Study Hiroshima 1958–60. Cardiovascular project report 4. Cardiovascular disease in relation to exposure to ionizing radiation. ABCC TR 22–62, 1962.

62. Shimizu K, Watanabe M, Ito S, *et al.* Heart diseases among A-bomb survivors in Hiroshima city. *J Hiroshima Med Ass* 1962; **15**: 1125–30.

63. Robertson TL, Shimizu Y, Kato H, *et al.* Incidence of stroke and coronary heart disease in atomic bomb survivors living in Hiroshima and Nagasaki, 1954–74. RERF TR 12–79, 1979.

64. Kodama K, Shimizu Y, Sawada H, *et al.* Incidence of stroke and coronary heart disease in the Adult Health Study sample, 1958–78. RERF TR 22–84, 1984.

65. Angevine DM, Jablon S, Matsumoto YS. ABCC-JNIH pathology studies Hiroshima and Nagasaki: report 1, October 1950-September 1962. ABCC TR 14–63, 1963.

66. Beebe GW, Yamamoto T, Matsumoto YS, *et al.* ABCC-JNIH pathology studies Hiroshima and Nagasaki: report 2, October 1950-December 1965. ABCC TR 8–67, 1967.

67. Yamamoto T, Moriyama I, Asano M, *et al.* RERF pathology studies, Hiroshima and Nagasaki,

report 4: the autopsy program and the Life Span Study, January 1961-December 1975. RERF TR 18–78, 1978.

68. Matsushita H, Hamada T, Ishida S. Statistical studies on heart disease of the pathological autopsy cases in the Atomic Bomb Hospital, Hiroshima. Proceedings of the 15th Meeting of the Late Atomic Bomb Effects Research Meeting. Hiroshima: Hiroshima Atomic Bomb Casualty Council, 1975; 42–6.

69. Sawada H, Kodama K, Shimizu Y, *et al.* Adult Health Study report 6: results of six examination cycles, 1968–80, Hiroshima and Nagasaki. RERF TR 3–86. 1986.

70. Takayama S, Ishibashi S, Nakano K, *et al.* Study on arteriosclerosis among atomic bomb survivors. *Nagasaki Med J* 1988; **63**: 729–33.

71. Mito K, Matsumoto Y, Kato M, *et al.* Study on pulse wave velocity among A-bomb survivors. *Nagasaki Med J* 1986; **61**: 489–93.

72. Takayama S, Ito Y, Okusaki K, *et al.* Study on arteriosclerosis among atomic bomb survivors (second report). *Nagasaki Med J* 1990; **43**: 502–5.

73. Ueda S, Yano K. Cardiovascular studies Hiroshima 1958–60 report number 1: electrocardiographic findings in relation to the aging process, formulation of the problem. ABCC TR 07–61, 1961.

74. Yano K, Ueda S. ABCC-JNIH Adult Health Study Hiroshima 1958–60, cardiovascular project report 2: electrocardiographic findings related to aging. ABCC TR 20–62, 1962.

75. Uraki J, Yuuki I, Osafune M, *et al.* Electrocardiographic studies on atomic bomb survivors. *J Hiroshima Med Ass* 1954; **7**: 81.

76. Uraki J, Yoshinaka T, Yuuki I, *et al.* Studies on the sequelae and after-effects of the atomic bomb (2nd report): electrocardiograpic studies on atomic bomb survivors. *J Hiroshima Med Ass* 1955; **8**: 382–7.

77. Miyanishi M, Yoshida M, Furonaka H, *et al.* Cardiovascular changes in atomic exposed survivors in terms of aging with special reference to electrocardiographic findings. *J Hiroshima Med Ass* 1971; **24**: 1183–95.

78. Hasegawa K, Kumazawa T, Ito C. Effects of atomic bomb radiation on the cardiovascular system. *J Hiroshima Med Ass* 1984; **37**: 401–4.

79. Tadehara F, Oyama H, Okusaki K, *et al.* Study on mass survey for cardiovascular diseases - analyzed using the electrocardiography in atomic bomb survivors. *J Hiroshima Med Ass* 1990; **65**: 700–8.

80. Sasaki H, Kodama K, Kitano K, *et al.* Secular trends of blood pressure in A-bomb survivors. *Nagasaki Med J* 1986; **61**: 442–8.

81. Kamada N, Yuzaki M, Yamamoto H, *et al.* Comprehensive medical research on survivors from the atomic bomb hypocenter — the results of the last ten years. *J Hiroshima Med Ass* 1982; **35**: 1084–98.

82. Sasaki T. Radiation effects on cold pressor test. *J Hiroshima Med Ass* 1962; **15**: 1013–5.

83. Sasaki H, Yamada M, Sawada H, *et al.* Study of cardiac performance of A-bomb survivors (using the mechanocardiogram). *Nagasaki Med J* 1984; **59**: 554–9.

84. Takemoto M, Higaki A, Kobayashi M, *et al.* An echocardiographic study of the cardiac function in the much elderly subjects. *J Hiroshima Med Ass* 1988; **41**: 508–9.

85. Ishibashi S, Tokunaga Y, Takayama S, *et al.* Study on cardiac function in atomic bomb survivors using the dual echocardiography. *J Hiroshima Med Ass* 1988; **41**: 504–7.

86. Ishibashi S, Takayama S, Nakano K, *et al.* Study on cardiac function on atomic bomb survivors, using pulsed doppler method. *Nagasaki Med J* 1988; **63**: 719–23.

87. Dear HD, Beebe GW, Sawayama T, *et al.* Rheumatic heart disease in the adult Japanese population. ABCC TR 14–68, 1968.

88. Dear HD, Beebe GW, Sawayama T, *et al.* Congenital heart disease in adult Japanese. ABCC TR 15–68, 1968.

8

Respiratory Diseases

8.1 PULMONARY FIBROSIS

INTRODUCTION

In pulmonary fibrosis the main site of inflammatory reaction is in the lung's alveolar wall or peripheral supporting tissue, and the disease is virtually synonymous with interstitial pneumonia. The fibroid shadows on chest X-rays are diffuse, and histologically the disease is characterized by the development of diffuse fibrosis in the pulmonary tissue.

As shown in Table 1[1], many causes have been advanced for pulmonary fibrosis, including inorganic dust, medication, physical and chemical agents, infection, granulomatous disease, and collagen disease, etc., but even today most causes are unknown[2]. Interstitial changes occurring during the fibrosis process are believed to be those shown in Fig. 1[2]. Figure 1(a) shows normal pulmonary alveolar walls and interstitial spaces; the alveolar walls consist of type I and type II respiratory epithelial cells, and are in contact via the basement membrane with blood vessels and supporting tissue (in the interstitial tissue). Figure 1(b) shows distortions in the interstitial thickness, due to clumping of inflammatory cells such as T-lymphocytes and macrophages etc., which occurs with sarcoidosis etc. Figure 1(c) shows the situation with idiopathic interstitial pneumonia, in which type I respiratory

Table 1   Diffuse interstitial pneumonia by cause of illness[1]

I Unknown causes
1. Idiopathic interstitial pneumonia (IIP) (diffuse interstitial pneumonia of unknown cause), usual interstitial pneumonia (UIP), Hamman-Rich syndrome (acute form), including the chronic form of IIP
2. Bronchiolitis obliterans interstitial pneumonia (BIP)
3. Desquamative interstitial pneumonia (DIP)
4. Lymphoid interstitial pneumonia (LIP)
5. Giant cell interstitial pneumonia (GIP)

II Known causes and those related to systemic diseases
1. Inoganic dust, asbestos, silica, tar, beryllium, tungsten carbide, cadmium, etc.
2. Medications: nitrofurantoin, busulfan, bleomycin, methotrexate, hexamethonium, aminobenzyl penicillin, gold, etc.
3. Other physical and chemical agents: X-rays, cobalt, oxygen, paraquat, mercury vapor, and parachloroethylene
4. Infectious agents: viruses, microplasma, mildly toxic bacteria
5. Granulomatous diseases (granulomatous interstitial pneumonia)
   (a) Extrinsic allergic alveolitis (hypersensitivity pneumonitis): farmer's lung, sugar cane lung, bird breeder's lung, etc.
   (b) Granulomatous disease of unknown cause: sarcoidosis, histicytosis X
6. Collagen diseases and related diseases: systemic lupus erythematosis, progressive systemic sclerosis, rheumatic fever, chronic rheumatoid artyhritis, dermatomyositis, polymyositis, polyarteritis nodosa, Sjögren's syndrome, etc.
7. Metabolic disorders: cholesterin pneumonia, uremic lung etc.
8. Circulatory disorders: chronic hypertension of the pulmonary vein, and other pulmonary congestion
9. Phacomatosis: tuberous sclerosis, Recklinghausen's disease etc.
10. Others: idiopathic lung hemosiderosis, Goodpasture's syndrome etc.

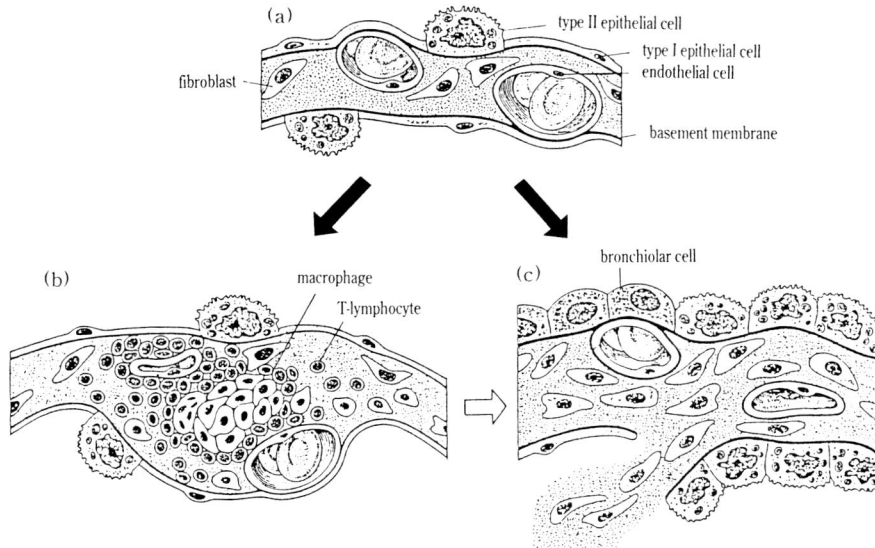

Figure 1   Development of fibrosis[2]

epithelial cells are damaged, and are replaced by type II cells and bronchiolar epithelial cells. There is marked proliferation of fibroblasts, with the interstitial components migrating into the alveolar epithelium. Viruses, autoimmunity and heredity etc. are believed to cause this series of changes, but the true situation has not been clarified.

The diagnostic criteria for pulmonary fibrosis are shown in Table 2[3]. The most important factors in diagnosis are pathological observations and chest X-ray observations that accompany the development of fibrosis (distribution and properties of shadows, and shrinkage of the lung field).

1. PULMONARY FIBROSIS AND RADIATION EXPOSURE

Thoracic irradiation with X-rays or ^{60}Co may cause radiation damage to the lung, leading to fever, coughing, chest pain, and dyspnea, etc., with various shadows observed in chest X-rays corresponding to the radiation field[4]. This reaction is generally termed radiation pneumonitis, and frequently occurs 2–10 weeks following irradiation[5]. With regard to clinical concepts, Groover et al[6] in 1923 were the first to report the development of radiation pneumonitis following radiotherapy for breast cancer. Several reports later appeared on experimental and clinical radiation pneumonitis.

Reports on the frequency of the disease were not uniform, varying from 5.4% (Engelstad[7]) to 91.8% (Ross[8]). In the general procedure, involving irradiation 5 days a week with single doses consisting of 1.50–3.50 Gy, the minimum depth dose which may cause development of the disease is believed to be 20–30 Gy[1]. Irradiation with 60 Gy over a 5–6 week period almost invariably leads to radiation pneumonitis[9]. However, there are large individual variations even for identical

Table 2   Diagnostic criteria[3]

I   Main symptoms and scientific observations
 1. Dry cough
 2. Dyspnea (greater than Hugh-Jones grade II level)
 3. Finger clubbing

II   Chest X-ray findings
 1. Shadow distribution (diffuse and scattered, lower lung field > upper lung field, marginal dominant distribution)
 2. Physical properties of shadow (granular, granular + small ring type, multiple ring type)
 3. Shrinkage of lung field (diaphragm elevation, shrinkage of lower field)

III   Pulmonary function observations
 1. Decreased respiratory volume (decreased vital capacity, %VC; decreased total lung capacity, %TLC)
 2. Decreased diffusing capacity of the lung (%D_{LCO}, %D_{LCO}/VA)
  (%D_{LCO} = diffusing capacity of the lung for carbon monoxide; %D_{LCO}/VA = volume of alveolar gas)
 3. Hypoxemia (decreased Pa_{O_2}, increased A-aD_{O_2})
  (Pa_{O_2} = partial pressure of oxygen in arterial blood); A-aD_{O_2} = difference in partial pressure between oxygen in alveolar gas and in arterial blood)

IV   Hematologic and immunologic observations
 1.   Increased erythrocyte sedimentation rate
 2.   Increased lactate dehydrogenase, LDH
 3.   Positive findings in rheumatoid arthritis (RA) test

V   Pathological (autopsy, pulmonary biopsy) observations

Pathological findings consistent with idiopathic interstitial pneumonia
I   A diagnosis of pulmonary fibrosis can only be made if the following diseases can be excluded: pneumoconiosis, pulmonary tuberculosis, diffuse panbronchioilitis, pneumonia, lung cancer, sarcoidosis, collagen diseases, hypersensitivity pneumonitis, radiation pneumonitis, drug-induced pneumonitis.

If the above diseases can be excluded, then:
II   Diagnosis is confirmed upon fulfillment of 3 of the above categories, including category II, or by fulfillment of the requirements of categories II and V.
III   Diagnosis is suspected upon fulfillment of 2 of the above categories, including category II.

---

doses, and clinically radiation damage to the lung depends not only on the total received dose but also the size of the irradiated field, i.e. the irradiated volume exerts a large effect[5]. Figure 2 shows the relationship between radiation dose, irradiated volume and pulmonary damage reported by Umegaki *et al*[10] during radiotherapy for breast cancer. Although a dose of 30 Gy can be withstood when the irradiated field is small, serious damage may result with a large irradiated field (e.g. a whole lung) with even a 15 Gy dose.

When radiation pneumonitis develops and advances, pulmonary fibrosis develops within 6 months to 1 year of irradiation, diffuse reticular and reticulonodular shadows appear in the lung field, and the lung shrinks considerably. With regard to the mechanism by which pulmonary fibrosis develops via radiation pneumonitis, Kojima[4] stated that autopsy data suggested the disease be classified into three histologic types (alveolar infiltrating type, interstitial type, and mixed type), and stressed the allergic mechanism shown in Fig. 3. In the alveolar infiltrating type there is marked infiltration of the pulmonary alveoli by edema and formation of vitreous membranes with a strong reaction by the alveolar epithelium, leading to fibrosis in the pulmonary alveoli. In the interstitial type infiltration is slight, mainly involving interstitial changes such as

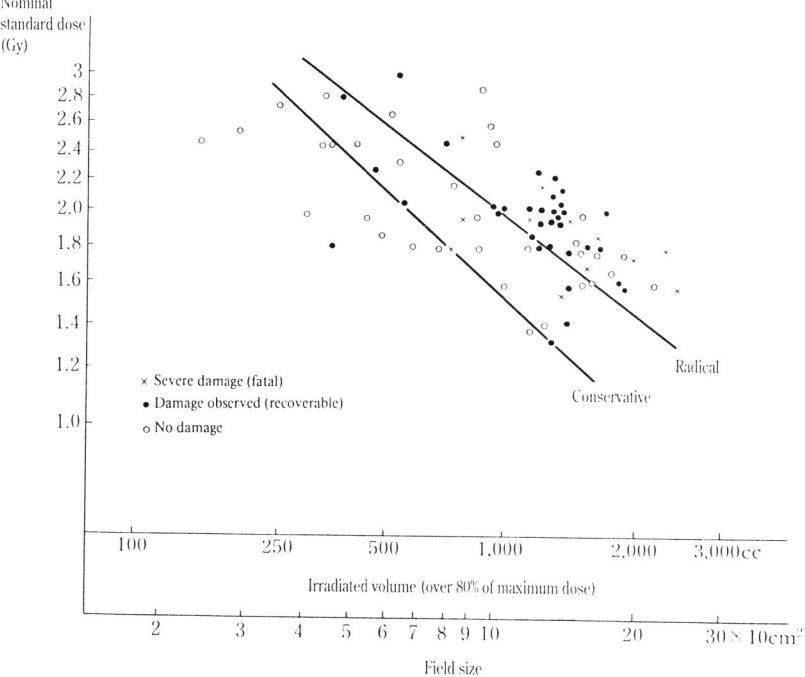

Figure 2   Radiotherapy of pulmonary cancer: relationship between irradiated volume, dose and pulmonary damage[10]

edematous fibrotic thickening of the interstitial spaces. The mixed type combines the characteristics of both types. The type produced depends on the degree of vascular damage; considerable vascular damage results in the alveolar infiltrating type, and slight damage leads to the interstitial type. Comparatively few analyses have been performed on radiation-caused changes in humoral factors that cause these histologic phenomena, but Kyomura *et al*[11] reported that mice experiments suggested the participation of increased intrapulmonary lipoperoxide due to radiation exposure.

2. PULMONARY FIBROSIS AND EXPOSURE TO THE ATOMIC BOMB

Studies on pulmonary fibrosis as a late effect of exposure to the atomic bomb were not performed until recently. From the results of thoracic examinations on 9,253 atomic bomb survivors, Tokunaga *et al*[12] found that the pulmonary fibrosis prevalence tended to be high among the directly and proximally exposed population. In studies by Okusaki *et al*[13] on 16,956 subjects, chest X-ray examinations also tended to show a high prevalence among the directly and proximally exposed, with males having a higher prevalence than females (1.82% versus 0.41%), and the prevalence increasing with age. The population was expanded to 42,728 subjects, and the prevalence of pulmonary fibrosis due to causes other than known ones such as pneumoconiosis,

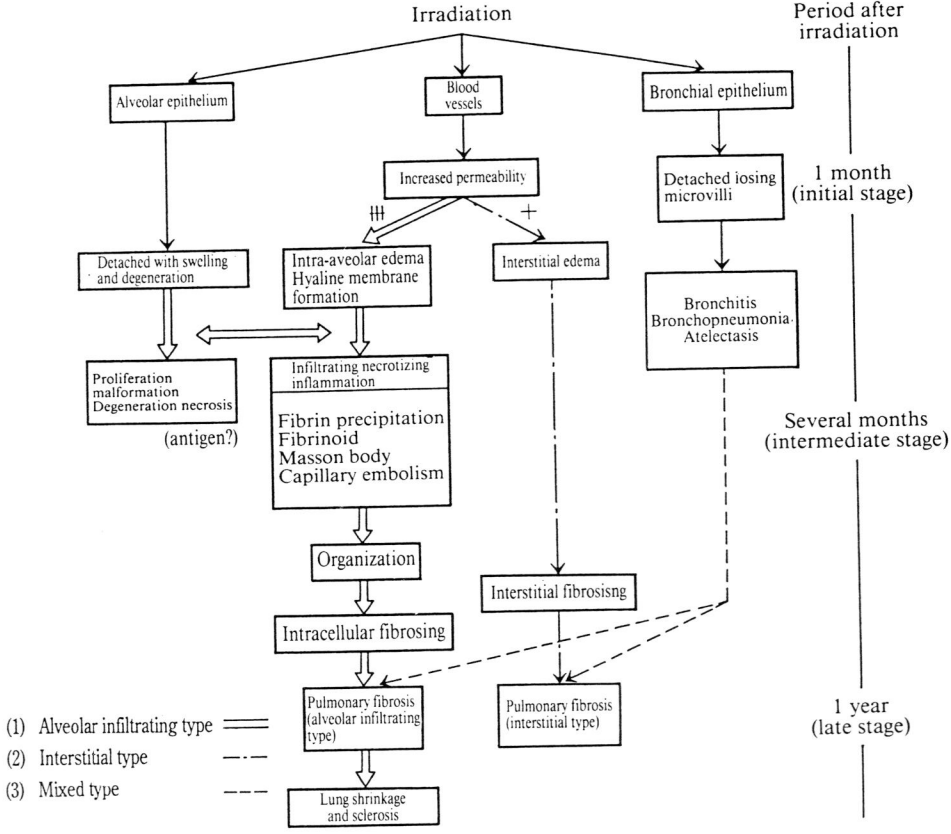

Figure 3 Development of radiation pneumonitis[4]

sarcoidosis and collagen disease etc. classified according to sex and age (Fig. 4), and also by age and exposure status (Fig. 5). The prevalence was high among males, increased with age, and was rather high among the directly and proximally exposed population. Also, the tendencies were more pronounced among the elderly.

There are many important differences between atomic bomb survivors and radiotherapy patients besides those of total received dose (1 : 100) and period between exposure and development of pulmonary fibrosis (100 : 1), including the scope of internal exposure and type of radiation. It is extremely difficult to consider the pulmonary fibrosis which appears as a late effect of atomic bomb exposure to be a form of pulmonary fibrosis developing from radiation pneumonitis. However, decreased immunocompetence has been reported among heavily exposed individuals, and a relationship may exist between pulmonary fibrosis and atomic bomb exposure. Further detailed studies are required.

(*Michio Yamakido, Ken Okusaki*)

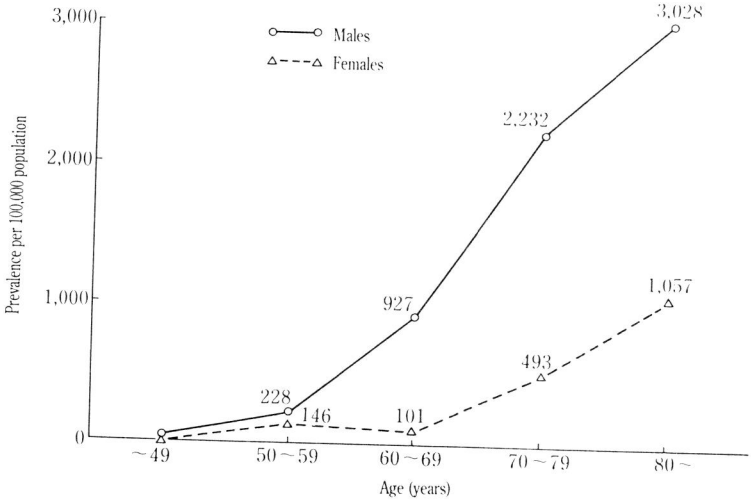

Figure 4   Prevalence of pulmonary fibrosis by sex and age

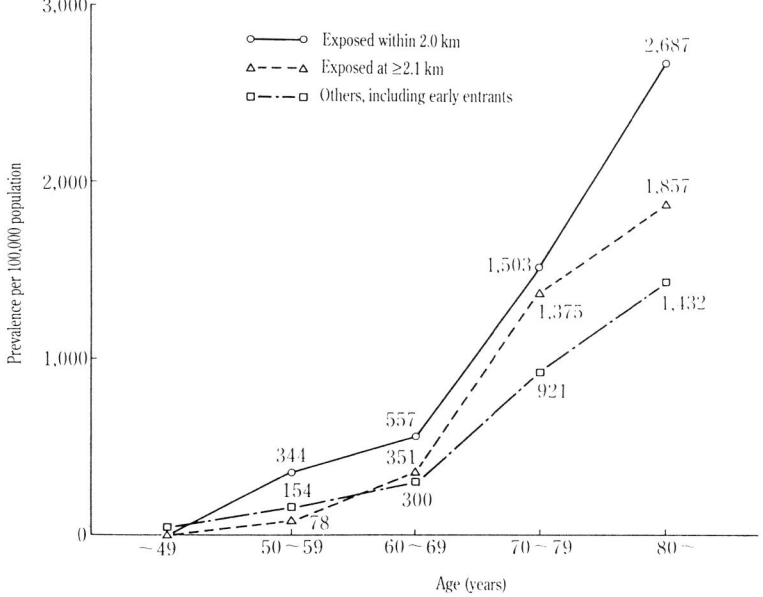

Figure 5   Prevalence of pulmonary fibrosis by age and distance from hypocenter

REFERENCES

1. Ueda H, Takeuchi J. *Naikagaku* (Internal Medicine), 3rd ed. Tokyo: Asakura Shoten, 1986: 415–21. (*In Japanese*)
2. Wyngaarden JB, Smith LH. Cecil textbook of medicine. 18th ed. Philadelphia: WB Saunders, 1988: 421–35.
3. Mikami R, Suzuki M, Tamura M, *et al.* Diagnostic criteria for 11P. *1985 nendo mashitsusei haishikkan chousa kenkyuu* (Investigation of Interstitial Lung Disease in 1985). 1985; 27–30. (*In Japanese*)
4. Kojima K. Radiation pneumonitis. *J Clin and Exp Med* 1967; **60** (11): 591–6. (*In Japanese*)
5. Takijima T, Yamabayashi H, Takizawa T, *et al*, editors. *Rinshou kokyuubyou kouza* (Clinical respiratory tract disease) Vol. 2 1st ed. Osaka: Kanehara Shuppan, 1978: 167–75. (*In Japanese*)
6. Groover TA, Christie AC, Meritt EA. Intrathoracic changes following roentgen treatment of breast carcinoma. *Am J Roentgenol* 1923; **10**: 417–26.
7. Engelstad RB. Pulmonary lesions after roentgen and radium irradiation. *Am J Roentgenol* 1940; **43**: 676–81.
8. Ross WM. Radiotherapeutic and radiological aspects of radiation fibrosis of lungs. *Thorax* 1956; **11**: 241–8.
9. Takahashi M, editor. *Hisshu Houshasen Igaku* (Required radiation medicine), 1st ed. Tokyo: Nankoudou, 1983: 178–209. (*In Japanese*)
10. Umegaki Y, Sakura M, Tsuboi E, *et al.* Results of radiotherapy of the lung cancer. *Japan J of Cancer Clinics* 1975; **21** (14): 1229–37. (*In Japanese*)
11. Hashimura T, Kono M, Imajo Y. Experimental studies on mechanisms and prevention of radiation pneumonitis. *Nippon Act Radio* 1989; **49** (3): 335–43. (*In Japanese*)
12. Tokunaga Y, Ito C, Mitsuyama T, *et al.* Study on pulmonary fibrosis. 1st report. Relationship between atomic bomb survivor and pulmonary fibrosis. *J Hiroshima Med Ass* 1988; **41** (7): 1235. (*In Japanese*)
13. Okusaki K, Ishibashi S, Takayama S, *et al.* Pulmonary fibrosis in atomic bomb survivor. *J Hiroshima Med Ass* 1990; **43** (3): 466–9. (*In Japanese*)

9

Hepatic Disorders

9 HEPATIC DISORDERS

INTRODUCTION

Acute damage of hepatic cells by ionizing radiation was reported in 1924 by Case and Warthin[1], who stated that the liver had a comparatively low radiosensitivity and that liver necrosis resulted from irradiation with over 40 to 50 Gy.

Later, however, radiation became extensively employed in therapeutic and diagnostic techniques, and it was found that rather low doses of ionizing radiation caused hepatic disorders such as hepatomegaly, ascites, and jaundice etc., frequently accompanied by increased alkaline phosphatase levels and decreased blood platelets. Observed pathological changes included congestion, bleeding, and progressive atrophy of hepatic cells accompanying dilation of the central veins of the liver[2-4].

With regard to the development of radiation-induced chronic liver disease, Thorotrast (thorium-232 oxide, an alpha-ray emitting contrast medium used in angiography), is a well-known carcinogen. However, it has been reported that Thorotrast not only causes malignant tumors but also leads to increased non-malignant liver disease such as cirrhosis of the liver and liver fibrosis etc. 20–40 years following administration[5,6].

Also, Miyoshi and Kumatori[7] performed clinical observations on subjects exposed to radioactivity in the Bikini atoll and found cases of hepatomegaly, jaundice and bromosulfophthalein (BSP) retention etc.; in addition, liver biopsies revealed various hepatic cell lesions e.g. presence of hyaline bodies, swelling of Kupffer cells, etc[7].

This chapter considers chronologically the advances in knowledge concerning the development of hepatic disorders in the atomic bomb survivors and its relationship with radiation.

1. HEPATIC DISORDERS AMONG ATOMIC BOMB SURVIVORS

A. Acute Period

Several reports appeared concerning hepatic disorders in the initial period following the atomic explosion, and it is clear that some liver disease was observed among atomic bomb survivors[8-10]. Kobayashi[8] reported hepatic disorders in 30 out of 36 subjects within 2–6 months of the explosion; Fukuda[9] stated that the large majority of survivors suffering radiation-caused hepatic disorders returned to normal within 10 weeks of the bombing; and Okura[10] reported that liver function damage among many atomic bomb survivors was observed until 6 months after the explosion, but that liver function recovered after 1 year.

B. 1950–69

In 1959, fourteen years after the atomic bombing, the Research Society for the Late Effects of the Atomic Bombs was inaugurated, and research into the late effects became more systematic. In the first symposium, Uraki[11] reported that studies on atomic bomb survivors resident in Kure and Otake showed no difference between exposed and non-exposed subjects with regard to rates of liver function damage, and that no liver function damage was observed which could be attributed to the atomic explosion[11]. However, Shigefuji[12] and Yokota[13] found liver disease to be the second most common complaint among patients hospitalized at the Atomic Bomb Hospital, clearly demonstrating it to be a major medical problem among atomic bomb survivors. In particular, it is noteworthy that hepatic disorders was common among anemia cases. In 1962 Shimizu *et al*[14] conducted a statistical study of applications for treatment of atomic bomb-related diseases in Hiroshima city, and found that the frequency of liver disease was almost 3 times greater than in the national health survey, with the tendency particularly marked among proximally exposed subjects.

Studies of autopsy data have also been performed, but consistent results have not been attained[15,16]. Yasuhi *et al*[15] found that Nagasaki University documents showed the frequency of liver cirrhosis to be higher than the national average in the Nagasaki area, as was the case with liver cancer complications, but hypothesized that the liver cirrhosis was due to a factor other than the atomic bomb since no difference was observed with the non-exposed population. However, Schreiber *et al*[16] found a significant relationship between liver cirrhosis and ionizing radiation when studying 143 liver cirrhosis autopsy cases in the Life Span Study sample of the Atomic Bomb Casualty Commission (ABCC). A similar tendency was particularly evident among Hiroshima females, and also suggested among Hiroshima males. The prevalence of primary hepatoma in the same population over the period 1961–67 was 3 times greater in Nagasaki than in Hiroshima, but no correlation was found between liver cancer and radiation[17].

C. After 1970

Ishida[18] conducted a variety of clinical investigations on Atomic Bomb Hospital patients, and found a high prevalence of hepatic disorders among atomic bomb survivors proximally exposed within 2.0 km of the hypocenter. Using examination records from the Atomic Bomb Survivors Health Clinic, Orimen[19] also found a high rate of liver disease among atomic bomb survivors; some of the results at first appear to suggest this was a direct effect of the bombing, but since liver disease in atomic bomb survivors is complex, it was difficult to conclude that primary liver disease is a chronic effect of radiation.

On the other hand, it is known that in Japan the hepatitis virus plays a major role in liver disease. Hepatitis B surface (HBs) antigen and antibody were twice investigated in the ABCC Adult Health Study, in 1969–70 (5,561 subjects) and 1971 (961 subjects)[20,21]. The positive rate of HBs antigen results tended to be high among heavily exposed atomic bomb survivors, but no statistical significance with respect to the degree of exposure was observed for positive determinations of either antigen or antibody. This is believed to have been due to the small number of cases in survivors exposed to ≥ 1 Gy. Kato *et al*[22] therefore studied all members of the Adult Health Study sample who had received ≥ 1 Gy over a 2-year period starting in 1975; the control population consisted of an equal number of subjects selected from the 0–0.9 Gy population who were matched in terms of sex, age, and dates of examination. The positive rates for HBs antigen and antibody were then determined for a total of 2,566 subjects. As with the previous studies, no difference between the two populations was observed with respect to the positive rate of HBs antibody findings, which are believed to indicate the exposure to the HB virus or the possibility of infection. However, the positive rate of HBs antigen results among the ≥ 1 Gy population was significantly higher than in the control population (3.4% versus 2.0%), with the tendency more pronounced among young people aged ≤ 20 at the time of bombing. It is believed that these positive HBs antigen findings suggest decreased immunocompetence among the heavily exposed population.

Pathological studies have also been performed on liver diseases. Hamada[23] investigated autopsy cases at the Hiroshima Atomic Bomb Hospital over the period 1951–80 and found that the frequency of liver cirrhosis was higher for females only, the same result obtained by Schreiber *et al*. Also, Asano *et al*[24] performed a pathological study on primary hepatoma and liver cirrhosis among autopsy cases in the expanded population of the Life Span Study sample at the Radiation Effects Research Foundation (RERF) over the period 1961–75. Orcein and aldehyde fuchsin staining was performed in all cases, and HBs antigen was also investigated. Liver cirrhosis was found to be 74.8% posthepatitic, 16.3% postnecrotic, 5.3% nutritional, and 3.7% other types. The liver cirrhosis prevalence was 5.8% in Hiroshima and 7.2% in Nagasaki; although the Nagasaki figure was slightly higher, the difference was not statistically significant. For both cities, an association was indicated between radiation dose and liver cirrhosis prevalence. On the other hand, although the primary hepatoma incidence in Nagasaki was double that of Hiroshima, no correlation with radiation was seen in either city. The rate of positive HBs antigen tests exhibited no correlation with radiation dose for either liver cirrhosis or primary hepatoma. However, among patients with no clear liver disease the HBs antigen was present in the liver 2.3 times more frequently in Nagasaki than in Hiroshima, suggesting that the high cancer incidence in Nagasaki was primarily due to infection by the HB virus. (Figure 1).

Recently the results of epidemiological studies on the long-term follow-up fixed cohort at the Radiation Effects Research Foundation have been summarized[25,26,27]. A mortality study on non-malignant disease in the Life Span Study sample over the period 1950–85 found a clear increase with radiation dose for digestive tract diseases, especially liver cirrhosis, with the tendency apparently becoming more pronounced recently among survivors exposed at a comparatively young age. Analysis of incidence among the Adult Health Study sample also suggests a correlation between radiation exposure and the development of chronic hepatitis and liver cirrhosis[26]. An analysis using the rather more reliable tumor registry data pertaining to the Life Span Study sample for the first time showed a significant correlation between primary hepatoma and radiation[27].

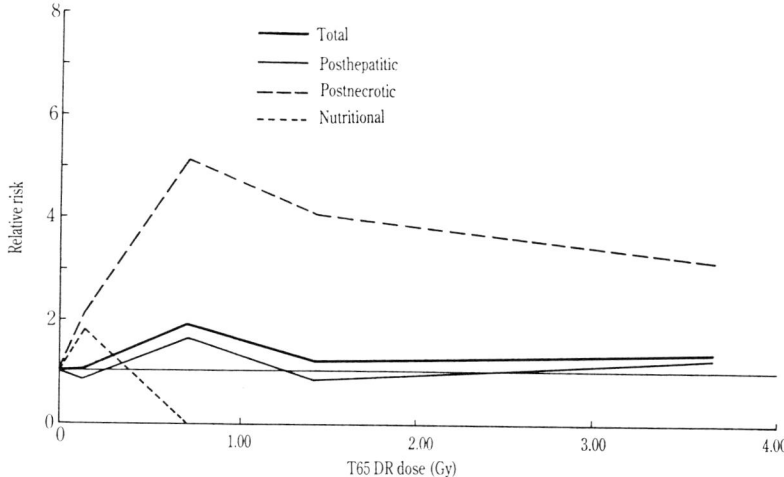

Figure 1   Relative risk of liver cirrhosis by dose and histologic type (Hiroshima and Nagasaki combined)[24]

CONCLUSION

Several clinicians reported hepatic disorders among atomic bomb survivors immediately following the bombing. A high rate of hepatic disorders was also observed later in atomic bomb survivors, posing a significant medical problem. Numerous clinical, pathological and epidemiological studies were performed, but it has not been clarified whether these liver diseases were caused by radiation. However, it is noteworthy that recent results have suggested a correlation with radiation for chronic hepatitis, liver cirrhosis and primary hepatoma. Nevertheless, many causes of hepatic disorders are known, including viruses and nutrition, and in the future it is necessary to perform further studies in order to determine whether the correlation is due to the direct action of radiation, or whether the radiation acts indirectly through the effects of these causative agents.

(Mitoshi Akiyama, Hideo Sasaki)

REFERENCES

1. Case JT, Warthin AS. The occurrence of hepatic lesions in patients treated by intensive deep roentgen radiation. *AJR* 1924; **12**: 27.
2. Ogata K, Hizawa K, Yoshida M, *et al.* Hepatic injury following irradiation, a morphologic study. *Tokushima J Exp Med* 1963; **9**: 240–51.
3. Ingold JA, Reed GB, Kaplan HS, *et al.* Radiation hepatitis. *AJR* 1965; **92**: 200–8.
4. Reed GB, Cox AJ. The human liver after radiation injury, a form of venoocclusive disease. *Am J Pathol* 1966; **48**: 597–612.
5. Da Silva Horta J, Da Silva Horta ME, *et al.* Malignancies in Portuguese Thorotrast patients. 1978; **32**: 135–7.
6. Kato U, Mori T, Kumatori T. Thorotrast dosimetric study in Japan. *Environ Res* 1979; **18**: 32–36.
7. Miyoshi K, Kumatori T. Clinical and hematological observations on subjects exposed to radioactivities in the Bikini atoll. *Japan J Hematol* 1955; **18**: 379–406. (*In Japanese*)

8.   Kobayashi T. Liver and capillary function disorders in atomic bomb-related diseases. Report on atomic bomb disaster investigation. 1953; **1** (Suppl): 704. (*In Japanese*)
9.   Fukuda T. Liver function of the patients with atomic bomb-related disease. Report on atomic bomb disaster investigation. 1953; **2** (Suppl): 707. (*In Japanese*)
10.   Okura I. Liver function tests performed in the Nagasaki patients with atomic bomb-related disease. Report on atomic bomb disaster investigation. 1953; **2** (Suppl): 1204. (*In Japanese)*
11.   Uraki J. Liver function of atomic bomb survivors. *Hiroshima J Med Sci* 1959; **12**: 955–7. (*In Japanese*)
12.   Shigeto F. General treatment for the late effects of atomic bomb. *Hiroshima J Med Sci* 1959; 12: 995–1002. (*In Japanese*)
13.   Yokota M. Clinical observations of atomic bomb survivors. *Nagasaki Med J* 1960; **36**: 589–95. (*In Japanese*)
14.   Shimizu K, Watanabe M, Ito S. Statistical observations of liver disease in Hiroshima atomic bomb survivors. *Hiroshima J Med Sci* 1962; **15**: 1007–12. (*In Japanese*)
15.   Yasuhi S, Yokouchi H, Uemura S, *et al.* Epidemiological, clinical, and pathological studies on liver cirrhosis and hepatoma with regards to atomic bomb exposure in Nagasaki area (report 1). *Hiroshima J Med Sci* 1962; **15**: 951–5. (*In Japanese*)
16.   Schreiber WM, Kato H, Robertson JD. Cirrhosis of the liver, Hiroshima-Nagasaki, 1 October 1961–31 December 1967. ABCC TR 17–69, 1969.
17.   Schreiber WM, Kato H, Robertson JD. Primary carcinoma of the liver in Hiroshima and Nagasaki, Japan. *Cancer* 1970; **26**: 69–75. (ABCC TR 15–69).
18.   Ishida S. Hepatic disorders - from the view of clinical medicine. *Hiroshima J Med Sci* 1970; **23**: 1089–103. (*In Japanese*)
19.   Orimen A. Liver function disorders. *Hiroshima J Med Sci* 1970; **23**: 1139–46. (*In Japanese*)
20.   Belsky JL, King RA, Ishimaru T, *et al.* Hepatitis-associated antigen in atomic bomb survivors and nonexposed control subjects: seroepidemiologic survey in a fixed cohort. *J Inf Dis* 1973; **128**: 1–6. (ABCC TR 30–71).
21.   Belsky JL, Okochi K, Ishimaru T, *et al.* Hepatitis-associated antigen and antibody in A-bomb survivors and nonexposed subjects, Hiroshima and Nagasaki. ABCC TR 12–72, 1972.
22.   Kato H, Mayumi M, Nishioka K, *et al.* The relationship of HBs antigen and antibody to radiation in the Adult Health Study sample, 1975–77. RERF TR 13–80, 1980.
23.   Hamada T. Liver cirrhosis and primary carcinoma of the liver among atomic bomb survivors. Study of autopsy cases. *Nagasaki Med J* 1979; **55**: 661–76 (*In Japanese*)
24.   Asano M, Kato H, Yoshimoto, *et al.* Primary liver carcinoma and liver cirrhosis in atomic bomb survivors, Hiroshima and Nagasaki, 1961–75, with special reference to HBs antigen. JNCI 1982; **69**: 1221–7. (RERF TR 9–81, 1981).
25.   Shimizu Y, Kato H, Schull WJ, *et al.* Studies of the mortality of A-bomb survivors. 9. Mortality, 1950–1985: part 3. Non-cancer mortality based on the revised doses (DS 86). *Radiat Res* 1992; **130**: 249–66. (RERF TR 2–91, 1991).
26.   Wong FL, Yamada M, Sasaki H, *et al.* Non-cancer disease incidence in the atomic bomb survivors: 1958–1986. *Radiat Res* 19993; **135**: 418–30. (RERF TR 1–92, 992).
27.   Thompson DE, Mabuchi K, Ron E, *et al.* Cancer incidence in atomic bomb survivors. Part II: Solid tumors, 1958–87. *Radiat Res* 1994; **137**: S17–67.

10

Gynecologic
Diseases

10 GYNECOLOGIC DISEASES

INTRODUCTION

The ovaries are considered to be the most radiosensitive organs, and hence obviously suffered damage when exposed to atomic bomb radiation. A study of the damage inflicted on the female reproductive tract had already begun around September 1945, with the details presented in the "Collection of the Reports on the Investigation of the Atomic Bomb Casualties"[1,2]. Several reports subsequently appeared, including several at the Atomic Bomb Casualty Commission (ABCC), commencing in 1949[3]. This chapter concentrates mainly on the effects of atomic bomb radiation on menstruation, fertility and childbirth.

1. EFFECTS ON MENSTRUATION

A discussion of the effects on menstruation includes post-bombing amenorrhea, and the ages at menarche and menopause, etc.

Detailed studies were performed by Tokyo University on 504 cases in Hiroshima between early September and November 1945, comparing the menstrual disorder rates with respect to distance from the atomic bomb[2]; the rates were found to range from 61.7 to 100% within 2.5 km of the hypocenter (Table 1). The amenorrhea rate was inversely proportional to the distance from the hypocenter, with many cases observed immediately after exposure, and with ovary damage being serious and soon manifested. Table 2 shows the recovery observed by March 1946; overall 78.4% had

Table 1 Relationship between type of abnormality and distance from the hypocenter (subjects studied by November 1945)[2]

Type / Distance from hypocenter (km)	Normal Type I	Abnormal					Total
		Type II	Type III	Type IV	Type V	No. and percentage of abnormalities (%)	
~ 0.5	0	1	2	0	1	4 (100.0%)	4
0.5 ~ 1.0	6	20	4	2	2	28 (82.3%)	34
1.0 ~ 1.5	28	73	24	4	9	110 (79.7%)	138
1.5 ~ 2.0	42	81	31	6	16	134 (76.1%)	176
2.0 ~ 2.5	39	35	13	3	12	63 (61.7%)	102
2.5 ~ 3.0	19	8	1	2	5	16 (45.7%)	35
3.0 ~ 3.5	5	2	1	1	0	4 (44.4%)	9
3.5 ~ 4.0	1	1	0	0	0	1	2
4.0 ~ 4.5	1	0	1	0	0	1	2
4.5 ~ 5.0	2	0	0	0	0	0	2
Total	143 (28.3)	221	77	18	45	361 (71.7%)	504

I : Normal
II : Amenorrhea immediately following bombing
III : One post-bombing menstrual cycle, followed by amenorrhea
IV : Two post-bombing menstrual cycles, followed by amenorrhea
V : Menstruatio praecox, menstruatio tarda, and metrorrhagia

Table 2   Relationship between recovery and both type of abnormality and distance from the hypocenter (until March 1946)[2]

Distance from hypocenter (km)	Normal Type I	Abnormal							Total
		Type II	Type III	Type IV	Type V	Number of abnormalities	Percentage of recoveries		
~ 0.5									
0.5 ~ 1.0	3	10 (3)	1 (0)	2 (2)	2 (1)	15 (6)	(40.0)		18
1.0 ~ 1.5	10 S1	20 (16) S1	9 (6)		3 (2)	32 (24)	(75.0)		42 S2
1.5 ~ 2.0	15	25 (24) S2	11 (9) S1	1 (1)	6 (6)	43 (40)	(93.0)		58 S3
2.0 ~ 2.5	24 S1	10 (8)	6 (5)	1 (1)	8 (8)	25 (22)	(88.0)		49 S1
2.5 ~ 3.0	6	4 (3)	1 (0)	1 (1)	3 (2)	9 (6)	(66.7)		15
3.0 ~ 3.5	2	1 (0)				1 (0)			3
3.5 ~ 4.0	1								1
4.0 ~ 4.5	1								1
4.5 ~ 5.0	1								1
Total	63 S2	70 (54) S3	28 (20) S1	5 (5)	22 (19)	125 (98)	(78.4)		188 S6

Numbers in paratheses indicate the number of cases of recovery
S = no. of pregnant cases

recovered, but the recovery rate worsened with increasing proximity to the hypocenter, i.e. the recovery rate decreased with an increase in radiation dose.

Sawada[3] studied 880 survivors directly exposed within 2.0 km of the hypocenter who were examined at the ABCC between 1949 and 1957, and found that approximately half had exhibited amenorrhea immediately after exposure, with the amenorrhea rate being high among women aged ≥ 40 at the time of bombing (ATB). Among the women who exhibited symptoms of acute radiation illness, the rate of amenorrhea was 69.0%, whereas among the survivors who did not display the symptoms the figure was 33.7%. The rate was thus clearly high among the population exhibiting acute symptoms.

Tabuchi[4,5] conducted a study starting in 1951 on exposed female survivors in the cities of Hiroshima, Otake and Kure (Table 3). Compared to the studies performed immediately following the atomic bombing, the frequency of amenorrhea had decreased, but was over 13 times greater than in the control population. The average duration of amenorrhea was 4–5 months, which was then followed by a resumption of menstruation. All reports state that in many cases ovary function was clearly harmed by exposure to radiation, but that this damage was temporary, with rapid recovery and recommencement of menstruation. However, as will be mentioned later, this marked the start of menopause in some females aged ≥ 40 ATB.

The ovaries suffer temporary damage from radiation exposure, but a problem exists with regard to how this affects the age at menarche. Shoji and Kariya[6] reported in 1946 that the age at menarche was postponed, but Mitani[7,8] reported in a later study on 21,792 exposed girls covering 1947 to 1953 that no definite correlation existed between the age at menarche and distance from the hypocenter. Applying the Kaplan-Meier method, Sawada[3] calculated the average age at menarche for 1,007 girls exposed

Table 3   Menstrual cycle of exposed females[5]

Location of study, and authors	Date of study	Post-bombing amenorrhea			Menarche		Menopause	
		No. of cases	No. of amenorrhea cases	Period of amenorrhea (months)	No. of cases	Average age (yrs.)	No. of cases	Average age (yrs.)
Otake (Nishida)	Aug. 1953	217	92 (42.4%)	4.07 ± 0.78	60	14.08 ± 0.27		
Otake (Mizuno)	Aug. 1956	138	42 (30.4%)	4.4	5	14.10	24	49.2
Hiroshima University (Hamaoka, Akagi)	Jan. 1954				32	13.6		
Kure	Sep. 1955	167	57 (34.7%)	5.37	34	14.91	14	49.0
ABCC patients	Aug. 1954	54	20 (37.0%)	5.2	5	16.4	8	47.5
ABCC (Kadota)	Aug. 1955 Jan. 1951~ Dec. 1954				556	14.45 ± 1.16		
Controls (non-exposed subjects)	Aug. 1954	161	4 (2.4%)		77	13.66 ± 0.36		

within 2.0 km of the hypocenter and also for a control population of 993 girls; no difference was found between the two populations, the ages at menarche being 14.71 years in the exposed population and 14.57 years for the non-exposed girls.

Tabuchi[5] found that radiation had no effect on the average age at menopause. However, Sawada[3] performed a detailed analysis of females undergoing regular examination at the Hiroshima ABCC during the period 1949–54, and found that the age at menopause was low among atomic bomb survivors, especially among those who had exhibited symptoms of acute radiation illness at the time of bombing. The average age at menopause in this latter population was 45.90 years, and 48.55 years among those not displaying the symptoms, figures which were clearly lower than in the control population (49.30 years). Furthermore, of those females who entered menopause immediately following the atomic bombing, the rate was clearly higher among the proximally exposed survivors who exhibited acute radiation illness symptoms.

However, no definite relationship was observed between the frequency of females experiencing early menopause at < 40 years of age and the occurrence of acute radiation illness symptoms. Figure 1 shows a comparison by calendar year of the frequency of menopausal females in the 40–44 and 45–49 year old age groups. Both populations exhibited a conspicuously high maximum in 1945, and it was found that among these, the subjects who displayed acute radiation illness symptoms at the time of bombing exhibited a clearly higher frequency than either the control population or those survivors who did not display the symptoms. Although it is not possible to conclude that this was only due to the direct effect of radiation on the ovaries, the effect is nonetheless believed to be considerable.

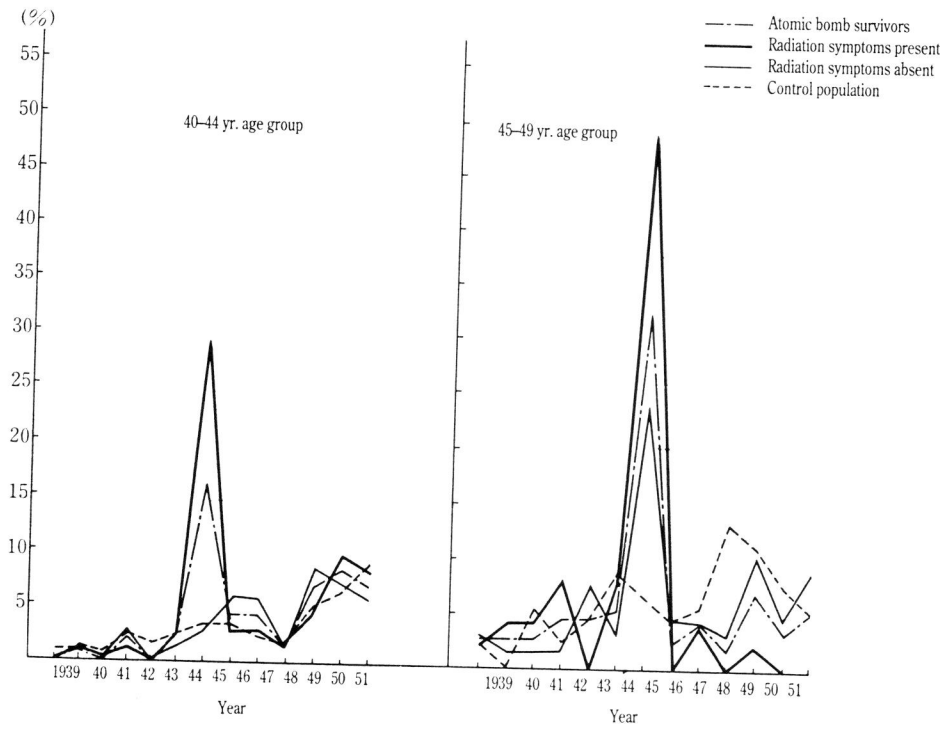

Figure 1   Onset of menopause as a function of year[3]

2. EFFECTS ON PREGNANCY AND CHILDBIRTH

With regard to fertility, in an analysis of delivery rates during 1948–53, Neel et al[9,10] found no difference between atomic bomb survivors and a control population. In an analysis of family registers, Siegel[11] also found no difference between the two populations with respect to either marital age or distance from the hypocenter. Also, the studies by Seto[12] (carried out in 1953 and reported in 1954) of birth and stillbirth registrations in the cities of Hiroshima and Otake, and by Tabuchi[5] in Otake and Kure, both failed to find evidence of high infertility rates among atomic bomb survivors.

An ABCC study by Blot and Sawada[13] over the period 1962–64 also found no definite correlation between radiation dose and female infertility or number of nulliparas; also, among heavily exposed atomic bomb survivors, no evidence was found of high mean pregnancy rates, high birth rates, or long time periods between first pregnancy and first delivery.

With regard to childbirth, although many pregnant females in Hiroshima were evacuated, this occurred with few pregnant atomic bomb survivors. Table 4 shows the results of a study performed on 309 cases up until May 1946[2]. It was found that excluding artificial abortion cases, the miscarriage and stillbirth rate was 6.8% (21

Table 4   Relationship between pregnancy and parturation with distance from the hypocenter[2]

Distance from hypocenter (km)	No. of cases	Effects immediately following bombing	Pregnancy and parturition			
			Incipient abortion	Abortion	Still-births	Term infant
0 ~ 0.5						
0.5 ~ 1.0						
1.0 ~ 1.5	16	1 case of premature birth (at 9 months) 2 cases of incipient abortion (at 3 and 5 months)	6	1		15
1.5 ~ 2.0	49	2 cases of premature birth (at 8 and 9 months) 2 cases of incipient abortion (at 6 and 9 months)	9	3	1	45
2.0 ~ 2.5	85		7	4 (2)	1	80
2.5 ~ 3.0	68		7	3	3	62
3.0 ~ 3.5	20		2	2	1	17
3.5 ~ 4.0	23		2	3		20
4.0 ~ 4.5	18		1			18
4.5 ~ 5.0	14		2		1	13
5.0 ~ 6.0	9					9
6.0 ~ 7.0	7					7
Total	309	3 cases of premature birth, 4 cases of incipient abortion	36	16 (2)	7	286

Number in parentheses indicate number of artificial terminations

cases), which was not high in comparison to the national average, and thus it was concluded that there was no special effect due to radiation exposure.

With respect to the later periods following radiation exposure, Nishida[14] investigated the birth rates among females exposed within 2.0 km of the hypocenter by examining birth and death registers, but also found no difference between exposed females and the control population (Table 5).

In a 1957 study (reported in 1959) Hamaoka[15] investigated infertility (those who experienced spontaneous abortion on two or more occasions during the same stage of gestation) among exposed females. As shown in Table 6, the infertility rate among 643 exposed was 1.24%, against 2.51% in 955 controls, with no difference thus observed between the two groups.

Table 5   Third trimester birth rates among female atomic bomb survivors (per 1,000 female population)[14]

Year	1951		1952		1953		1954		1955 (until Aug. 31st)	
Exposure status Birth rates	Exposed females	Controls	Exposed females	Controls	Exposed females	Controls	Exposed females	Controls	Exposed females	Controls
Female population	9,003	139,808	8,958	146,492	8,904	153,985	8,868	160,101	8,834	172,790
No. of births	347	6,136	339	5,766	350	5,950	292	5,553	152	3,201
Birth rates	38.542	43.888	37.843	39.360	39.308	38.640	32.927	34.684	17.206	18.525

Table 6   Frequency of infertility among female atomic bomb survivors[15]

Location of study	No. of subjects studied	No. of females believed to be capable of pregnancy	No. of infertile females	Overall infertility rate (No. of infertile cases/no. believed capable of pregnancy)	Primary infertility	Secondary infertility
Otake	481	357	2	0.56%	2 (0.28%)	1 (0.28%)
Kure	226	150	4	2.64%	2 (1.32%)	2 (1.32%)
Umida	160	96	1	1.04%	1 (1.04%)	0
Hiroshima	79	40	1	2.50%	0	1 (2.50%)
Total	946	643	8	1.24%	4 (0.62%)	4 (0.62%)
Controls	1,106	955	24	2.51%	10 (1.04%)	14 (1.46%)

CONCLUSION

The gynecologic effects of exposure to atomic bomb radiation can be summarized as follows:

1)   Temporary amenorrhea was observed among survivors exhibiting acute symptoms immediately following exposure, and was common among heavily exposed individuals. The recovery rate from amenorrhea was inversely proportional to the received dose.

2)   Most studies found no difference between the exposed and control populations with respect to the age at menarche.

3)   The age at menopause was clearly lower among atomic bomb survivors who exhibited acute radiation illness symptoms than among those who did not display the symptoms or those in the control population. Furthermore, among those females reaching menopause immediately following the atomic bombing, the rate was clearly higher among those proximally exposed survivors who exhibited acute radiation illness symptoms. However, even though it cannot be concluded that this was only due to the direct effect of radiation on the ovaries, it is nonetheless believed that the effect on the ovaries was considerable.

4)   No difference was observed between the exposed and control populations with respect to fertility, abortion, premature birth, and stillbirth.

(Chikako Ito)

REFERENCES

1.   Mitani Y, Ito M, Nozu S, *et al.* Effects of atomic bomb exposure on female sexual function. *Genshibakudan saigai chousa houkokushu* [Collection of the reports on the investigation of the atomic bomb casualties] Vol. 1. Tokyo: Japan Society for the Promotion of Science, 1953: 735–8. (*In Japanese*)

2.   Mitani Y, Ito M, Nozu S, *et al.* Effects of atomic bomb exposure on female sexual function. *Genshibakudan saigai chousa houkokushu* [Collection of the reports on the investigation of the

atomic bomb casualties] Vol. 2. Tokyo: Japan Society for the Promotion of Science 1953: 738–46. (*In Japanese*)

3. Sawada H. Sexual function of female atomic bomb survivors. *J Hiroshima Med Ass* 1960; **13**: 1158–70. (*In Japanese*)
4. Tabuchi A. Obstetrical and gynecological survey of atomic bomb survivors. *J Hiroshima Med Ass* 1955; **8**: 322–4. (*In Japanese*)
5. Tabuchi A. Obstetrical and gynecological survey of atomic bomb survivors. *J Hiroshima Med Ass* 1959; **12**: 958–65. (*In Japanese*)
6. Shoji T, Kariya Y. Effects of atomic bomb on menstruation of female students. *Obst and Gyn* 1947; **14**: 45–51. (*In Japanese*)
7. Mitani Y. Survey of menarche among female students in Nagasaki, especially effects of the atomic bomb. *J Jap Obst & Gyn* 1953; **5**: 84–90. (*In Japanese*)
8. Mitani Y. Survey of menarche among female students in Nagasaki, especially effects of the atomic bomb (report 2). *Clin Gyn and Obst* 1954; **8**: 71–5. (*In Japanese*)
9. Neel JV, McDonald DJ, Morton NE, *et al.* The effect of exposure to the atomic bombs on pregnancy termination in Hiroshima and Nagasaki. *Science* 1953; **118**: 537–41.
10. Neel JV, Morton NE, Schull WJ, *et al.* The effect of exposure of parents to the atomic bombs on the first generation offspring in Hiroshima and Nagasaki. *Jpn J Genetics* 1953; **28**: 211–8.
11. Seigel DG. Frequency of live birth among survivors of the atomic bombs Hiroshima and Nagasaki. *Radiat Res* 1966; **28**: 278–88.
12. Seto N. Fertility of atomic bomb exposed female survivors. *J Hiroshima Med Ass* 1954; **2**: 864–96.
13. Blot WJ, Sawada H. Fertility among female survivors of the atomic bombs, Hiroshima and Nagasaki. ABCC TR 26–71, 1971.
14. Nishida S. Life span of the atomic bomb survivors. Report 3 for latter period, 1951–55, on birth and stillbirths of the survivors. *J Hiroshima Med Ass* 1957; **10** (Suppl): 35–69.
15. Hamaoka H. Sterility and infertility of women exposed to the atomic bomb. *J Hiroshima Med Ass* 1959; **12** (Suppl): 96–111.

11

Dermatologic Effects

11 KELOIDS

INTRODUCTION

Burns caused by the atomic bomb were characterized by their covering large areas of the body surface, with almost all being second or third degree burns. Mortality rates were extremely high, but even if the victim were fortunate enough to recover, the burns were far greater in size than in usual burn cases, and instead of being restricted to one site, scars formed over various parts of the body. Keloids rose from the skin surface in irregular shapes, copper-colored and shining, with a rubber-like consistency and slight elasticity, and were accompanied by stinging pain and itching[1] (Fig. 1). One to four months after the atomic bomb burns had apparently recovered, scars swelled and keloids developed.

The burn scars in atomic bomb survivors can be classified into scars appearing in the initial period following the bombing and those forming 10 or more years later during the non-active phase[2].

a) INITIAL PERIOD SCARS

The results of studies on initial period scars were:

1. In a series of Tokyo University studies, Hatano and Watanuki[3] reported that initial period scars occurred in 60–70% of burn cases; Harada[4] reported that

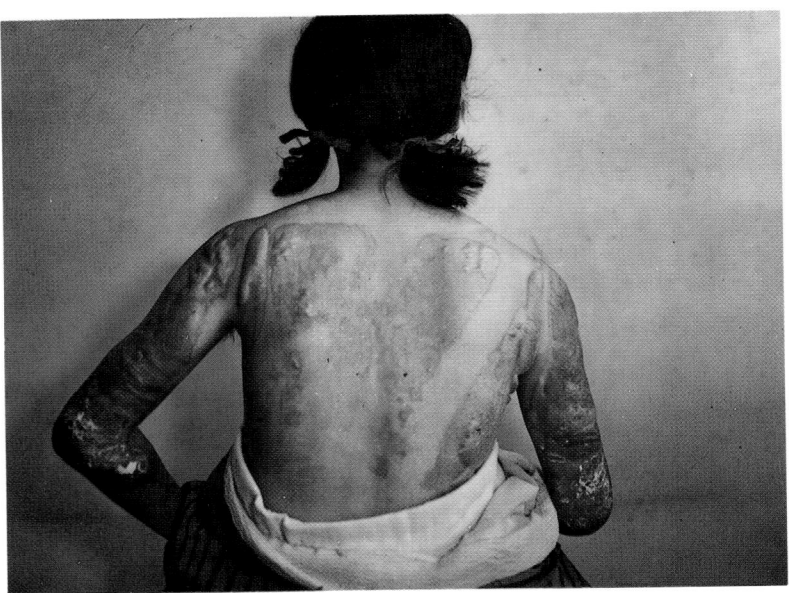

Figure 1   Keloids observed 2 years after exposure

59% had either hypertrophic scars or keloid protrusions of 3 mm or more. These figures are high in comparison with normal burns.

2. The keloid incidence with respect to distance from the hypocenter was at a maximum of 68% among survivors at a distance of 1.4–2.0 km, followed by 50% at 2.0–2.5 km, and 47% at 1.0–1.4 km. The percentage of survivors who suffered bomb burns was greatest at a distance of 1.0–2.5 km, but the point of special interest is that keloids or hypertrophic scars were formed in 50–70% of cases.

3. Keloids frequently occurred on the forearms, upper arms, shoulders, and legs etc., but not often on the hips, back, or thighs; this is thought to be due to clothing cover. Instead of frequent occurrence at particular sites, keloid formation was observed over the whole body.

4. No correlation was observed between keloid incidence and either sex or age.

5. Despite point #4, it has also been reported that keloids frequently occurred among subjects who received burns to 6–15% of the body surface, who were aged 16–20 years, and who required 6–8 months for recovery i.e. individuals burned over a large area and who barely recovered after a long period.

6. Keloid formation was most widespread during 1946–47.

7. When initial period scars underwent early surgery such as resection, recurrence of keloids from the surgical scars was extremely frequent (approximately 80% of cases).

b) NON-ACTIVE PHASE SCARS

Non-active phase scars are those remaining 10 years after the atomic bombing. Studies have shown that:

1. Such scars can be morphologically classified as keloid, hypertrophic, strand-shaped, and contracted scars.

2. Although initial period scars with prominent protrusions of medium or greater size (≥ 33 mm) partially exhibited keloidal type scars during the non-active phase, the majority became reduced to hypertrophic or strand-shaped scars.

3. Post-operative recurrence rates following surgical resection during this period were extremely low ($\leq 25\%$).

Records of the characteristic observations 30–40 years after keloid formation can not be found, but today, approximately half a century after the bombing, burn scars can be observed during examinations; however, most are either slight protrusions or exhibit almost no protrusions, with many having a colored and bleached, mottled condition. However, according to the atomic bomb survivors the burn scars may sometimes display extreme itchiness and stinging pain. When this occurs, the fading scar site is generally said to temporarily possess a definite coloration with the scar boundary becoming distinct. As was mentioned in Chapter 1–8, skin cancers have begun to appear at these thermal burn scar sites.

(Nanao Kamada)

REFERENCES

1. Wells W, Tsukifuji N. Scars remaining in atomic bomb survivors. *Surg Gynec Obstet* 1952; **65**: 129–41.
2. Harada T. Characteristics of keloid induced by A-bomb and its treatment. *Proceedings of the First Meeting of the Research Society for Late Effects of Atomic Bomb*; 1959 June 13–14; Hiroshima. Hiroshima: Research Society for Late Effects of Atomic Bomb. 1959: 15–7.
3. Hatano S, Watanuki K. Report on effects of A-bomb in Hiroshima, with special reference to keloid formation. *Medical Report on Atomic Bomb Effects*, compiled by the Special Committee for the Investigation of the Effects of the Atomic Bomb, National Research Council of Japan, Japan Society for the Promotion of Science. Tokyo; 1953: 621–31.
4. Harada T. Burns and scars induced by A-bomb, with special reference to keloid formation. *Proceedings of the 7th Meeting of the Research Society for Late Effects of Atomic Bomb*; 1965 Oct 16–17; Hiroshima. Hiroshima: Research Society for Late Effects of Atomic Bomb. 1959: 199–203.

12

Musculo-Skeletal
Diseases

12 MUSCULO-SKELETAL DISEASES

INTRODUCTION

In the 4th week after conception the rudiments of the upper and lower limbs appear as mesenchymal tissue protrusions and at approximately 3 months have the external human shape, at which point ossification commences. Longitudinal growth occurs due to proliferation, growth and ossification of the epiphyseal cartilage in the long bone, and this continues until puberty. After the longitudinal growth of bone has ceased, metabolism continues to vigorously perform the cycle of bone formation, maintenance and resorption.

Since bone continues rapid growth until puberty, the effect of radiation on the skeletal system and the damage which is later observed depends on the age at which exposure occurs.

Few reports have appeared concerning musculo-skeletal diseases in atomic bomb survivors. This chapter discusses bone tumors, and considers the effects of radiation exposure with respect to the period of life at which exposure occurred (the fetal period, the period to the end of puberty, and the adult period).

1. BONE TUMORS

The development of radiation-induced bone tumors can be classified into those produced by external irradiation and those caused by long-term internal irradiation from substances that selectively target bone tissue such as radium, plutonium and strontium etc. A famous case involving occupational exposure occurred in 1929 when the development of osteosarcoma was observed in an employee at a factory in which radium etc. was used in the manufacture of luminous watches[1]. The development of osteosarcoma following X-ray therapy was first reported in the 1920s; many reports later appeared concerning the effects of external irradiation. It was reported that osteosarcomas are induced by large doses (≥ 10 Gy) of external X-ray irradiation[2]. However, it was recently reported that an increased incidence also occurred in a population who as children received comparatively low doses of X-rays during treatment for benign diseases[3].

With regard to bone tumors among atomic bomb survivors, Yamamoto and Wakabayashi[4] studied 2,526 autopsy cases in the Atomic Bomb Casualty Commission (ABCC) Life Span Study sample during the period 1950–65, but only 1 case of osteosarcoma was observed, and that occurred in a non-exposed individual. An analysis was also performed based on the death certificates for the mortalities occurring in 1950–85 among the approximately 76,000 subjects in the Life Span Study sample of the ABCC (later the Radiation Effects Research Foundation, RERF); however, this also failed to show a relationship between bone cancer and radiation exposure[5]. The mortality rate in Japan due to cancer of the bone or joints is 0.4 per 100,000; i.e. it is a rare form of cancer[6]. One reason why atomic bomb exposure effects are not observed is that the number of cases is insufficient for a statistical analysis.

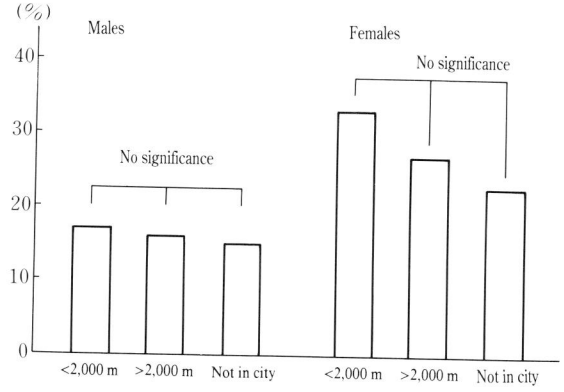

Figure 1   Brachymesophalangism in prenatally exposed children and non-exposed children (from data in Ref. 7)

2. EFFECTS OF PRENATAL EXPOSURE ON BONE TISSUE

Animal experiments have proved that fetal skeleton systems are sensitive to radiation. Since microcephaly among prenatally exposed atomic bomb survivors is discussed in detail in another chapter, the discussion here will be on deformities related to the skeletal system.

In 1951–52, Sutow and West[7] performed an X-ray study in Nagasaki on the skeletal systems of 74 prenatally exposed children and a control population of 91. Neural arch defects, and various bone abnormalities such as those in hand bones, ribs and lumbar-sacral bones, as well as multiple abnormalities, were investigated; however, no difference was observed between the exposed children and the control population. A study was also conducted in Hiroshima on 219 prenatally exposed individuals and a control population of children; bone maturity and the percentages of polydactyly, syndactyly and brachydactyly were investigated, but there were no differences with respect to bone maturity or the rate of finger malformation[8] (Fig. 1). However, both of these studies were performed 6 to 8 years after exposure, and it is possible that abnormalities occurred in fetuses which were aborted or stillborn, and among those who died as infants.

3. EFFECTS OF PRE-PUBERTY EXPOSURE ON BONE TISSUE

It is well-known that bone growth damage results from radiation exposure prior to puberty, a period of vigorous bone growth. For growth development and damage suffered by atomic bomb survivors, see, Chapter 17.

4. EFFECTS OF ADULT EXPOSURE ON BONE TISSUE

Damage produced by adult exposure to a large radiation dose was reported in 1927 in a case in which bilateral hip fractures occurred following radiotherapy for uterocervical carcinoma[9]. Later, Stampfki and Kerr[10] reported that hip fractures occurred in 0.87% of patients 1–3 years after receiving approximately 26 Gy of pelvic irradiation during treatment for malignant gynecologic tumors. Biopsies of the irradiated sites revealed that the trabecula had narrowed and osteoporosis developed, and it was believed that the bone mass had decreased due to radiation-caused damage to the blood circulation and bone cells.

Recently it has become known that in aged patients also osteosclerosis, osteonecrosis and compression fractures are frequently observed side effects following irradiation for malignant gynecologic tumors or irradiation of para-aortic lymph nodes. Rosenthal et al[11] used a computed tomography (CT) scan to measure the spinal bone of a 40-year old male 4 years after undergoing radiotherapy for myeloma, and found that the bone mass in the irradiation field had decreased by approximately 26% relative to other parts. By CT scanning, Hamada et al[12] measured the lumbar vertebrae bone mass of an individual who had undergone irradiation for a malignant gynecologic tumor, and found that the bone mass began to decrease after exposure to 20 Gy, decreasing to approximately 50% after exposure to 50 Gy, with bone metabolism damage indicated soon after irradiation.

With regard to atomic bomb survivors, Blackard and Siegel[13] in 1963 observed osteoporosis during an X-ray study on the femur, hand bones, and vertebrae of 264 individuals under observation at the Hiroshima Atomic Bomb Casualty Commission (ABCC). Although osteoporosis was frequent among females aged 50 or over who were exposed less than 2 km from the hypocenter, the number of subjects was too small for a comparison to be made with various other populations (Table 1).

Fujiwara et al[14] studied approximately 14,000 subjects in the RERF Adult Health Study sample who received chest X-ray examinations between 1958 and 1986, and determined the incidence of thoracic vertebral fractures diagnosed as a result of X-ray examination. No difference was observed between incidence and dose (Table 2).

5. RHEUMATOID ARTHRITIS AND GOUT

Rheumatoid arthritis is the main joint lesion and is a chronic inflammatory disease which frequently involves the connective tissue of the whole body, and is accompanied by immunologic abnormalities. Wood et al[15] performed diagnoses

Table 1   Prevalence of osteoporosis[13]

	Age	Less than 2 km from hypocenter			3.0 ~ 3.5 km from hypocenter or not in city		
		No. of patients	No. of subjects	Prevalence (%)	No. of patients	No. of subjects	Prevalence (%)
Males	< 50 yr.	0	24	0	1	15	6.7
	≥ 50 yr.	1	25	4.0	1	21	4.8
Females	< 50 yr.	2	44	4.5	1	57	1.8
	≥ 50 yr.	14	43	32.6	4	36	11.1

Table 2   Age-adjusted incidence of thoracic vertebral fractures[14]

	Dose (Gy)	Age-adjusted incidence (per 1,000 person years)
Males	0–0.004	2.66
	0.005–0.09	2.87
	0.10–0.99	2.71
	1.00–1.99	2.10
	2 +	2.77
Female	0–0.004	4.09
	0.005–0.09	3.89
	0.10–0.99	4.93
	1.00–1.99	3.78
	2 +	4.02

of rheumatoid arthritis based on the diagnostic criteria proposed by the American Rheumatoid Association on approximately 16,000 subjects examined at the ABCC during the period 1958–64. The prevalence of confirmed rheumatoid arthritis was 0.24% among the population exposed at less than 1,400 m from the hypocenter, 0.36% among the population exposed at $\geq$ 1,400 m, and 0.46% among those not in the city; thus, no significant difference was observed. Furthermore, in order to perform diagnoses of rheumatoid arthritis among subjects examined by the ABCC in Hiroshima and Nagasaki in the period 1965–67, Kato et al[16] additionally took patient histories and tested for rheumatoid factor and syphilis, but these results also showed no difference in prevalence with respect to distance from the hypocenter (Fig. 2). Studying rheumatoid arthritis in inpatients and outpatients, Matsuo et al[17] found no difference between atomic bomb survivors and non-exposed subjects with regard to functional damage and bone changes diagnosed by X-ray examination.

Kato et al.[16] considered gout, but the effect of exposure was not investigated since out of 7,449 subjects in Hiroshima only 3 gout cases were diagnosed.

CONCLUSION

Bones are said to be resistant to radiation; it has been reported that effects result from high-dose irradiation, but at the present time there have been no reports of musculo-skeletal damage among atomic bomb survivors.

There are few cases of musculo-skeletal disease being a direct cause of death, but such disease is related to aging and occurs frequently among old people. With the average age of the atomic bomb survivors already over 60, it is anticipated that the number of people with these diseases will increase, and further research is required.

(*Saeko Fujiwara*)

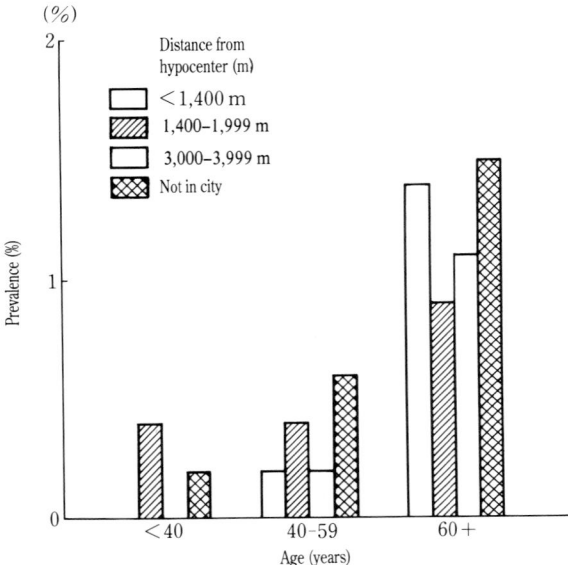

Figure 2   Prevalence of confirmed rheumatoid arthritis (Hiroshima; totals of males & females) (from data in Ref. 16)

REFERENCES

1. Martland HS. Occupational poisoning in manufacture of luminous watch dials. *JAMA* 1929; **92**: 466–73.
2. Tucker MA, D'Angio GJ, Boice JD, *et al.* Bone sarcomas linked to radiotherapy and chemotherapy in children. *New Engl J Med* 1987; **317**: 588–93.
3. Ron E, Modan B, Boice JD. Mortality after radiotherapy for ringworm of the scalp. *Am J Epidemiol* 1988; **127**: 713–25.
4. Yamamoto T, Wakabayashi T. Bone tumor among atomic bomb survivors, Hiroshima-Nagasaki. *Acta Path Jpn* 1969; **19**: 201–12.
5. Shimizu Y, Kato H, Shull WJ. Life Span Study. Report 11. Part 2. Cancer mortality in the years 1950–85 based on the recently revised doses (DS86). *Radiat Res* 1990; **121**: 120–41.
6. Ministry of Health and Welfare. Mortality statistics for malignant neoplasms, 1972–84. (*In Japanese*)
7. Sutow WW, West E. Studies on children exposed *in utero*, Nagasaki: a roentgenological survey of the skeleton system. *J Hiroshima Med Ass* 1953; **16**: 1092–103. (*In Japanese*)
8. Pryde AW, Kitabatake T. Brachyphalangism and brachymetapodia of the hand: a radiological study. ABCC TR 18–59.
9. Baensh W. Knöckenschädigung nach Röntgenbestrahlung. Forschr a.d., *Geb. d. Röntgenstrahlen* 1927; **36**: 1245.
10. Stampfli WP, Kerr HD. Fractures of the femoral neck following pelvic irradiation. *Am J Roentgenol* 1947; **57**: 71–83.
11. Rosenthal DI, Hayes CW, Rosen B, *et al.* Fatty replacement of spinal bone marrow due to radiation: demonstration by dual energy quantitative CT and MR imaging. *J Computer Ass Tomography* 1989; **13**: 463–5.
12. Hamada K, Hori R, Shigekawa K, *et al.* The early changes in bone mineral metabolism due to

radiation measurement of bone mineral density in lumbar vertebra by quantitative computed tomography. *Acta Obst Gynec Jpn* 1991; *43*: 1–7. (*In Japanese*)

13. Blackard WG, Seigel DG. Peripheral osteoporosis. ABCC TR 17–63.
14. Fujiwara S, Mizuno S, Ochi Y, *et al.* The incidence of thoracic vertebral fractures in a Japanese population, Hiroshima and Nagasaki, 1958–86. *J Clin Epidemiol* 1991; **44**: 1007–14.
15. Wood JW, Kato H, Johnson KG, *et al.* Rheumatoid arthritis in Hiroshima and Nagasaki, Japan: prevalence, incidence, and clinical characteristics. *Arthritis Rheumat* 1967; **10**: 21–31.
16. Kato H, Duff IF, Russell WJ, *et al.* Rheumatoid arthritis and gout in Hiroshima and Nagasaki, Japan. A prevalence and incidence study. *J Chron Dis* 1971; **23**: 659–79.
17. Matsuo K, Shikaya T, Mukai H, *et al.* A comparative study between A-bomb survival group with rheumatoid arthritis and non-exposed group with same disease. *Nagasaki Med J* 1989; **63**: 755–8. (*In Japanese*)

13

Prenatal Exposure

13.1 MICROCEPHALY

INTRODUCTION

Epidemiological and experimental evidence testifies to the harmful effects of ionizing radiation exposure on the developing fetal brain. It is known that actively dividing cells are more sensitive to ionizing radiation than cells which have completed division or differentiated cells which seldom undergo cell division. Based on this fact, studies of great interest were performed on individuals who were exposed to radiation prenatally, when cellular growth is rapid[1,2]. In order to identify and describe the characteristic effects of ionizing radiation on the growth of the embryo and the fetus, the Atomic Bomb Casualty Commission (ABCC) and its successor, the Radiation Effects Research Foundation (RERF), have conducted various studies over many years. Accordingly, the documentation of the deleterious effects of ionizing radiation exposure on human brain development rests largely on the many reports concerning those survivors who were exposed prenatally to the atomic bombs in Hiroshima and Nagasaki[3-7].

Radiation exerts a great effect in causing microcephaly and mental retardation, but in the case of children with small head size without mental retardation, no evidence other than retardation of growth and development was observed[8,9]. Small head size is defined as a head circumference which is more than two standard deviations below the sex- and age-specific mean head size for the entire clinical study population. Microcephaly is a condition of poor development of the brain in which the cranium and cerebral hemisphere are abnormally small. Since it is generally difficult to determine brain size, the relationship with developmental retardation of the brain was investigated by measuring head size. Craniostenosis due to early cranial accretion is usually considered separately (craniostenosis is a condition in which the head remains small due to the skull not becoming large, and although it externally resembles microcephaly, there is no abnormality in the brain). Besides hereditary microcephaly (true microcephaly), other causes of developmental brain damage include exposure during fetal development to oxygen deprivation (embryonic or fetal hypoxemia), toxication, irradiation, infectious diseases (e.g. rubella or cytomegalovirus infection), and maternal environment abnormalities, etc. Microcephaly is frequently accompanied by retardation of mental development and seizures.

1. BRAIN DEVELOPMENT AND GESTATIONAL AGE

The gestational age of prenatally exposed atomic bomb survivors is the most important factor in determining the nature of the insult to the developing brain from exposure to ionizing radiation. Different functions of the primate central nervous system are localized in different structures, with the differentiation of these taking place at different stages of development and over different time periods. Generally the embryonic stage in humans is considered to be the period up to the 8th week

230

after fertilization, and the fetal stage the period from the beginning of the 9th week after fertilization. The formation of human organs is complete by the 8th week after fertilization. However, cerebral development occurs in two phases, with rapid cerebral cortex formation at 8–15 weeks after fertilization (Fig. 1). In fact, Dobbing and Sands[10] reported that the normal number of neurons in the cerebral neocortex of the human adult is generally constant at about the level reached at 16 weeks after fertilization. Therefore, the gestational ages in weeks were grouped so as to reflect the known phases in normal development of the brain. That is, development was classified into four periods from the presumed day of fertilization, i.e., 0–7 weeks, 8–15 weeks, 16–25 weeks, and ≥26 weeks. By the end of the first period, the precursors of the neurons and neuroglia (the principal cells that make up the central nervous system) are mitotically active. In the second period, a rapid increase in the number of neurons occurs, with immature neurons that lose their capacity to divide migrating from the proliferation zone and becoming perennial cells. In the third period, *in situ* cellular differentiation accelerates, the synaptogenesis that commences about the 8th week after fertilization increases, and definitive cyto-architecture of the brain unfolds. The final period consists mainly of continued cytoarchitectural development, cellular differentiation and synaptogenesis.

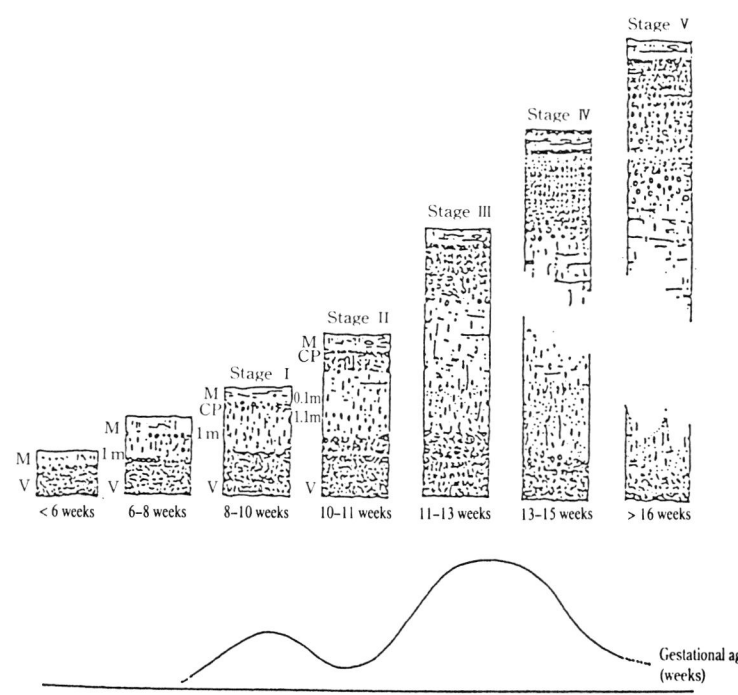

Figure 1   Cortical development of the human cerebrum. The curve at the bottom indicates two waves of cell migrations to the neocortex.

2. STUDY POPULATION OF PRENATALLY EXPOSED ATOMIC BOMB SURVIVORS

The first ABCC population of prenatally exposed atomic bomb survivors was established from materials of the genetic study conducted at the ABCC from 1948 to 1953. It was created in Hiroshima in 1953 and in Nagasaki in 1955, based on the records of births occurring before May 31st 1946 but after the atomic bombing (August 6th 1945 in Hiroshima, August 9th 1945 in Nagasaki)[7]. Due to the importance of clinical and epidemiological studies on this population, the Hiroshima and Nagasaki clinical sample of prenatally exposed atomic bomb survivors was established. The sample was selected on the basis of birth records in the 1950 census and ABCC master files, and taken from all survivors exposed within 2,000 meters of the atomic bomb who were residing within the contact area in Hiroshima and Nagasaki as of October 1st 1950. The comparison groups were matched by sex and age (trimester), and were randomly selected from distally exposed survivors (3,000–4,999 m) and non-exposed survivors ($\geq$ 10,000 m) residing within the contact area. The schoolchildren study population consisted primarily of prenatally exposed schoolchildren enrolled in Hiroshima elementary schools in 1956. Data concerning seizures placed "seizures", "epilepsy" and "convulsions" in the same category. The first examinations were conducted in 1948, with the large majority of the population re-examined at 2-year intervals up until 1964.

3. RESEARCH ON BRAIN DAMAGE AND MICROCEPHALY IN PRENATALLY EXPOSED ATOMIC BOMB SURVIVORS

Early reports referring to research prior to 1970[3-5] indicate an increase in mental retardation and microcephaly with increasing radiation dose, and confirmed the specific biological risk that follows prenatal exposure. However, the early studies were made at a time when it was not possible to assign individual absorbed doses for embryos and fetuses. Subsequently, the estimated fetal absorbed doses became available, and important advances have recently been made in the understanding of the sequence and timing of the presented events culminating in the formation of the human brain[2,10-12].

In 1987 it became possible to use DS86 dose estimates for prenatally exposed survivors[13]. The values referred to in this discussion are based on the DS86 uterine absorbed dose estimates. The former T65DR dosimetry system[14] values for fetal absorbed doses were merely estimates of the maternal shielded kerma multiplied by correction factors averaged over all stages of fetal development[15]. However, the DS86 estimated doses are individually calculated without using average correction factors; thus they allow better for the scattering of radiant energy that occurs within tissues. The DS86 doses can still not be used for the actual fetal doses, and therefore these reports were based on the estimated maternal uterine absorbed doses. Kerr[15] confirmed that there is not a great difference between the fetal dose and estimated maternal uterine dose.

Consideration must be given to the criteria adopted by the ABCC and RERF for determination of severe mental retardation. The selection of severely retarded cases was made on the basis of clinical observations performed at the ABCC clinical facility and not on the basis of intelligence quotient (IQ) scores. The criteria for clinical diagnosis of severe mental retardation were if the child proved "unable to perform simple calculations, to make simple conversation, to care for himself or herself, or if he or she was completely unmanageable or had been institutionalized"[3].

Besides a report on severe mental retardation believed related to brain damage[16], ABCC-RERF reports have also appeared concerning IQ[17], school performance[18] and seizures[19]. An evaluation will be made of the risk to development of the brain, and of the relationship with microcephaly in the low dose range.

Evaluation of data pertaining to prenatally exposed atomic bomb survivors in Hiroshima and Nagasaki concerning the development of severe mental retardation with or without microcephaly, intelligence quotient (IQ), school performance, and seizures, revealed that radiation had a significant effect on brain growth among the survivors exposed prenatally at 8–15 weeks and 16–25 weeks. In particular, severe radiation-related mental retardation occurred in 80% of those exposed prenatally at 8–15 weeks (Fig. 2). A study of the development of unprovoked seizures also found a marked radiation effect at a gestational age of 8–15 weeks (Fig. 3).

Thirty cases of severe mental retardation were clinically detected before they reached 17 years of age. Of these 30 cases, 18 (60%) presented complications of small head size more than two standard deviations below the mean value, and 10 cases (33%) of small head size more than three standard deviations below the mean value. Here, small head size accompanied by severe mental retardation will be broadly considered as microcephaly. Fifteen of the 18 microcephaly cases (83%) were among

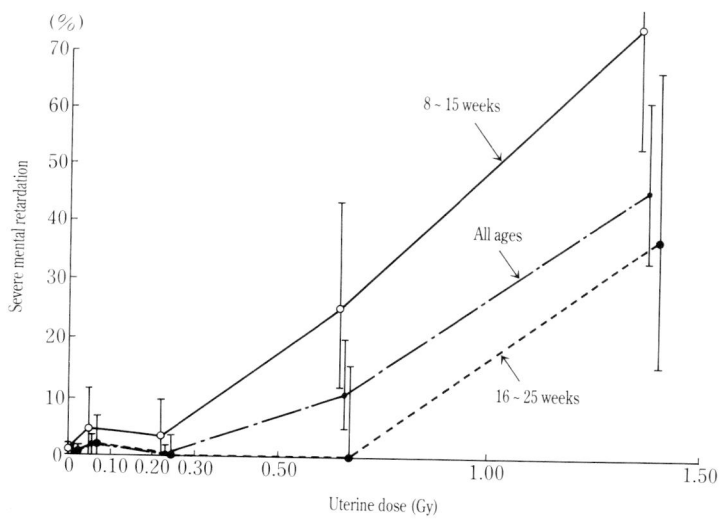

Figure 2   Frequency of severe mental retardation and 90% confidence limits by DS86 uterine absorbed dose and gestational age[29]

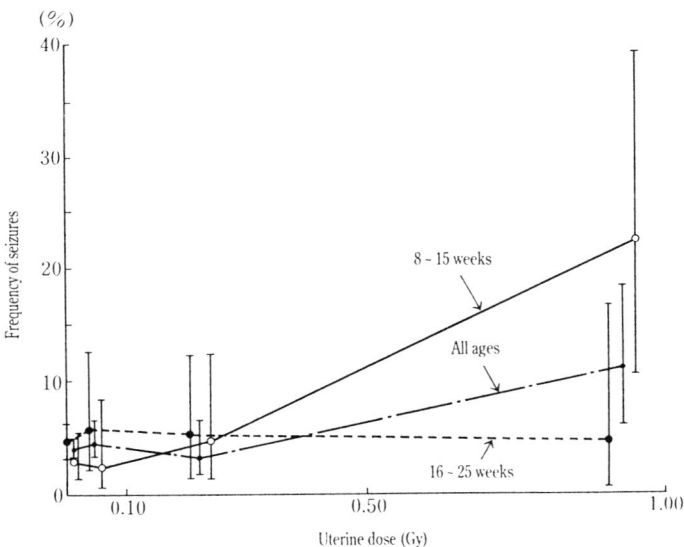

Figure 3   Frequency of seizures and 90% confidence limits by DS86 uterine absorbed dose and gestational age[29]

the survivors exposed at 8–15 weeks after fertilization, the period of maximum radiosensitivity. For a radiation dose of ≥ 0.01 Gy, microcephaly was observed in 15 of the 17 severely mentally retarded cases (88%) in the 8–15 week group, and in 2 of the 4 severely mentally retarded cases (50%) in the 16–25 week group. IQ data was collected in 1955–56 at the Hiroshima and Nagasaki ABCC clinical facilities for prenatally exposed atomic bomb survivors and non-exposed survivors (those over 10,000 meters from the hypocenter). The examinees were 10–11 years old at the time. Of the study subjects, 11 were severely mentally retarded cases, of whom 8 (73%) had an IQ of less than 70, the cases ranging from 56 to 64[17]. In the 8–15 week group (the group clinically found to be at the greatest risk of severe mental retardation) the estimated decrease in IQ score was 21–29 points per 1.0 Gy of DS86 uterine absorbed dose.

School performance data was based on school records of 1st to 4th grade schoolchildren enrolled at 44 elementary schools in Hiroshima city in August and September 1956, including a school for the blind and an orphanage. The prenatally exposed children were aged 10–11 at the time, with the majority having completed 4th grade, and included 14 severely mentally retarded cases. A significant decline in average school performance was observed in the populations prenatally exposed at 8–15 weeks and 16–25 weeks, with the tendency most pronounced in the lower grades. As in the case of severe mental retardation and IQ data, no evidence of a radiation effect on school performance was observed in the children exposed prenatally at gestational ages of less than 8 weeks or more than 26 weeks[18].

Seizures are a common after-effect of developmental damage of the brain, and would therefore be expected to occur more frequently among children suffering radiation-related brain damage than in children without brain damage. Health records pertaining to seizures were procured during regular examinations conducted at 2-year intervals from the age of 2. Seizures were not recorded for atomic bomb survivors exposed prenatally at 0–7 weeks after fertilization, even for exposure to ≥ 0.10 Gy. Their frequency was greatest among the children exposed at 8–15 weeks. Excluding the 22 severely mentally retarded cases, the only significant increase in seizures was found to be in unprovoked seizures[19].

Many studies on brain damage and microcephaly among prenatally exposed atomic bomb survivors in Hiroshima and Nagasaki have reported the harmful effect of radiation exposure. Evaluation of data for the prenatally exposed survivors in Hiroshima and Nagasaki with regard to the development of severe mental retardation (in both the presence and absence of microcephaly)[16], IQ[17], and school performance[18] have shown that the effect of ionizing radiation on brain growth is most significant among those individuals exposed at 8–15 weeks and 16–25 weeks after fertilization. A study on unprovoked seizures[19] also found a marked radiation effect in the same 8–15 week group. Of the 30 cases clinically diagnosed as severely mentally retarded by the age of 17, small head complications were observed in 18 (60%). Microcephaly and mental retardation are prone to induction by radiation, but mentally retarded cases with small head size (i.e. microcephaly) had an average IQ of 63.8 ± 8.5 compared to a score of 68.9 ± 11.9 for mentally retarded cases without small head circumference. The score for small head size without mental retardation was 97.1 ± 20.3, and the average IQ score for the entire study population was 107.8 ± 16.4. Thus no difference was observed between the first two average IQ scores above (i.e. for those with mental retardation), but a large significant difference was observed between these two and children with small head circumference only[20]. Furthermore, other studies revealed a significant decrease in anthropometric measurements (e.g. height, body weight, sitting height, and chest circumference) in children with a small head size in comparison with children who did not have a small head size.

The clinical study population at 18 years of age exhibited a significant linear decrease with increasing dose for each parameter associated with head size, height and body weight[21]. The bones forming the cranial vault are known to develop in close relation with the growth of the brain and dura mater. Dobbing[22] also investigated the relationship between the developing brain and the development of a small head size, with or without the presence of mental retardation. However, it is unknown to what extent microcephaly is a symptom independent of severe mental retardation, and by what mechanism radiation-related damage is caused.

The above risk estimate includes several uncertainties. It is limited by the data available, and in particular the small number of heavily exposed survivors. Besides radiation, other factors can inflict damage on the central nervous system of the embryo and fetus, such as nutritional deprivation, genetic variation, and bacterial and viral infections during pregnancy, for there is substantial evidence to suggest that the cerebrum and its adnexa are especially sensitive to oxygen deprivation[23,24]. Nevertheless, even if these factors are present the prudent course would be to assume that the dose-dependency is not materially altered except additively by these confounders. Due to the various uncertainties, in the determination of the dose-response relationship it would be best to postulate that the risk of nervous system damage is additional, and that there is no dose dependence. Furthermore, no evidence has been found so far suggesting permanent loss of reproductive ability in prenatally exposed atomic bomb survivors[25,26].

CONCLUSION

The developmental process and morphological characteristics of histogenesis of the human cerebral cortex are said to be basically the same as in other mammals. It is of great interest that the period of high susceptibility of the cerebral cortex to developmental damage noted in epidemiological studies on prenatally exposed atomic bomb survivors is consistent with experimental results involving irradiated mice[27].

The estimation of a threshold for atomic bomb survivors exposed prenatally to low doses is also of interest from the viewpoint of radiation protection. In the recent series of analyses based on DS86 uterine absorbed doses, data pertaining to severe mental retardation with or without microcephaly, IQ, and school performance show radiation to have a definite deleterious effect on the brain only in the case of individuals exposed prenatally at a gestational age of 8–15 weeks or 16–25 weeks. However, excluding the severely mentally retarded cases, the frequency and risk of seizures are unclear. The occurrence of severe mental retardation in these populations seems to suggest a threshold for the DS86 uterine absorbed dose in the low-dose region. It is still unclear whether a threshold exists for those exposed at 8–15 weeks after fertilization, but of the 19 severely mentally retarded cases belonging to this population, excluding two probable non-radiation-related cases of Down's syndrome, who were respectively exposed to DS86 doses of 0.29 Gy and 0.56 Gy, the estimated threshold under DS86 dosimetry ranged from 0.39 Gy (with a 95% lower bound of 0.12 Gy) to 0.46 Gy (95% lower bound = 0.23 Gy), both of which differ significantly from zero. A regression analysis of IQ and school performance data indicates a linear relationship, although variations in the means of the IQ and school performance scores in the low dose region resemble those in the control group, particularly for doses of ≤ 0.10 Gy. On the other hand, the risk of severe mental retardation among survivors exposed at 16–25 weeks after fertilization is related linear-quadratically or quadratically to the uterine absorbed dose for the population for whom DS86 doses were available. Using a linear model, the threshold value for this period has an estimated 95% lower bound in the neighborhood of 0.21 Gy. With respect to determination of thresholds for a radiation effect on the developing central nervous system, it is necessary to perform further systematic studies involving animal experiments etc. that consider the relationship between the stage of cranial formation and the gestational age at exposure, and the brain site and type of damage produced, etc.

(*Masanori Otake*)

REFERENCES

1. United Nations Scientific Committee on Effects of Atomic Radiation (UNSCEAR). Genetic and somatic effects of ionizing radiation. New York: United Nations, 1986: 263–366.
2. International Committee for Radiological Protection. Developmental effects of irradiation on the brain of the embryo and fetus. ICRP publication 49. Oxford: Pergamon Press, 1986: 1–43.
3. Wood JW, Johnson KG, Omori Y, *et al.* Mental retardation in children exposed *in utero*, Hiroshima and Nagasaki. *Am J Public Health* 1967; **57**: 1381–90. (ABCC TR 10–66).
4. Blot WJ. Review of thirty years study of Hiroshima and Nagasaki atomic bomb survivors. II. Biological effect. C. Growth and development following prenatal and children exposure to atomic radiation. *J Radiat Res* 1975; **16** (Suppl): 82–8.
5. Miller RW, Mulvihill JH. Small head size after atomic irradiation. *Teratology* 1956; **14**: 355–8.
6. Otake M, Schull WJ. *In utero* exposure to A-bomb radiation and mental retardation. A reassessment. *Brit J Radiol* 1984; **57**: 409–14. (RERF TR 1–83).
7. Schull WJ, Otake M. Effects on intelligence of prenatal exposure to ionizing radiation. RERF TR 7–86, 1986.
8. Wood JW, Johnson KG, Omori Y. *In utero* exposure to the Hiroshima atomic bomb. An evaluation of head size and mental retardation; 20 years later. *Pediatrics* 1967; **39**: 385–92. (ABCC TR 9–65).
9. Tabuchi A, Hirai T, Nakagawa S, *et al.* Clinical findings on *in utero* exposed microcephalic children. ABCC TR 28–67, 1967.
10. Dobbing J, Sands J. Quantitative growth and development of human brain. *Arch Dis Child* 1973; **48**: 757–67.
11. Rakic P. Cell migration and neuronal ectopias in the brain. In: Bergsma D, editor. Morphogenesis and malformation of the face and brain. New York: Alan Liss, 1975: 95–129.
12. Kameyama Y. High vulnerability of the developing fetal brain to ionizing radiation and hyperthermia. *Environmental Med* 1989; **33**: 1–17.
13. Roesch WC, editor. Reassessment of atomic bomb radiation dosimetry in Hiroshima and Nagasaki. Final Report, Vol. 1 and 2. Hiroshima: Radiation Effects Research Foundation, 1987.
14. Milton RC, Shohoji T. Tentative 1965 radiation dose estimation for atomic bomb survivors, Hiroshima and Nagasaki. ABCC TR 1–68, 1968.
15. Kerr GD. Organ dose estimates for the Japanese atomic bomb survivors. *Health Physics* 1979; **37**: 487–508.
16. Otake M, Yoshimaru H, Schull WJ. Severe mental retardation among the prenatally exposed survivors of atomic bombing of Hiroshima and Nagasaki: a comparison of the T65DR and DS86 dosimetry systems. RERF TR 16–87, 1987.
17. Schull WJ, Otake M, Yoshimaru H. Effect on intelligence test score of prenatal exposure to ionizing radiation in Hiroshima and Nagasaki: a comparison of the T65DR and DS86 dosimetry systems. RERF TR 3–88, 1988.
18. Otake M, Schull WJ, Fujikoshi Y, *et al.* Effect on school performance of prenatal exposure to ionizing radiation in Hiroshima: a comparison of the T65DR and DS86 dosimetry systems. RERF TR 2–88, 1988.
19. Dunn K, Yoshimaru H, Otake M, Schull WJ. Prenatal exposure to ionizing radiation and subsequent development of seizures. *Am J Epidemiol* 1990; **131**: 114–23.
20. Otake M, Schull WJ. Radiation-related small head sizes among prenatally exposed A-bomb survivors. *Int J Radiat Biol* 1993; **63**: 255–270.
21. Ishimaru T, Nakajima E, Kawamoto S. Relationship of height, weight, head circumference, and chest circumference at age 18, to gamma and neutron doses among *in utero* exposed children, Hiroshima and Nagasaki. RERF TR 19–84, 1984.
22. Dobbing J. The pathogenesis of microcephly with mental retardation. In: European Atomic Energy Community-8067. Effects of prenatal irradiation with special emphasis on late effects. 1984: 199–212.
23. Winick M. Malnutrition and brain development. In: Winick M, editor. Nutrition: pre- and postnatal development. New York: Plenum Press, 1979: 41–59.

24. Mole RH. Consequences of prenatal radiation exposure for postnatal development: a review. *Int J Radiat Biol* 1982; **42**: 1–12.

25. Blot WJ, Moriyama IM, Miller RW. Reproductive potential of males exposed *in utero* or prepubertally to atomic radiation. ABCC TR 39–72, 1972.

26. Blot WJ, Shimizu Y, Kato H, *et al.* Frequency of marriage and live birth among survivors prenatally exposed to the atomic bomb. *Am J Epidemiol* 1975; **102**: 128–36.

27. Hoshino K, Kameyama Y. Development-stage-dependent radiosensitivity of neural cells in the ventricular zone of telencephalon in mouse and rat fetuses. *Teratology* 1988; **37**: 257–62.

28. Sidman RL, Rakic P. Neuronal migration, with special reference to developing human brain: a review. *Brain Res* 1973; **62**: 1–35.

29. Otake M, Yoshimaru H, Schull WJ. Prenatal exposure to atomic radiation and brain damage. *Cong Anom* 1989; **29**: 309–20.

13.2 MORTALITY RATES AND CANCER INCIDENCE IN PRENATALLY EXPOSED ATOMIC BOMB SURVIVORS

INTRODUCTION

In addition to radiation, the atomic bomb caused physical injury due to the bomb blast and heat emission, which together with wartime socioeconomic impoverishment (and food shortages in particular) adversely affected the health of pregnant women and their fetuses[1]. However, it is difficult in the case of fetal exposure to the atomic bomb to accurately clarify pregnancy-terminating abnormalities such as abortions and stillbirths etc. due to insufficient data resulting from the postwar confusion.

Examinations performed up to the age of 17 showed increased brain damage among prenatally exposed atomic bomb survivors. In particular, approximately two-thirds of the 30 cases of severe mental retardation were observed among those exposed at a gestational age of 8–15 weeks[2]. It is known that atomic bomb radiation inhibited brain development during the embryologically important period in which neurons proliferate and migrate from the proliferative zones to the cerebral cortex.

The late effects of atomic bomb radiation on mortality rates and cancer incidence among liveborn prenatally exposed atomic bomb survivors have not yet been clarified[3,4]. However, there will be interest in whether an increase occurs in the rates after middle age. For mortality rates, as with other atomic bomb survivors, studies are being carried out to verify whether life spans are being reduced by specific and non-specific fatal diseases. It was feared that the survivors who were aged under 40 at the time of bombing (ATB) and who were exposed to high doses (≥ 2.0 Gy) would exhibit an increased mortality rate from non-malignant diseases starting from 20 years following the bombing[5].

Fairly concrete evidence exists of the carcinogenic effect of prenatal irradiation. Increased childhood cancer is frequently observed following irradiation of the pregnant mother for diagnostic purposes[6]. Radiation-induced tumors (in the lung and pituitary gland etc.) have been observed with mouse fetuses irradiated in the late uterine stage[7], and it has been suggested that prenatal irradiation of mice generally increases the likelihood of tumor development (e.g. in the lung) due to postnatal exposure to chemical substances[8].

This chapter considers mortality rates and cancer incidence in prenatally exposed atomic bomb survivors. In particular, emphasis will be placed on comparisons with the survivors exposed at a young age (< 10 years ATB), who are generally believed to face a greater risk of radiation-induced cancer.

1. POPULATION STUDIED IN THE "MORTALITY STUDY OF CHILDREN EXPOSED *IN UTERO*"

The Radiation Effects Research Foundation (RERF) defines prenatally exposed atomic bomb survivors as individuals who were exposed to atomic bomb radiation while in the womb and who were born during the period between the atomic explosion (August 6th 1945 in Hiroshima, and August 9th 1945 in Nagasaki) and May 31st 1946[9]. Of the approximately 2,800 subjects in the mortality study, this review will not consider those children who were not present in either city at the time of bombing; the subject population therefore consists of approximately 1,800 individuals (Table 1). The mortality data for the first 5 years of life is limited to 1,263 subjects selected from birth records. Apart from birth records, prenatally exposed survivors were also selected from the RERF master file and from data in the 1960 Atomic Bomb Survivors Survey.

The overwhelming majority were prenatally exposed survivors from Hiroshima (1,534 subjects, 85.7%), with few from Nagasaki. The mortality rates and cancer incidence were investigated with respect to the trimester of pregnancy at exposure based on the date of birth, i.e. first trimester (date of birth February–May 1946), second trimester (November 1945–January 1946), and third trimester (August–October 1945).

Since the new DS86 dosimetry system does not provide an estimate of fetal absorbed dose, the total maternal uterine absorbed dose of neutrons and gamma rays was used. Although the uterine dose seems to be close to the fetal dose during the third trimester, the value in the first trimester may be excessive. The 0 Gy population consisted of 772 subjects; the significantly exposed population ($\geqslant 0.01$ Gy) was composed of 1,019 subjects, with an average dose of 0.302 Gy.

2. REASONS FOR THE LOW NUMBER OF PRENATALLY EXPOSED ATOMIC BOMB SURVIVORS IN NAGASAKI

The original population for the "Mortality Study of Children Exposed *In Utero*" consisted of approximately 5,300 survivors prenatally exposed within 10 km of the hypocenter (the total area of the former city boundaries) (Table 2), with the Hiroshima : Nagasaki ratio being 1.30 : 1.00[9]. However, the number of prenatally exposed

Table 1   Subjects in the population of the Mortality Study of Children Exposed *In Utero*

Number of subjects		1,791 (1,630)
City	Hiroshima	1,534 (1,401)
	Nagasaki	257 (229)
Sex	Male	852 (765)
	Female	939 (865)
Data source	Birth records	1,263 (1,102)
	Others	528 (528)
Pregnancy trimester	1st trimester	574 (532)
(at the time of bombing)	2nd trimester	687 (622)
	3rd trimester	530 (476)
Maternal uterine dose	0 Gy	772 (710)
	$\geqslant 0.01$ Gy	1,019 (920)
		[0.302 Gy]

(   ) : Number of survivors in October 1950
[   ] : Average dose $\geqslant 0.01$ Sv

Table 2 Comparison by city of prenatally exposed atomic bomb survivors and female survivors aged 20–39 at the time of bombing (ATB)

Prenatally exposed survivors					Female survivors (aged 20–39 ATB)				
Distance from hypocenter (km)	Total	Hiroshima (H)	Nagasaki (N)	Ratio of Hiroshima/ Nagasaki (km)	Distance from hypocenter (km)	Total	Hiroshima (H)	Nagasaki (N)	Ratio of Hiroshima/ Nagasaki H/N
< 1.50	471	398	73	5.45	< 1.00	273	204	69	2.96
1.50–1.99	647	541	106	5.10	1.00–1.39	1,455	1,138	317	3.59
2.00–2.99	1,267	822	445	1.85	1.40–1.99	1,3,640	2,916	724	4.03
3.00–9.99	2,988	1,279	1,709	0.75	2.00–2.49	3,035	2,199	836	2.63
Total	5,373	3,040	2,333	1.33					

1. Prenatally exposed survivors amended from the ABCC TR 13–66 report. For distances greater than 2 km, figures include subjects not selected in the prenatally exposed survivor mortality study sample.
2. Female survivors amended from the ABCC TR 15–63 report. For distances greater than 2.5 km, figures are omitted due to the method of selection. The report states that the numbers of proximally exposed subjects (> 2.5 km) in Hiroshima and Nagasaki were respectively 21,339 and 6,803; the Hiroshima: Nagasaki ratio was therefore 3 : 1.

survivors in Nagasaki receiving proximal exposure was exceedingly small. Table 1 reflects the fact that the population of the above study was selected from those survivors prenatally exposed within 4 km of the hypocenter in such a way as to reflect the ratio of proximally exposed survivors (those exposed within 1.5 km of the bomb) observed between the two cities.

The number of proximally exposed atomic bomb survivors in the RERF Life Span Study sample (those exposed within 2.0 km) was approximately 3 times greater in Hiroshima than in Nagasaki (see notes in Table 2)[10], with a higher value observed for survivors exposed both proximally and prenatally. For female survivors aged 20–39 ATB, the ratio between Hiroshima and Nagasaki exceeded 3.0 for the population exposed at 1.00–1.99 km from the hypocenter (Table 2)[10], but this is an inadequate explanation for the inter-city difference regarding prenatally exposed survivors. The explanation probably lies in the bias observed between the cities in the selection of the proximally exposed subjects of the Life Span Study sample, or in differences between the cities with respect to the number of pregnant women evacuated before the bombing, the geographical distribution of residential areas, and socioeconomic factors.

3. MORTALITY STUDIES

Confirmation of whether subjects were alive or dead was obtained from Japanese family registers, with the causes of death ascertained from death certificates. For individuals with Japanese nationality, confirmation of death was possible in 99% of cases.

The first attempts to study the causes of death among prenatally exposed atomic bomb survivors were carried out retrospectively in the 1960s[10]. Consequently, it was not possible to ascertain the cause of death for 50 (31%) of the total of 161 individuals who were identified from birth records but who died between 1945 and September 1950. Although many of the unknown causes of death occurred among infants, no cancer deaths were confirmed until 1950.

As shown in Fig. 1, the total number of deaths to date is 237, of whom 43.9% (104 subjects) died during infancy (under 1 year old)[4]. The most recent mortality rate data for prenatally exposed atomic bomb survivors covered up to 1984 (when the subjects were aged 39 years), and was summarized in a 1988 RERF report on cancer incidence. In comparison with the 0 Gy maternal uterine dose population, the ≤ 0.60 Gy population exhibited high mortality rates both as infants and in the 15–39 age range (even excluding cancer deaths).

The observed infant mortality rate in the ≥ 0.60 Gy population was 3 times greater than in the 0 Gy population (i.e. a relative risk of 3) (Table 3). Unfortunately, during the immediate postwar period the confusion surrounding population movement and mortality statistics made accurate ascertainment of the causes of death during infancy extremely difficult. However, up to 12 of the 18 infant deaths in the ≥ 0.60 Gy population occurred among survivors exposed during the third trimester, indicating the possibility that instead of an increase in specific fatal diseases due to the atomic bomb radiation, the increase in infant mortality was due to physical injuries inflicted by the bomb.

With regard to the mortality rate in the 15–39 age bracket in the ≥ 0.60 Gy population, the number of deaths is still low, and no causal relationship has been established between atomic bomb radiation and specific causes of death. Also, although a definite increase due to atomic bomb radiation can be observed in the frequency of severe mental retardation among prenatally exposed survivors, there is no evidence indicating a relationship between the mortality rate among these cases and an increase in mortality rate in the 15–39 age bracket for the same population.

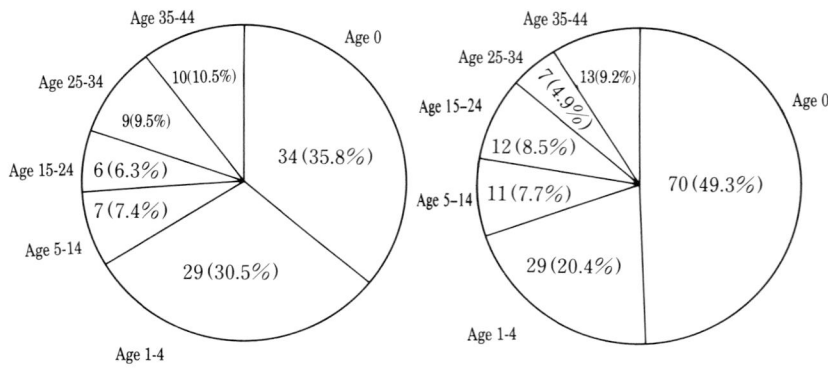

95 deaths observed in 772 subjects (100%)   142 deaths observed in 1,019 subjects (100%)

Figure 1   Number of deaths among prenatally exposed atomic bomb survivors by age at the time of death (1945–89)

Table 3 Infant mortalities (under age 1) among prenatally exposed survivors identified from birth records

	Maternal uterine dose (GY)				
	0	0.01–0.29	0.30 ~ 0.59	≥ 0.60	Total
Subjects	510	542	112	99	1,263
Infant mortalities	34	43	9	18	104
Expected infant mortalities	39.8	41.7	8.8	6.9	97.2
Relative risk	1.00	1.21	1.20	3.05*	

Expected number of infant mortalities calculated from mortality rates for all Japan.
*Null hypothesis: the ratio of observed to predicted numbers = 1, $P < 0.01$.

Two of the deaths in the 15–39 age bracket among the ≥ 0.60 Gy population occurred in severely mentally retarded cases (the causes of death being meningitis and renal insufficiency), but further investigation will be required to determine whether the increase was accidental, the result of confounding factors other than radiation (such as socioeconomic factors etc.), or due to the adverse health effects of atomic bomb radiation.

4. CANCER INCIDENCE STUDIES

The cancer incidence among prenatally exposed atomic bomb survivors was first reported in 1967 as part of a study on leukemia in the children of atomic bomb survivors[11]. A 1970 report[12] described the cancer mortality rate among prenatally exposed survivors aged under 10, with further results appearing in another study on leukemia among children of atomic bomb survivors (1981)[13]. These leukemia and mortality studies showed no increased cancer incidence among prenatally exposed survivors as a result of atomic bomb radiation.

Cancer cases are currently confirmed from the cause of death listed on the death certificates and from the tumor registries supervised by the medical societies of Hiroshima and Nagasaki. Although ascertainment of fatal cancer cases is possible for all time periods and for all regions of Japan, ascertainment of non-fatal cancer cases is restricted to those individuals within the tumor registry areas after 1958, the date when compilation of the registries commenced. It was assumed that the frequency at which the reporting of "overlooked" tumors (due to migration) did not correlate with parental radiation doses.

The cancer incidence among prenatally exposed atomic bomb survivors in the period 1950–84 was reported in 1988 (Table 1), and included cases in the above-mentioned mortality and leukemia studies. Table 4 summarizes those results. Thirteen cancer cases in the 6–38 year old age bracket were confirmed in the ≥ 0.01 Gy population, and 5 cases in the 0 Gy population. The increase in total cancer incidence among prenatally exposed survivors with increasing radiation dose was found to show marginal statistical significance (p = 0.03), but no particular relation-

Table 4 Cancer risk for prenatally exposed survivors and survivors exposed site young (under 10 years at the time of bombing, ATB)

	Prenatally exposed survivors cancer incidence (1950–84)		Survivors exposed while young cancer mortalities (1950–85)	
	Maternal uterine dose (Gy)		Kerma dose (Gy)	
	0	≥ 0.01	0	≥ 0.01
Subjects	710	920	6,901	8,994
Cancer cases	5 (0)	13 (2)	49 (7)	93 (24)
Relative risk at 1 Gy	All cancer sites	3.77	Leukemia	17.1
			Other cancers	2.35
Excess absolute risk	All cancer sites	6.57	Leukemia	2.93
			Other cancers	2.29

Figures in parentheses indicate number of leukemia cases.
Excess absolute risk is calculated per 10,000 person years per 1 Gy.

ship was observed between the cancer cases and the stage of pregnancy at which exposure occurred.

The study found only 2 cases of childhood cancer (at ages of under 15 years) among the prenatally exposed, both of whom were exposed to a maternal uterine dose of ≥ 0.30 Gy. The first was a 6-year-old with liver cancer who was reported to have severe mental retardation; the mother is believed to have received a uterine dose of 1.39 Gy during the first trimester of pregnancy (at 8 weeks after fertilization). The second was a Wilms tumor patient aged 14 whose mother is believed to have received a uterine dose of 1.56 Gy during the second trimester.

Only 2 leukemia cases were observed, with both mothers estimated to have received uterine doses of ≤ 0.05 Gy. One was an 18-year-old girl with acute myelocytic leukemia whose mother was exposed during the third trimester; the other was a 29-year-old man with acute lymphocytic leukemia whose mother was exposed during the first trimester.

A comparison of cancer incidence between prenatally exposed survivors and survivors exposed immediately after birth (aged 0–1 ATB) would provide precise data regarding the relationship between radiosensitivity and the development of cancer. However, no data concerning cancer incidence among survivors aged 0–1 ATB has yet been published. Table 4 shows a comparison with cancer mortality for survivors exposed while young (aged under 10 ATB). A consideration of the relative and absolute risks shows that the cancer risk from prenatal exposure is at most of the same order as for survivors exposed at under 10 years ATB.

If it is supposed that cancer is also induced by prenatal exposure to radiation, then it is believed that the primary factor for leukemia is the latency period for the particular type of leukemia[14], and that the primary factor for solid tumors is the age at which solid tumors frequently occur at a specific site. No specificity is currently observable among cancer cases in prenatally exposed survivors with respect to either cancer site or the trimester in which exposure occurred. It is expected that at least one-fifth of the ≥ 0.01 Gy population who are still alive will eventually develop cancer. Consequently, the cumulative total of 13 cancer cases as of 1984 would be less than 10% of the final cumulative lifetime total, and the epidemiological data presently available is still inadequate. It is therefore important to carry out further studies on the cancer incidence among prenatally exposed atomic bomb survivors.

CONCLUSION

Due to their uniqueness, the number of prenatally exposed atomic bomb survivors is small. In order to evaluate the effect of atomic bomb radiation on the mortality rates and cancer incidence among prenatally exposed survivors after reaching adulthood, it is important to make comparisons with survivors exposed at a young age, and particularly those exposed during infancy. Figure 2 summarizes various characteristics for the different pregnancy trimesters and for the first 10 years of life[15,16].

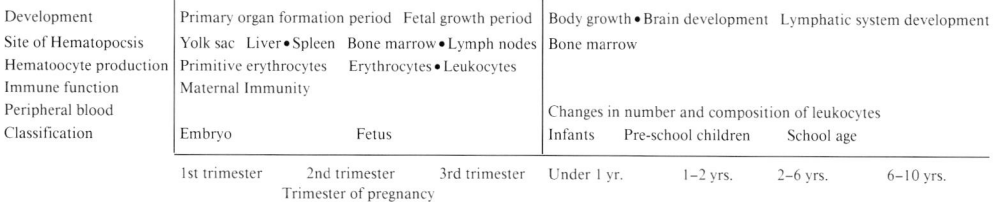

Development	Primary organ formation period	Fetal growth period	Body growth • Brain development	Lymphatic system development
Site of Hematopocsis	Yolk sac Liver • Spleen	Bone marrow • Lymph nodes	Bone marrow	
Hematoocyte production	Primitive erythrocytes	Erythrocytes • Leukocytes		
Immune function	Maternal Immunity			
Peripheral blood			Changes in number and composition of leukocytes	
Classification	Embryo	Fetus	Infants Pre-school children	School age

1st trimester	2nd trimester	3rd trimester	Under 1 yr.	1–2 yrs.	2–6 yrs.	6–10 yrs.
	Trimester of pregnancy					

Figure 2 Characteristics observed during pregnancy and up until age 10

It is well known that a fierce debate ensued when the cancer risk coefficient for childhood cancers induced by prenatal radiation was estimated from data related to diagnostic radiation exposure and found to be too high in comparison with data for prenatally exposed atomic bomb survivors[12].

Survivors exposed while young changed their residence more often than older atomic bomb survivors, a fact that also applies to prenatally exposed survivors. Consequently, ascertainment concerning data relating to cancer patients who moved outside the areas covered by the tumor registries is limited, and it is thus possible that the value of absolute cancer risk is too low.

Atomic bomb survivors exposed at under 15 years ATB characteristically developed radiation-induced leukemia 5–10 years after the bombing[14], and thus it is not believed that an increase in leukemia will be observed among prenatally exposed survivors in the future.

(*Yasutiko Yoshimoto*)

REFERENCES

1. Yamazaki JN, Schull WJ. Perinatal loss and neurological abnormalities among children of the atomic bomb: Nagasaki and Hiroshima revisited, 1949–1989. *JAMA* 1990; **264**: 605–9.
2. Otake M, Yoshimaru H, Schull WJ. Severe mental retardation among the prenatally exposed

survivors of the atomic bombing of Hiroshima and Nagasaki: a comparison of the T65DR and DS86 dosimetry systems. RERF TR 16–87, 1987.

3.   Yoshimoto Y, Kato H, Schull WJ. Risk of cancer among *in utero* children exposed to A-bomb radiation. 1950–84. *Lancet* 1988; **2**: 665–9. (RERF TR 4–88, 1988).

4.   Yoshimoto Y, Soda M, Mabuchi K. Cancer risks among the *in utero* children and the survivors of < 10 yr age exposed to A-bomb radiation, 1946–89. Proceedings of the 34th Annual Meeting of the Japan Radiation Research Society; 1991 Nov; Tokyo. Japan Radiation Research Society, 1991: 241. (*In Japanese*)

5.   Shimizu Y, Kato H, Schull WJ, *et al.* Life Span Study report II, part 3, Noncancer mortality, 1950–85, based on the revised doses (DS86). RERF TR 2–91, 1991.

6.   Mole RH. Childhood cancer after prenatal exposure to diagnostic X-ray examinations in Britain. *Br J Cancer* 1990; **62**: 152–68.

7.   Sasaki S, Kasuga T, Sato F, *et al.* Late effects of fetal mice X-irradiated at middle or late intrauterine stage. *Gann* 1978; **69**: 167–77.

8.   Nomura T. Induction of persistent hypersensitivity to lung tumorigenesis by *in utero* X-radiation in mice. *Environ Mutagen* 1984; **6**: 33–40.

9.   Kato H, Keehn RJ. Mortality in live-born children who were *in utero* at time of the atomic bombs. ABCC TR 13–66, 1966.

10.   Jablon S, Ishida M, Yamasaki M. JNIH-ABCC Life Span Study, Hiroshima and Nagasaki. Report 3, Mortality, October 1950–September 1960. ABCC TR 15–63, 1963.

11.   Hoshino T, Kato H, Finch SC, *et al.* Leukemia in offspring of atomic bomb survivors. *Blood* 1967; **30**: 719–30. (ABCC TR 3–67).

12.   Jablon S, Kato H. Childhood cancer in relation to prenatal exposure to A-bomb radiation. *Lancet* 1970; **2**: 1000–3. (ABCC TR 26–70).

13.   Ishimaru T, Ichimaru M, Mikami M. Leukemia incidence among individuals exposed *in utero*, children of atomic bomb survivors, and their controls. Hiroshima and Nagasaki, 1945–79. RERF TR 11–81, 1981.

14.   Ichimaru M, Ishimaru T, Mikami M, *et al.* Incidence of leukemia in a fixed cohort of atomic bomb survivors and controls, Hiroshima and Nagasaki, October 1950–December 1978. RERF TR 13–81.

15.   Timiras PS. Developmental physiology and aging. New York: Macmillan, 1972: 1.

16.   Wintrobe MM. Clinical hematology. 8th ed. Philadelphia: Lea & Febiger, 1981: 35.

14

Chromosomal Aberrations

14.1 DIRECTLY EXPOSED SURVIVORS

a) CHROMOSOMAL ABERRATIONS IN PERIPHERAL BLOOD LYMPHOCYTES

INTRODUCTION

Chromosomes, whose basic chemical component is deoxyribonucleic acid (DNA), are contained in cell nuclei and usually exist in an amorphous form known as chromatin. At the beginning of DNA synthesis (which precedes cell proliferation) the chromatin is transformed into two chromatids. At the start of mitosis the chromatids undergo condensation and become short. At metaphase, each chromosome takes on a distinct identifiable form; during this period it can be seen that a chromosome is formed from two chromatids, with each chromosome possessing individual characteristics. In human somatic cells there are 46 individual chromosomes (23 pairs), which have a length of 1–10 μm. Each possesses a characteristic configuration (a specific pattern in the banding technique), length, and centromere location. Chromosomal analysis is performed by microscopic observation of metaphase cells.

After metaphase, mitosis is complete when the respective chromatids divide, producing two daughter cells. The period between division and the next DNA synthetic phase (the S phase) is known as the DNA presynthetic phase, gap 1 (the G_1 phase), and the period between the S phase and mitosis is referred to as the postsynthetic phase, gap 2 (the G_2 phase). The cell cycle is important when analyzing chromosomal behavior.

Cell division is observed in tissue undergoing vigorous proliferation, especially in fetuses, hematopoietic tissue cells in bone marrow, and in male gonads (testes). As mitosis proceeds and cell differentiation occurs, there is no further DNA synthesis. In other words, the nuclei of cells which have undergone differentiation (e.g. neurons) remain in the G_1 state, the condition being termed the G_0 phase. Small mature lymphocytes in peripheral blood are also in the G_0 phase, and differ from mature differentiated cells in that upon contact with antigens they undergo transformation into undifferentiated cells and synthesize DNA.

1. CHROMOSOMAL ABERRATIONS

A. Mechanism of Aberration Formation

Ionizing radiation causes the chromatin (i.e. DNA) to break. After breakage, repair takes place between the break points with the chromatin reconstituting its original state. However, if the radiation dose is large the number of break points also becomes large, and it is possible for repair to occur between different break points, resulting in structural rearrangements. Abnormalities due to misrepair are termed "exchange-type aberrations," with typical examples shown in Fig. 1. In some cases repair does not occur after breakage, and the abnormality thus produced is termed a "break."

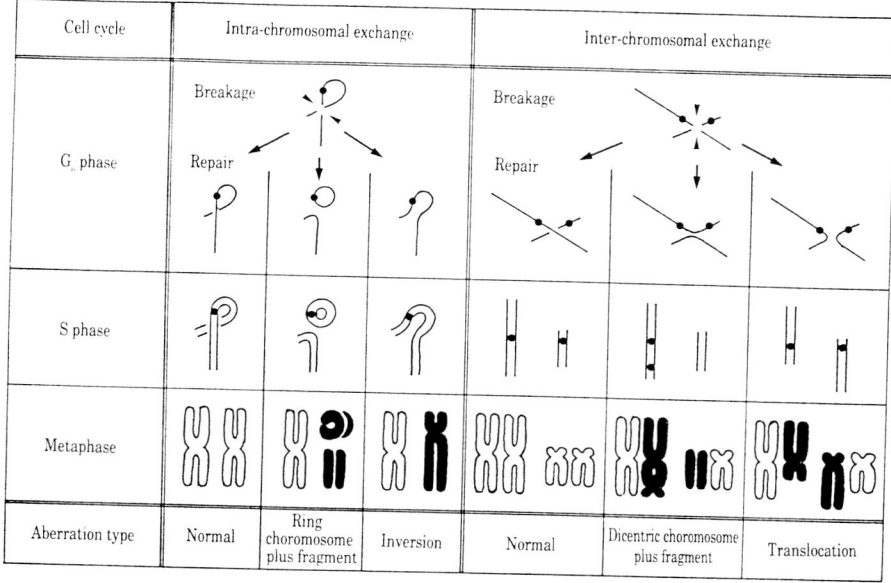

Figure 1   Types of radiation-induced chromosomal aberrations

Besides ionizing radiation, studies are also being carried out on various mutagenic substances that induce breaks and exchange-type aberrations in chromosomes. Many mutagens act on chromosomes to produce chromatid aberrations, thus creating various aberrations in either one of the two chromosomes. On the other hand, radiation-produced chromosomal aberrations are determined by the cell cycle at the time injury is inflicted. In the DNA presynthetic phase (the G_1 phase) breakage and exchange is induced before chromatid formation and the anomalies are referred to as "chromosome-type aberrations." When the cells are exposed to ionizing radiation during the period between the late S and G_2 phases, the chromatids have already been synthesized, and there is thus an increased probability of aberrations in one of the two chromatids. For this reason they are called "chromatid-type aberrations," and exhibit the same structural anomalies as those caused by exposure to various mutagens such as chemical agents. After induction of an abnormality, mitosis proceeds and when the next division occurs these anomalies appear as chromosome-type aberrations. Since the formation process is different from that of true chromosome-type aberrations, they are known as "derivative chromosome-type aberrations."

B. Radiation-Induced Chromosomal Aberrations in Lymphocytes

As previously mentioned, the lymphocytes circulate in the body's peripheral blood as mature and differentiated cells in the G_0 phase of the cell cycle. However, they possess the immunological characteristic that contact with foreign bodies such as antigens causes the lymphocytes to de-differentiate and undergo blastic transformation. In particular, it is known that addition of phytohemagglutinin (PHA) (a substance extracted from kidney beans) to cultures of lymphocytes produces a blastic change in the small lymphocytes and synchronous commencement of mitosis. This technique has become a routine cytogenetic procedure. It is impossible to analyze chromosomes in human somatic cells without the use of peripheral blood lymphocytes.

This technique, known as the blood culture method, allows chromosomal analysis of many individuals at one time due to the use of extremely small quantities of blood. The method involves the use of 1–2 ml of blood (greater or smaller quantities pose no problem) containing a small amount of the anticoagulant "heparin," a culture medium (e.g. RPMI 1640), PHA, and a small amount of fetal calf (or bovine) serum. The blood is cultured for 48 hours at 37°C; following treatment of the culture with colchicine (or colcemid) to arrest the cells at metaphase prevent mitosis, the cells are treated with hypotonic solution and fixed. The cells suspended in the fixative solution are dropped on to a microscopic slide to flatten and spread the metaphase chromosomes. After drying, the metaphase chromosomes are stained with Giemsa solution. The procedure itself is extremely simple.

Another characteristic of peripheral blood lymphocytes is that not all the lymphocytes circulating around the body are in the G_0 phase; some survive for a long period of time, possibly even decades. Therefore, when structural rearrangements are produced in lymphocyte chromosomes due to radiation exposure, then providing the damage is not fatal, the damaged cells containing the aberrations persist in the body for many years. The presence or absence of late effects of radiation can be confirmed from the presence or absence of chromosomal aberrations in the lymphocytes of the irradiated persons.

Studies on the chromosomal aberrations in the lymphocytes of atomic bomb survivors (discussed below) have utilized the characteristics of lymphocytes *in vivo*. However, the greatest advantage of lymphocytes is that they can be used in *in vitro* irradiation experiments; the results pertaining to lymphocyte aberrations can be extrapolated for the the evaluation of radiation effects in individuals irradiated *in vivo*.

C. Types of Chromosomal Aberrations

Typical examples of radiation-induced "chromosome-type aberrations" are shown in Fig. 1. As previously mentioned, the lymphocytes are in the G_0 phase, and thus radiation-induced chromosomal aberrations are without exception of chromosome type. There are two kinds, i.e. abnormalities due to exchanges between two break points within the same chromosome (intra-chromosomal exchange), and aberrations due to exchanges between breaks in different chromosomes (inter-chromosomal exchange). Intra-chromosomal exchange is represented by a ring chromosome (hereafter abbreviated to "r"), and an inverted chromosome (hereafter abbreviated to "inv"); inter-chromosomal exchange is represented by dicentric ("dic") and translocated ("t") chromosomes. Theoretically, these pairs, i.e. (r and inv) and (dic and t), are each expected to be formed in a ratio of 1 : 1. However, both ring and dicentric chromosomes are accompanied by acentric fragments, and consequently they are extremely unstable in subsequent mitoses; they are therefore referred to as "unstable aberrations" (or "Cu-type aberrations"). In contrast, inversions and translocations do not suffer from such handicaps during mitosis, and since they undergo a normal mitotic process, they are often called "stable (Cs-type) aberrations." Normal chromosomes and various examples of chromosomal aberrations are shown in Figs. 2–5.

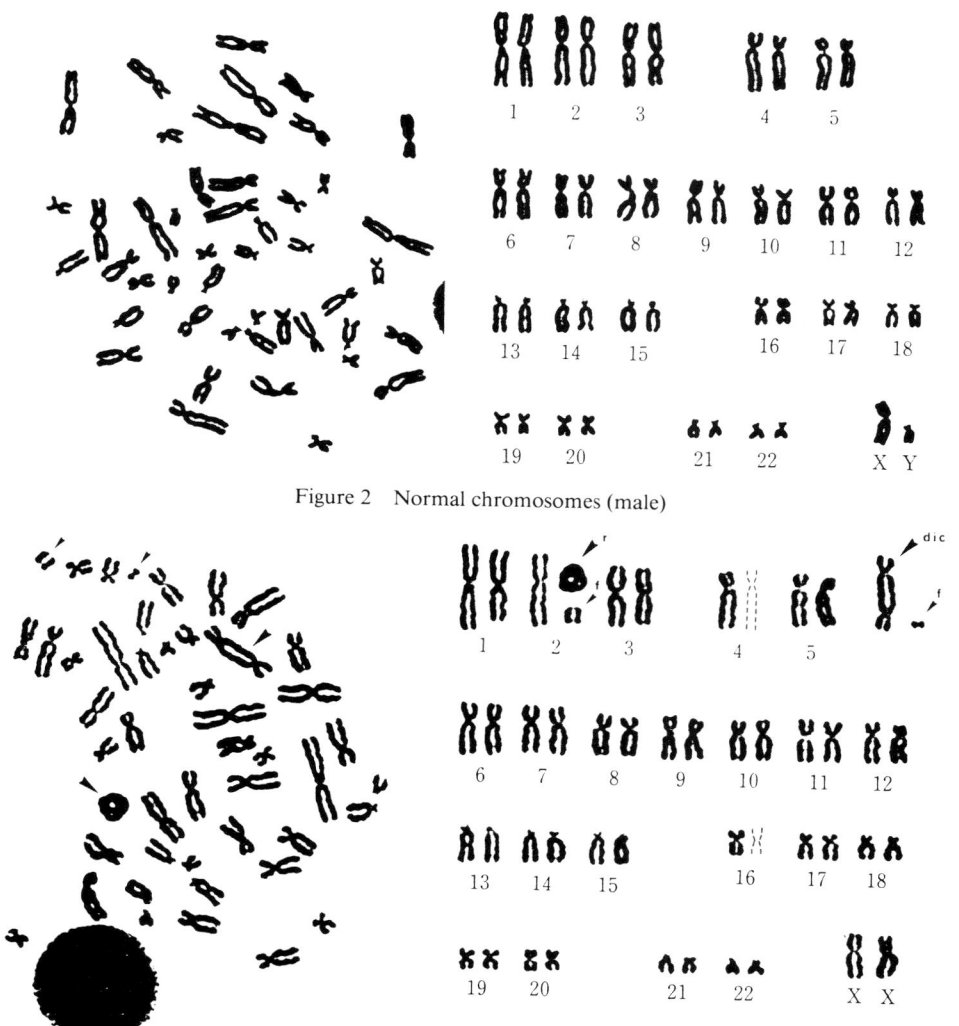

Figure 2   Normal chromosomes (male)

Figure 3   Ring chromosome (r) and dicentric chromosome (dic) in a female. (in both cases accompanied by a fragment, f)

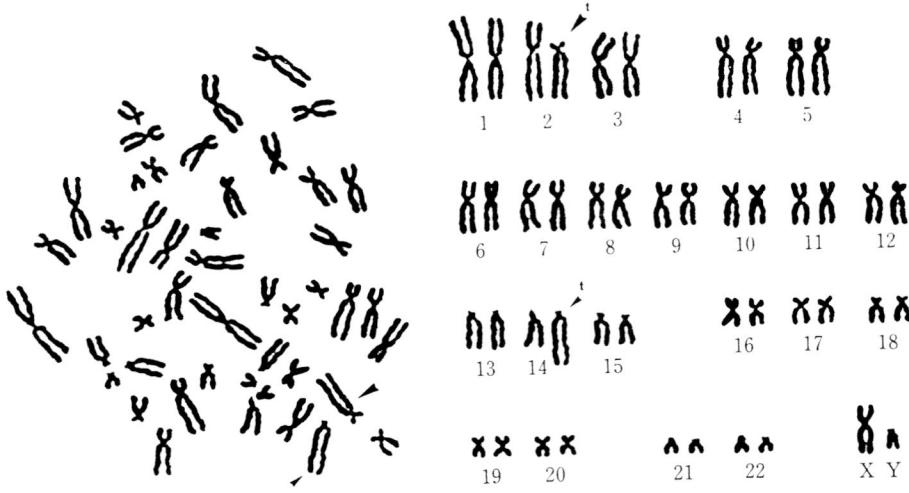

Figure 4   Translocation chromosomes (t) in a male

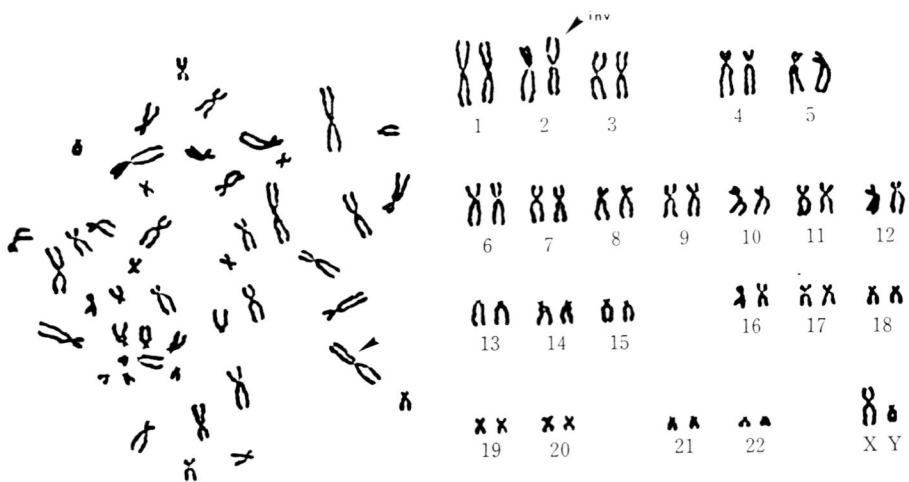

Figure 5   Inversion chromosome (inv) in a male

Due to the above specific structural characteristics, dicentric and ring chromosomes can be accurately and objectively identified. However, the identification of translocation and inversion chromosomes is often influenced by the experience of the observer, and it is difficult to compare their frequencies between different laboratories. Even though the ratio of (dic + r) : (t + inv) is 1 : 1, it has until recently been accepted that the identification rate of (t + inv) is almost 20% that of (dic + r). The accuracy of the dose-response relationship derived from the frequency of (t + inv) has been considered inconsistent. Since cells possessing dicentric or ring chromosomes suffer mitotic damage in the living body, they decrease with time, until finally they are present at a low but constant level. Accuracy in the dose-response relationship is lost 5 years after exposure, which means that immediate evaluation of radiation damage is desirable for use of Cu-type aberrations as indicators.

In vitro irradiation experiments using lymphocytes have yielded many results, some of the important ones being:

(1) For low linear energy transfer (LET) radiation (X-rays and gamma rays) the frequency of chromosomal aberration per unit dose is low, and the dose-response relationship obeys the linear-quadratic (L-LQ) model. Differences in dose rate effect are observed, with the biological effect of acute irradiation being double that of chronic irradiation.

(2) For high linear energy transfer (LET) radiation (neutrons and alpha rays) the dose-response relationship is linear (the L model), with a high frequency of aberrations per unit dose. A dose rate effect is not observed. These facts show that in comparison to low LET radiation, the relative biological effectiveness (RBE) of high LET radiation is high at low doses, but tends to decrease with increases in dose.

2. CHROMOSOMAL ABERRATIONS IN THE LYMPHOCYTES OF ATOMIC BOMB SURVIVORS

A. Directly Exposed Survivors

The chromosome study on the subjects in the Adult Health Study (AHS) sample at the Radiation Effects Research Foundation (RERF) has continued since 1967, yielding several important results[1-8]. In particular, the new dosimetry system (DS86)[9] was employed to analyze the estimated doses of individual survivors. Investigation of the relationship with dose is also being pursued at institutions outside RERF. The results obtained to date are summarized below:

1. *Differences in Dose-Response Relationship Between Hiroshima and Nagasaki*

Early results were yielded by a study based on a total of 1,431 subjects, consisting of atomic bomb survivors exposed to an estimated DS86 kerma dose of $\leqslant 4$ Gy (788 in Hiroshima, 457 in Nagasaki) and individuals who were not in the cities at the time of bombing (110 in Hiroshima, 76 in Nagasaki)[5]. Analyses were performed on 100 cells per individual, with 30 cells regarded as the minimum number acceptable for analysis. After examination, cancer patients and those with a history of radiotherapy were excluded.

The frequency of cells with chromosome aberrations was plotted against estimated radiation dose (here, the bone marrow dose) (Fig. 6). According to the L-LQ model for the relationship between dose and the frequency of abnormal cells, the coefficient of the dose-square term was greater in Nagasaki than in Hiroshima. However, Hiroshima displayed a linear dose-response relationship with a higher aberration frequency per 1 Gy than Nagasaki, which is due in part to the neutron dose in Hiroshima being greater than in Nagasaki. This is a major problem which needs to be examined in the future.

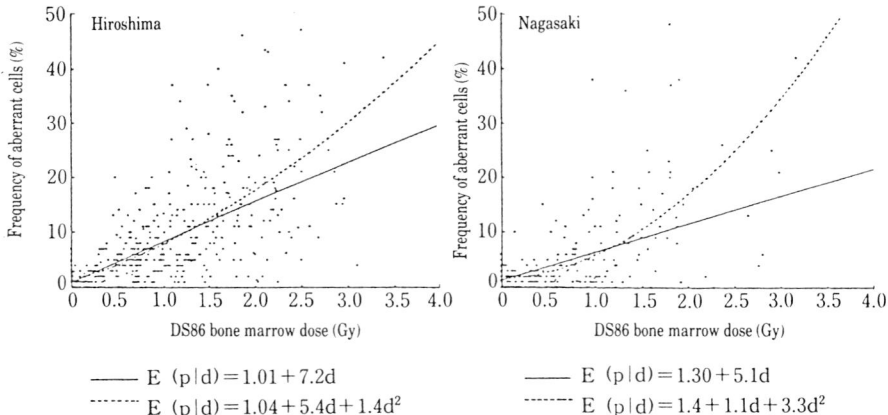

$$\text{Hiroshima} \qquad \text{Nagasaki}$$

—— E (p|d) = 1.01 + 7.2d   —— E (p|d) = 1.30 + 5.1d

······ E (p|d) = 1.04 + 5.4d + 1.4d²   ······ E (p|d) = 1.4 + 1.1d + 3.3d²

Figure 6   Frequency of cells with chromosomal aberrations by DS86 bone marrow dose, and application of linear model (solid line) and linear quadratic model (dotted line)

2. *Types of Chromosomal Aberration*

At the time the chromosome study commenced, over 20 years had already passed since the atomic bombing, and the majority of observed chromosomal aberrations were Cs type (translocation and inversion). In the initial studies (in the late 1960s) 95% of the aberrations were Cs type, with translocation aberrations accounting for 60% of these. Inversions and deletions (del) were also identified. The frequency of dicentric and ring chromosomes was extremely low (less than 5%), and consequently dose-response studies focused on stable aberrations. Although the frequency of (dicentric + ring) chromosomes was low, a correlation with dose was observed. The above results were common to both Hiroshima and Nagasaki.

The (dic + r) frequency in the non-exposed adult population has been estimated at 1.0–1.5 per 1,000 cells[13]. However, in the atomic bomb exposed population, the frequency of Cu-type aberrations was 2–3 times greater than in the non-irradiated adult population. Also, the frequency of (t + inv) Cs-type aberrations tended to be high at 1–2%. The reason for this has not yet been clarified, but one possibility is that the effect of diagnostic exposure to X-rays during gastro-intestinal fluoroscopy cannot be ignored. Since Cs-type aberrations are not eliminated, it is anticipated that the frequency of Cs aberrations rises with increasing age as a result of the cumulative effect.

Analysis of chromosomal aberrations by the G-banding method has afforded a basis of support for the possibility that the formation of exchange-type chromosomal aberrations is proportional to the amount of DNA in individual chromosomes, or chromosomal length. That is, the radiation-produced breaks in chromosomes are distributed in a random fashion, with the number of chromosomal aberrations formed on the basis of random breaks being proportional to the length of each chromosome. The same holds true for the elimination of aberrations. However, the possibility of breakages and aberrations being unevenly distributed at specific sites of certain chromosomes cannot be discounted, and certain reports support this view[12].

The question of whether or not the formation of aberrations is a random phenomenon still remains unresolved.

Observations in non-exposed adults tend to show a significantly high frequency of Cs-type aberrations in specific loci at chromomsomes 7 and 14. Since T-cell receptor (TCR) genes, which regulate T-lymphocyte activity, and immunoglobulins are assigned to these chromosomes, this may be a characteristic of T-lymphocytes.

3. *Variations in Aberration Frequencies – Discrepancies with regard to Dose*

As can be seen from Fig. 6, in both Hiroshima and Nagasaki there is a wide distribution in individual aberration frequencies within a given dose range. In many cases a low frequency is observed at high doses, or a high frequency seen at low doses. There are many possible causes for such discrepancies with respect to dose, such as (a) errors in the estimated doses, (b) differences in individual radiosensitivity, or (c) differences in the behavior of aberrant cells *in vivo*, and the fact that some individuals might have received high-dose radiotherapy. It is unlikely that differences in radiosensitivity produces such a discrepancy. It is already known that errors exist in the dose estimates for individual survivors[14], and there is a strong likelihood that such random errors in dose estimates are the primary cause of the inordinate variation in the distribution of aberration frequencies. A statistical analysis on the relationship between chromosome aberration frequency and epilation (a symptom of acute radiation illness) has shown that for an identical dose the aberration frequency was higher in cases of severe epilation than in cases of mild or no epilation[8]. Thus increasing importance is being placed on the use of chromosomal aberration data as a sensitive biological indicator for estimating absorbed radiation dose (so-called "biological dosimetry"), which can be regarded as an accurate technique for supplementing physical dose estimates of individual exposure.

4. *Clones of Aberrant Cells*

A clone of cells showing identical chromosomal aberrations can frequently be detected in one individual; without exception the aberrations are of Cs type. In order to define this as a cytogenetic clone, a minimum of 4 cells per 100 observed cells must contain an identical aberration. Clones originate from a cell with chromosomal damage induced in lymphocytic stem cells through preferential growth. The chromosome study on 300 atomic bomb survivors with chromosome aberrations who were exposed to a DS86 kerma dose of ≥ 1.0 Gy detected 10 clonal cases. Since no clonal cases were observed in survivors exposed to low doses, it can be concluded that the cytogenetic clones were due to exposure to atomic bomb radiation. Clones were also confirmed in a repeat examination.

As previously mentioned, the frequencies of Cu- and Cs-type aberrations are expected to be equal. However, because several decades have passed since exposure to the atomic bomb, the unstable Cu aberration frequency has decreased to 1/10 that of the stable Cs type. This means that Cu-type aberrations have been eliminated from the bodies of survivors, whereas Cs-type aberrations have been retained. Following induction of the aberration, cells with chromosome aberrations are selected through cellular proliferation, as a result of which abnormal cell clones are manifested. From the viewpoint of proliferation, it is possible that cells adapt to the *in vivo* environment with preferential development of clones. Detailed chromosomal analyses yielded no evidence of specific chromosomes contributing to the formation of clones. Elucidation of the relationship between clonal cell proliferation and the growth factor for cell proliferation is therefore an important area for research.

There are many unclarified points relating to the biological significance of clone cells and the role they play in the body. From the aspect of immunocompetence, the isolation of clones and various multidisciplinary studies are obviously needed.

B. Prenatally Exposed Survivors

Prenatally exposed survivors are defined as those individuals who were exposed *in utero* at the time of the atomic bombing and who were born after August 6th 1945 and before May 1946. Although shielded by maternal tissue, they are considered directly exposed atomic bomb survivors. Depending on gestational age at the time of bombing, undifferentiated cells in the course of development would have been exposed to atomic bomb radiation, and it was predicted that biological damage would have been considerable since exposure had occurred during a period of high radiosensitivity. The physical effects of atomic bomb radiation on prenatally exposed survivors (in particular with respect to brain development) are discussed in detail in other chapters and will not be mentioned here.

The results of the chromosome study performed by Bloom *et al*[15] in the late 1960s on prenatally exposed atomic bomb survivors in Hiroshima and Nagasaki are summarized below.

A comparison of 38 exposed cases and 48 controls revealed that most aberrations in the exposed population were Cu type, which occurred in 19 out of 3,643 cells (0.52%), with Cs-type aberrations accounting for only a small 0.08% (3 cells), whereas in the control population a mere 2 fragments (both Cu-type) were identified in the 4,678 cells examined. The aberration frequency in the exposed population was thus found to be significantly higher than in the control population. Since data analysis was based on the old T65D system of dosimetry, the estimated maternal doses in the exposed population tended to be rather high (although this will not be discussed in detail here). Aberrations identified in the study were included in the cell in the first mitotic division following induction of the aberration. This suggests the possibility that if the aberration had been created as a result of atomic bomb radiation, the lymphocytes with abnormalities induced in the fetus would have remained for over 20 years after exposure without undergoing mitosis. Also, there was a discussion of the possibility of the spleen being the organ producing these lymphocytes.

These observations in part contradict current findings e.g. the frequency of Cs-type aberrations is lower than for Cu type, and the aberration frequency in the control population is virtually zero. In particular, when aberrations are induced in the fetus (which is in a period of considerable cell proliferation), it is likely that clonal cells with Cs aberrations will be formed. The failure to observe a reduced frequency of Cu-type aberrations in these subjects due to elimination demands further investigation.

The RERF Adult Health Study sample was expanded in 1976 to include prenatally exposed survivors and their controls, and a cytogenetic re-evaluation has been conducted since 1985. In particular, detailed analyses using the G-banding method are being performed to determine the presence or absence of Cs-type aberrations.

CONCLUSION

Chromosome studies on survivors directly exposed to the atomic bomb have yielded a considerable amount of new data. In particular, due to the use of chromosomal aberrations in biological dosimetry, data have been accumulated that complement physical dose estimates. The frequency of unstable aberrations such as dicentrics and rings have become regarded as an important basis of biological dosimetry; however, it has been confirmed that, as in the case of the atomic bomb survivors, the dicentric and ring frequencies are unreliable when several decades have elapsed since exposure. Cells with Cs aberrations such as translocations and inversions persist at unaltered frequencies. Furthermore, the proportionality of the induction of aberrations to the amount of DNA for individual chromosomes proves that biological predictions were relevant and correct.

Since over 5 years have already passed since the Chernobyl accident, doubts remain concerning the use of dicentrics and rings as biological dose indicators. In contrast, the relevance of the use of Cs aberrations for dose estimations has been confirmed by studies on the atomic bomb survivors, thus demonstrating the future utility of this technique.

Since the chromosome studies began in 1967, the basic techniques of chromosomal research have not changed. Therefore by a direct comparison of observations made over a period of time, and with the possibility of analyzing the reproduciblity of data, a considerable amount of basic data pertaining to biological dosimetry has accumulated.

Following recent rapid advances in molecular biology techniques, a new technique (termed the "fluorescence in situ hybridization," FISH, or "chromosome painting" method) has been developed which allows identification of individual chromosomes[16]. The method is extremely useful for rapid and accurate screening of the reciprocal translocations predominantly seen in atomic bomb survivors. Using this technique, a homologous pair of targeted chromosomes can be painted yellow, whereas non-targeted chromosomes are stained red. Thus, a translocation between painted and unpainted chromosomes is unequivocally shown by a bi-color structure (partly yellow and partly red). Also, translocations can be identified not only in the metaphase but also in the interphase.

The FISH procedure is rather complex, but since it is easy to increase the number of metaphases more than tenfold in comparison with conventional methods, it is possible to increase the statistical precision regarding observed aberration frequency. Screening for Cs aberrations has only been performed in two or three research laboratories, and is a new practical technique for biological dosimetry which has attracted great interest.

Preliminary studies on the Hiroshima atomic bomb survivors conducted at RERF have made it clear that the dose-response regression derived from the translocational frequency obtained by use of the FISH method is in close agreement with data based on the Cs aberration frequencies determined by both the conventional and G-banding methods.

Since the FISH technique is also applicable to the identification of gene loci in specific chromosomes, it has become possible to explain somatic cell mutations as well as chromosomal changes occurring during the malignant transformation of cells.

The biological implications of stable chromosomal aberrations persisting in lymphocytes remain unclear. It is believed that these chromosomal mutations may have no effect on health, although they are perhaps an important biological model for the clarification of somatic cell mutations which can occur in other cell structures.

(Akio Awa)

REFERENCES

1. Awa AA. Review of thirty years study of Hiroshima and Nagasaki atomic bomb survivors. II. Biological effects. G. Chromosome aberrations in somatic cells. *J Radiat Res* 1975; **16** (Suppl): 122–31.

2. Awa AA, Sofuni T, Honda T, *et al.* Relationship between the radiation dose and chromosome aberrations in atomic bomb survivors of Hiroshima and Nagasaki. *J Radiat Res* 1978; **19**: 126–40.

3. Awa AA. Chromosomal aberrations in atomic bomb survivors. In: Takebe H, Utsunomiya J, editors. Genetics of human tumors in Japan. GANN Monograph on Cancer Research. Tokyo: *Jpn Sci Soc* 1988; **35**: 175–89.

4. Awa AA, Ohtaki K, Itoh M, *et al.* Chromosome aberration data for A-bomb dosimetry reassessment. *Proceedings of the 23rd Annual Meeting of NCRP*; Apr 8–9; 1987, Washington DC. Bethesda: National Council on Radiation Protection and Measurements, 1988: 185–202.

5. Preston DL, McConney ME, Awa AA, *et al.* Comparison of the dose-response relationships for chromosome aberration frequencies between the T65D and DS86 dosimetry. RERF TR 7–88, 1988.

6. Ohtaki K, Shimba H, Awa AA, *et al.* Comparison of type and frequency of chromosome aberrations by conventional and G-staining methods in Hiroshima atomic bomb survivors. *J Radiat Res* 1982; **23**: 441–9.

7. Awa AA. Review of forty-five years study of Hiroshima and Nagasaki atomic bomb survivors. II. Biological effects. Persistent chromosome aberrations in the somatic cells of A-bomb survivors, Hiroshima and Nagasaki. 1. *Radiat Res* 1991; **32** (Suppl): 265–74.

8. Sposto R, Stram DO, Awa AA. An investigation of random errors in the DS86 dosimetry using data on chromosome aberrations and severe epilation. RERF TR 7–90, 1990.

9. Roesch WC, editor. US-Japan joint reassessment of atomic bomb radiation dosimetry in Hiroshima and Nagasaki. Final Report, Vol. 1 and 2. Hiroshima: Radiation Effects Research Foundation, 1987.

10. Sasaki MS. Chromosomal approaches to the dose assessment in human exposures to ionizing radiation. *Berzelius Symp* 1988; **15**: 119–28, 1988.

11. Kamada N, Shigeta C, Kuramoto A, *et al.* Acute and late effects of A-bomb radiation studied in a group of young girls with a defined condition at the time of bombing. *J Radiat Res* 1989; **30**: 218–25.

12. Tanaka K, Kamada N, Ohkita T, *et al.* Nonrandom distribution of chromosome breaks in lymphocytes of atomic bomb survivors. *J Radiat Res* 1983; **24**: 291–304.

13. Bender MA, Awa AA, Brooks AL, *et al.* Current status of cytogenetic procedures to detect and quantify previous exposures to radiation. *Mutat Res* 1988; **196**: 103–59.

14. Jablon S. Atomic bomb radiation dose estimation at ABCC. ABCC TR 23–71, 1971.

15. Bloom AD, Neriishi S, Archer PG. Cytogenetics of *in utero* exposed subjects, Hiroshima and Nagasaki. ABCC TR 7–68, 1968.

16. Lucas J, Awa AA, Straume T, *et al.* Rapid translocation frequency analysis in humans decades after exposure to ionizing radiation. *Int J Radiat Biol* 1991; **62**: 53–63.

14.1   DIRECTLY EXPOSED SURVIVORS

b)   CHROMOSOMAL ABERRATIONS IN BONE MARROW CELLS

INTRODUCTION

Chromosomal aberrations in the peripheral blood T-cells and bone marrow cells of atomic bomb survivors are a directly observable radiation-induced effect, like radiation cataracts. Since peripheral blood T-cell chromosomal aberrations in atomic bomb survivors were discussed in the previous section, this chapter will deal with chromosomal aberrations in bone marrow cells. Chromosome analyses of human cells became possible in the latter half of the 1950s, but no observations of chromosomal aberrations were made immediately after the atomic bombing. The first reports concerning chromosomal anomalies in atomic bomb survivors appeared in the early 1960s. The acquisition of data pertaining to chromosomal aberrations can be broadly divided into two time periods according to the research techniques employed, i.e. the period before the banding method had been developed (1962–75), and the period after the technique became established (since 1975). This section reviews each of these periods.

1. NON-BANDING METHODS (1962–75)

A. Frequency of Chromosomal Aberrations in Bone Marrow Cells

Chromosomal aberrations in the bone marrow cells of atomic bomb survivors were first reported in 1964[1]. However, at that time no positive results were obtained, i.e. a comparison between 10 non-exposed subjects and a total of 20 exposed survivors (8 exposed at a distance of 1.0–1.5 km, 4 at 1.6–2.0 km, and 8 at 2.2–3.5 km) concluded that "at the present time there appears to be no significant difference between the two populations. It is hoped that future investigations will continue when the number of cases increases." Two years after that report, chromosomal examinations detected chromosomal aberrations in 22% and 36% of the bone marrow cells of 2 atomic bomb survivors respectively exposed at 550 m and 700 m from the hypocenter. It is thought that the reason for the previous report not detecting abnormalities was that no subjects exposed within 1 km of the hypocenter had been included in the study. A subsequent study focused on survivors proximally exposed at less than 1 km, investigating chromosomal aberrations in the bone marrow cells of 114 subjects exposed within 3 km of the hypocenter, including 21 within 500 m and 19 at 501–1,000 m (Table 1)[2]. Chromosomal aberrations were observed in an average of 21.5% of the cells in 19 of the 21 survivors in the ≤ 500 m population (90.5%), and in an average of 14.1 cells in 10 out of the 19 subjects exposed at 501–1,000 m (52.6%). As in the previous study, only an extremely low frequency of aberrations was observed in survivors exposed at distances greater than 1 km (2 cases out of 84).

All the chromosomal anomalies were stable aberrations, and had evolved into chromosomes capable of transmitting the same aberration to the next daughter cells

Table 1   Chromosomal aberrations in bone marrow cells

Distance from hypocenter (m)	No. of cases	No. of cells observed	Chromosomal aberrations		
			No. of cells (%)	No. of cases (%)	No. of clones
0 ~ 500	21	1,195	257 (21.5)	19 (90.5)	7
501 ~ 1,000	19	918	129 (14.1)	10 (52.6)	7
1,001 ~ 1,500	28	556	1 (0.2)	1 (6.2)	0
1.501 ~ 2,000	23	728	0	0	0
2,001 ~ 3,000	23	737	3 (0.4)	1 (4.2)	0
Non-exposed	17	624	0	0	0

through mitosis. The types of aberrations included deletions (44.9%), balanced reciprocal translocations (28.4%) and unbalanced reciprocal translocations (19.2%). A comparison of the frequency of aberrations in the various chromosome groups reveals that when chromosomes in the A, B and G groups underwent deletion, this occurred at double the anticipated rate. Abnormal clones were detected in 7 subjects in each of the ≤ 500 m and 501–1,000 m populations, with Bq-, + E, and Gq- clones being observed.

B. Comparison of Chromosomal Aberrations in Bone Marrow Cells and T-cells

Examination of cases of chromosomal abnormalities in the bone marrow cells and T-cells of atomic bomb survivors exposed within 1 km showed that in the ≤ 500 m population the average frequencies of aberration were 21.5% for bone marrow cells and 27.1% for T-cells, whereas the figures for the 501–1,000 m population were 14.1% and 23.0% respectively. In both populations the T-cell chromosomes exhibited a higher rate of abnormality than the bone marrow cells (Table 2). For the 44 subjects with a known received dose a comparison of the bone marrow and T-cell

Table 2   Frequency of chromosomal aberrations in T-lymphocytes and bone marrow cells

Frequency of chromosomal aberrations (%)	T-lymphocytes		Bone marrow cells	
	No. of exposed survivors			
	< 500 m	501 ~ 1,000 m	< 500 m	501 ~ 1,000 m
0 ~ 9.9	1	4	4	10
10 ~ 19.9	10	12	6	5
20 ~ 29.9	14	8	5	3
30 ~ 39.9	6	5	4	1
40 ~ 49.9	2	2	1	0
50 ~ 59.9	2	0	0	0
60 ~	1	1	1	0
No. of cases	36	32	21	19
No. of cells observed	2,679	2,394	1,195	918
Average frequency of aberrations	27.1	23.0	21.5	14.1

aberrational frequencies for the same individual revealed that for each population the rate of bone marrow abnormalities was approximately 3/4 that of the T-cells (Table 3). The types of T-cell aberrations were deletions (43.5%), translocations (45.6%), and inversions (10.8%); the types and frequencies of changes in bone marrow cells were approximately the same.

Table 3 Comparison by dose of frequency of chromosomal aberrations in bone marrow cells and T-lymphocytes

Dose (Gy)	No. of survivors	Frequency of chromosomal aberrations	
		Bone marrow cells (%)	T-lymphocytes (%)
≥ 4.0	13	32.1	43.1
2.0 ~ 3.99	17	21.8	27.4
≤ 1.99	14	8.6	11.7

C. Changes in Chromosomal Aberrations with Time

Observation of chromosomal aberrations in healthy atomic bomb survivors with respect to time shows that, whereas the frequency of T-cell abnormalities remains approximately constant, some variations are found with bone marrow chromosomal aberrations depending on factors such as bone marrow hematopoeitic condition and viral infection etc. Figure 1 shows a female exposed to a T65D dose of 6.39 Gy at a distance of 550 m from the hypocenter at the age of 15 and who developed breast cancer 35 years later. The abnormalities in the T-cells were found to be approximately constant, but in the bone marrow cells varied with each examination[3].

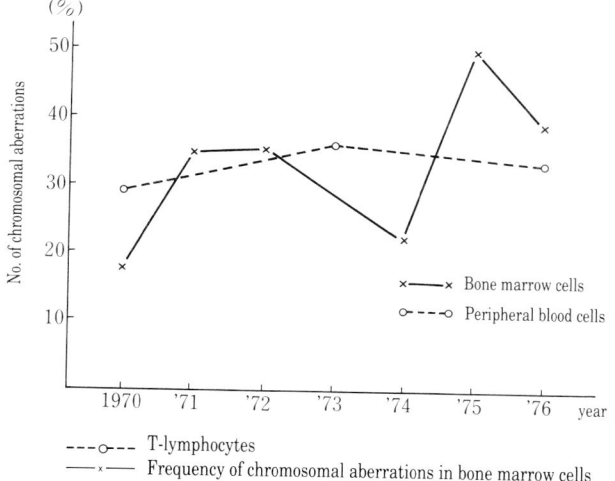

Figure 1   Sequential changes in chromosomal aberrations in the bone marrow cells and T-lymphocytes of an atomic bomb survivor exposed at 550 m from the hypocenter to a T65D dose of 6.39 Gy

Figure 2 shows changes in the abnormal clones in 4 healthy survivors; as seen with the + C clone in the lower left case and the Gq- clone in the bottom right case, the abnormal clones decreased and new clones appeared. The upper right case developed chronic myelocytic leukemia in 1980, but Gq- aberrations were detected in the bone marrow cells, reaching a maximum in 1970 [this was before the banding technique had been developed, and it is unclear whether this occurred in the Philadelphia (Ph[1]) chromosome].

2. BANDING METHODS (AFTER 1976)

Chromosomal banding techniques advanced greatly in 1970–75, with the development from the quinacrine (Q) banding method[4] of various methods such as the Giemsa (G) banding method[5], the R-banding method[6] and the C-banding method[7].

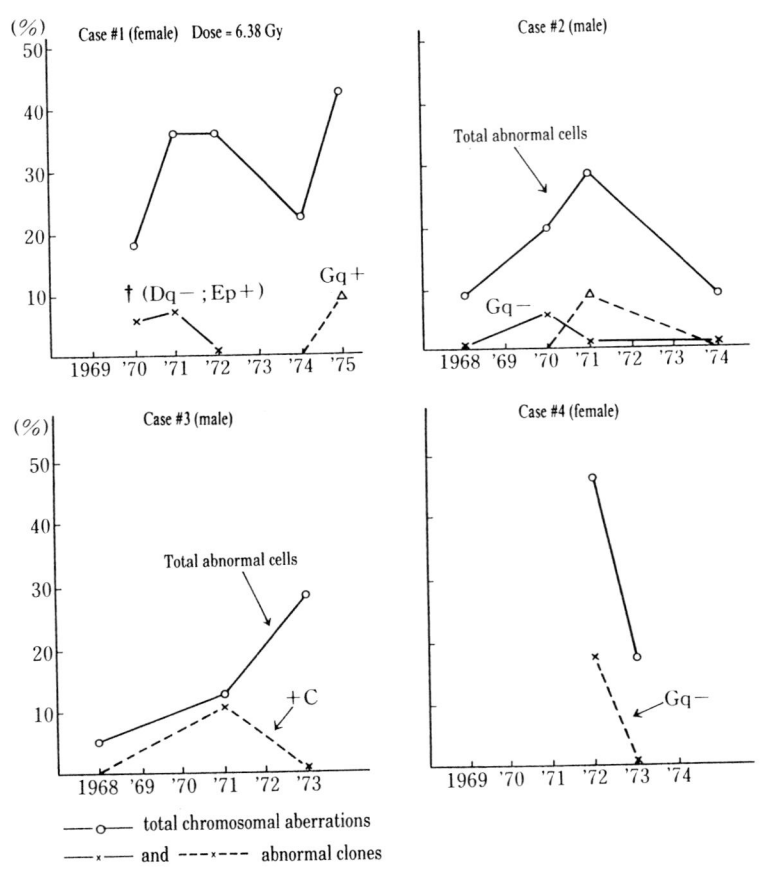

Figure 2   Sequential changes in chromosomal aberrations in the bone marrow cells of atomic bomb survivors exposed within 1 km of the hypocenter

Abnormalities in survivor bone marrow cells were observed using the G-banding technique, which permits the preservation of permanent specimens. The frequency of cases of chromosomal aberrations and the detection rate of abnormal cells do not differ greatly from the findings obtained to date, clarifying the nature of structural aberrations in chromosomes. In an analysis of bone marrow chromosomes in 13 survivors exposed within 1 km, 710 cells were observed with abnormalities detected in 121 (with 4.8%–34.8% of the aberrations seen in 11 subjects). Only 1 unstable abnormality (dicentric) was observed, the rest being stable; the types and frequencies of the structural abnormalities are shown in Table 4. Simple translocations between two chromosomes were the predominant aberration, occurring in 57 cells (47.1%), followed by inversions (14 cells, 11.6%) and deletions (6 cells, 5.0%). Complex abnormalities involving 3 or more chromosomal aberrations within a metaphase were observed in 34 cells (28.1%). Among these, two translocations were present simultaneously in the same cell in 13 cases (10.7%), with translocation and inversion occurring in 6 cases (5.0%); besides these there were 15 other cells (12.4%) which contained more than one aberration, with combinations such as translocation and inversion, translocation and insertion, and translocation and deletion. Also, among the structural anomalies 82.1% of cells possessed balanced abnormalities with the correct amount of chromosome material, and 17.9% had unbalanced abnormalities. Of the 121 cells with chromosomal aberrations shown in Table 4, 296 break sites were clarified by the banding method, with the distribution of these shown in Fig. 3. The break points were distributed throughout the chromosomes, but found to be concentrated in two or three chromosomes, and within certain regions of the chromosomes. The number of observed breaks per chromosome was compared with the number of expected breaks calculated from chromosome length, and statistical analysis performed using the x^2 test. Many breaks were observed in number 17 chromosome (p < 0.001) and number 1 chromosome (p < 0.01), but in contrast few

Table 4 Frequency of chromosomal aberrations by type

Type of rearrangement	No. and frequency of chromosomal aberrations in bone marrow cells (%)
Stable type	
Deletion	6 (5.0)
Interstitial deletion	1 (0.8)
Duplication	3 (2.5)
Translocation	57 (47.1)
Inversion	14 (11.6)
Complex translocation	5 (4.1)
2 translocations within metaphase	13 ⎫
Translocation + inversion within metaphase	6 ⎬ 34 (28.1)
Others	15 ⎭
Unstable type	
Dicentrics	1 (0.8)
No. of aberrant cells	121 (100)

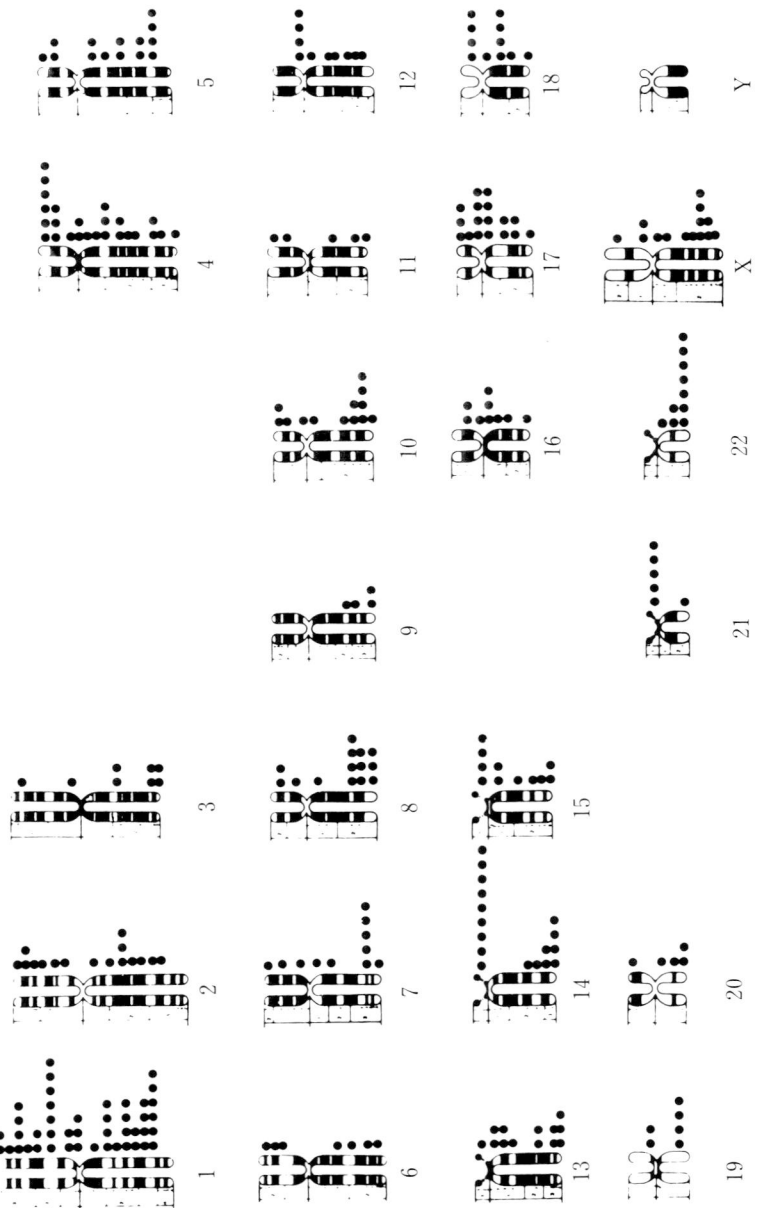

• = one break point

Figure 3   Break points in chromosome in the bone marrow cells of atomic bomb survivors exposed within 1 km of the hypocenter (exhibiting non-random distribution)

seen in number 3 chromosome (p < 0.001) or in chromosomes number 6, 9, and 11 (p < 0.05), thus indicating a non-random distribution. Reports to date on break points observed following exposure to radiation also refer to non-random distribution, but questions of specificity are as yet unresolved, e.g. regarding the points within a specific chromosome region at which breakage frequently occurs, and those at which it rarely occurs.

In conclusion, the results of chromosomal analysis by banding techniques have supported the findings of the non-banding methods, and have also clarified the types of chromosomal aberrations and their break points.

CONCLUSION

Chromosomal studies on atomic bomb survivors have been pursued on two fronts, using peripheral blood lymphocytes and bone marrow cells respectively, each approach having both advantages and disadvantages. Peripheral blood lymphocytes have the advantage that test specimens are easy to obtain, results are stable (the chromosomal aberrations are believed to have become constant 30 years after exposure), and it is also possible to estimate the doses which survivors received at the time of the atomic bombing. On the other hand, it is not easy to procure bone marrow specimens, and repeated bone marrow aspirations in particular are almost impossible to perform. However, the advantage of using chromosomal aberrations in bone marrow cells is that they realistically reflect the dynamic conditions within those cells, and it is possible to clarify the various stages in the development of leukemia. With the aging of the atomic bomb survivors in recent years, there has been a marked decrease in bone marrow cells, and in approximately 1/3 of the cases it has become impossible to obtain data for more than 20 metaphases. This tendency is expected to continue, making the study of bone marrow chromosomes in atomic bomb survivors much more difficult. Recently various molecular biology techniques have become available, and based on the results of previous chromosome studies, their adoption in the monitoring of the diseases occurring in atomic bomb survivors is likely to increase in importance.

(Nanao Kamada)

REFERENCES

1. Kamada N. Chromosome aberrations of bone marrow cells in atomic bomb survivors. *J Hiroshima Med Ass* 1964; **17**: 811–4. (*In Japanese*)
2. Kamada N, Yuzaki M, Yamamoto O, *et al.* Comprehensive medical research on survivors from the atomic bomb hypocenter. The results of the last ten years. *J Hiroshima Med Ass* 1982; **35**: 1084–98. (*In Japanese*)
3. Kamada N, Tanaka K. Cytogenetic background in radiation-exposed people and its relation to tumorigenesis. *Clinica* 1981; **8**: 1003–10. (*In Japanese*)
4. Caspersson T, *et al.* Analysis of the human metaphase chromosome set by aid of DNA-binding fluorescent agents. *Exptl Cell Res* 1970; **62**: 490–2.
5. Seabright M. A rapid technique for chromosomes. *Lancet* 1971; **2**: 971.
6. Dutrillausx B, Lejeune J. New technique in the study of human chromosomes: methods and

applications. In: Harris H, Hirshhorn K, editors. Advances in human genetics, Vol. 6. New York: Plenum Press, 1975: 119–26.

7. Sumner AT. A simple technique for demonstrating centromeric heterochromatin. *Exp Cell Res* 1972; **75**: 304–6.

8. Tanaka K, Kamada N, Kuramoto A, *et al.* Chromosome aberrations of bone marrow cells in heavily exposed atomic bomb survivors. Observation by means of banding method. *J Hiroshima Med Ass* 1986; **39**: 244–8. (*In Japanese*)

14.2 CHROMOSOMAL ABERRATIONS IN THE PERIPHERAL BLOOD LYMPHOCYTES OF EARLY ENTRANTS

INTRODUCTION

Atomic bomb radioactivity is classified into initial radiation and residual radiation. At the instant of the nuclear detonation of uranium-235 (^{235}U) in Hiroshima and plutonium-239 (^{239}P) in Nagasaki, neutron and gamma rays were released together with the flash, and within approximately one minute of the explosion beta and gamma rays were emitted from the products of nuclear fission. Alpha rays were also produced. Since alpha and beta rays have poor transmissibility and were absorbed in the air, it was the neutrons and gamma rays that affected the human body.

Residual radiation is observed at the earth's surface over a long period of time as induced radiation and radioactive fallout. Induced radiation is the radiation produced when large quantities of emitted neutrons collide with substances at the earth's surface to form new radioactive materials, which then release beta and gamma rays. [The radioactive materials and their half-lives are ^{24}Na (15 hours); ^{28}Al (2.3 minutes); ^{56}Mn (2.6 hours); ^{46}Sc (83.9 days); ^{60}Co (5.26 years); and ^{134}Cs (2.05 years)]. The products of radioactive fallout were formed by the nuclear fission of ^{235}U, ^{90}Sr, ^{137}Cs, ^{140}Ba and over 200 other nuclei, and also formed from radioactive materials contained in substances made radioactive in the atmosphere, in dust produced by impact, and in smoke from the fires. In contrast to the short half-life of induced radioactivity, the effects of the radioactive fallout products are longterm, due to the presence of ^{137}Cs (with a half life of 30 years) and ^{90}Sr (29 years).

If only the amount of induced radiation produced in the soil is calculated, the cumulative dose of gamma rays between 1 and 100 hours of the explosion at a point 1 meter above the hypocenter is said to have been approximately 1 Gy (the amount produced more than 100 hours after the explosion is believed negligible). The initial neutron radiation decreased sharply with increasing distance from the hypocenter, as did the induced radiation (approximately 0.20 Gy at 500 m, and 0.01 Gy at 1,000 m). It has been calculated that remaining in the vicinity of the hypocenter for 8 hours on August 7th would have led to an exposure of $\leqslant 0.10$ Gy[1]. It is believed that in addition to external exposure to this residual radiation, early entrants to the city would also have received internal bodily exposure due to inhalation, eating and drinking, and absorption through the skin.

1. RADIATION DOSE AND FREQUENCY OF CHROMOSOMAL ABERRATIONS

It has been known for about 30 years that on being irradiated the chromosomes in human bone marrow cells become adhesive and undergo condensation, and that the same changes are observed during *in vitro* experiments. The first report to describe radiation-induced chromosomal aberrations in human peripheral blood cells was in

1960 by Tough *et al*[2]. It was later demonstrated *in vitro* that there was a strong correlation between radiation dose and the frequency of chromosomal aberrations in peripheral blood lymphocytes[3,4]. Section 3 summarizes the method by which the biological dose estimates for early entrants were obtained by analysis of the chromosomes in peripheral blood lymphocytes[5].

2. CLASSIFICATION OF EARLY ENTRANTS

Out of a total of 40 subjects studied, 20 were members of the Kahokubutai (Kohgetsuchutai) volunteer corps from Kamo-gun in Hiroshima prefecture[6], who entered Hiroshima on the day after the bombing and remained for 4–7 days engaged in relief work etc. in the vicinity of the former Western Drill Ground (these individuals are thought to have been exposed to the greatest radiation dose of any entrants). The time of entry to the hypocenter area of the other 20 varied from immediately after the explosion to the 3rd day after the bombing. Virtually all of the Kahokubutai corps members followed the same patterns of activity after their early entry into the city, making it possible to very accurately estimate the doses received by all survivors who were early entrants and remained in the city for a long time. The subsequent medical exposure histories of these individuals were obtained in detail.

3. CHROMOSOMAL ABERRATIONS AND ESTIMATED DOSES OF EARLY ENTRANTS

Specimens of peripheral blood lymphocyte cultures were obtained according to the method of Moorhead *et al*[7], i.e. peripheral blood samples (10 ml) were taken, left standing at room temperature for 1 hour, and the buffy coat removed. The buffy coat was cultured for 52 hours with RPMI-1640 (8 ml), fetal calf (or bovine) serum (2 ml) and phytohemagglutinin [PHA, Wellcome Co.; 0.1 ml], with colcemid added for the final 2 hours. The most important difference from previous methods was that in this technique the observed metaphase is believed to be the first mitosis after the start of culturing. Observation is by the conventional method, whereby staining with 5% Giemsa solution is performed for 20 minutes, the widely dispersed metaphase is selected, and 200–500 cells are analyzed.

Forty early entrants were classified into 4 groups according to their length of stay near the hypocenter and medical radiation exposure histories (Table 1). Group A consisted of entrants who were present for a long time but had little medical exposure (10 individuals from the volunteer corps), group B was composed of entrants who

Table 1   Early entrants

Group A:	Long stay	
Group B:	Long stay and considerable medical exposure	Kahokubutai volunteer corps Every day after Aug. 7th
Group C:	Short stay	
Group D:	Short stay and considerable medical exposure	1 or 2 entries, Aug. 6th–9th

stayed for a long time and also received a considerable amount of medical exposure (10 individuals from the volunteer corps), group C consisted of entrants who remained only a short time and had little medical exposure (6 individuals), and group D was composed of entrants who stayed only a short time but received a considerable amount of medical exposure (14 individuals). The results of chromosomal analyses on these 40 subjects, together with details of their time of entry, medical exposure histories, and estimated T65D doses[8] are shown in Table 2. The chromosomal aberrations were divided into stable aberrations (which can persist for a long time without damage during mitosis) and unstable aberrations (which do not survive to the next generation).

The average ages at examination for the various groups were 63.9 years (group A), 64.9 years (group B), 68.8 years (group C), and 65.5 years (group D). The ages at the time of bombing were therefore 20–25 years, with almost no difference between the groups in this respect. The percentage of stable abnormalities observed was 0–2.0% for group A (average 1.06%), 0.5–5.0% for group B (average 1.80%), 0–1.0% for group C (average 0.50%), and 0–2.4% for group D (average 0.73%). The estimated doses were < 0.01 Gy–0.135 Gy for group A (average 0.048 Gy); < 0.01 Gy–0.712 Gy for group B (average 0.139 Gy); an average of < 0.01 Gy for group C; and < 0.01 Gy–0.212 Gy for group D (average 0.019 Gy).

The frequency of chromosomal aberrations for each group in Table 1 is shown in Fig. 1. A significant difference in frequency was not observed between groups C and D (the short-term populations) ($p > 0.24$), but large significant differences were seen between each of groups A and B ($p < 0.005$), A and C ($p < 0.005$), B and C ($p < 0.005$), and B and D ($p < 0.005$). These results are summarized in Table 3.

4. EARLY ENTRANTS AND THE PROBLEM OF MEDICAL EXPOSURE

The question of whether medical exposure aggravated the effects of atomic bomb radiation has already been investigated[9–11]. A marked individual difference can be observed among group D subjects, but is thought to be due to factors such as the use of medications that could produce chromosomal aberrations, and medical exposures which were not revealed to the examiners. For early entrants, differences in both length of stay and medical exposure were reflected in the frequency of chromosomal aberrations, with the order being (long stay + medical exposure, 0.139 Gy) > (long stay + no medical exposure, 0.048 Gy) > (short stay + medical exposure, 0.019 Gy) > (short stay + no medical exposure, $\leqslant 0.01$ Gy). Within each group there was a wide variation, but the cumulative dose due to atomic bomb radioactivity could be simply considered as $\leqslant 0.048$ Gy for the long-stay population and $\leqslant 0.01$ Gy for the short-stay population. The difference between these two populations regarding exposure to atomic bomb radioactivity was considerable, equal to about 0.038 Gy between these two populations (0.048 Gy for group A compared to 0.010 Gy for group C). On the other hand, the differences between the groups in exposure to medical radiation following the atomic bombing varied from 0.091 Gy (0.139 Gy for group B compared to 0.048 Gy for group A) to 0.009 Gy (0.019 Gy for group D compared to 0.010 Gy for group C). The Japan Broadcasting Corporation (Nippon Hoso Kyokai, NHK)[6] reported that Maruyama performed a complex physical calculation on

Table 2   Chromosomal aberatons and exposure status of early entrants

Case	Age (yrs)	Chromosomal aberrations			No. of observed cells	No. of stable cells	Estimated dose (Gy)	Dates of entry	Medical radiaton exposure history		
		Unstable	Stable	Total					Organ or disease	No. of exposures	Time of exposure (when known)
1	60	8	10	18	500	2.0	0.135		Stomach	1 time	5 yrs. before
2	65	4	9	13	500	1.8	0.096		Stomach	1 time	1 yr. before
3	60	8	9	17	500	1.8	0.096		—	—	—
4	64	6	9	15	500	1.8	0.096		Stomach	5 ~ 6 times	
5	59	10	8	18	500	1.6	0.058	Approx. 1 week starting Aug. 7th	Stomach	2 times	10 and 20 yrs. and before
Group A 6	59	3	4	7	500	0.8	< 0.01		Stomach	1 time	
7	67	7	3	9	500	0.4	< 0.01		Stomach	1 time	5 yrs. before
8	76	0	2	2	500	0.4	< 0.01		Stomach	1 time	5 yrs. before
9	60	5	0	5	500	0	< 0.01		Stomach	Approx. 5 times	—
10	69	1	0	1	500	0	< 0.01		Stomach	2 times	10 and 20 yrs. before
11	72	4	10	14	200	5.0	0.712		Stomach	> 10 times	
12	60	3	5	8	200	2.5	0.231		Stomach	> 10 times	
13	59	3	4	7	200	2.0	0.135		Stomach	> 10 times	
Group B 14	59	4	4	8	200	2.0	0.135	Approx. 1 week starting Aug. 7th	Stomach	2 times	CT
15	73	4	4	8	200	2.0	0.135		Stomach / Colon	3 times / 2 times	Colon
16	70	3	3	6	200	1.5	0.038		Brain		CT
17	60	2	2	4	200	1.0	< 0.01		Stomach	> 10 times	
18	60	2	2	4	200	1.0	< 0.01		Stomach	> 10 times	
19	62	1	1	2	200	0.5	< 0.01		Stomach	> 10 times	
20	74	0	1	1	200	0.5	< 0.01		Stomach	> 10 times	
21	69	5	5	10	500	1.0	< 0.01	Aug. 6th	Stomach	1 time	
22	63	0	3	3	500	0.6	< 0.01	Aug. 7th, 8th	Stomach	2 times	2 and 20 yrs. before
Group C 23	17	1	3	4	500	0.6	< 0.01	Aug. 7th	Stomach	2 times	10 and 20 yrs. before
24	58	0	3	3	500	0.6	< 0.01	Aug. 8th	Stomach	1 time	
25	87	0	1	1	500	0.2	< 0.01	Aug. 7th	Stomach	1 time	
26	65	1	0	1	500	0	< 0.01	Aug. 8th	Stomach	1 time	
27	66	0	12	12	500	2.4	0.212	Aug. 6th	Stomach	> 10 times	
28	63	1	8	9	500	1.6	0.058	Aug. 7th	Stomach	> 10 times	
29	56	3	5	8	500	1.0	< 0.01	Aug. 8th, 9th	Stomach	> 10 times	
30	59	0	4	4	500	0.8	< 0.01	Aug. 8th, 9th	Stomach	> 10 times	
31	57	0	4	4	500	0.8	< 0.01	Aug. 8th	Stomach	> 10 times	
32	69	0	4	4	500	0.8	< 0.01	Aug. 9th	Cholelithiasis	Thyroid cancer	
Group D 33	76	1	3	4	500	0.6	< 0.01	Aug. 8th	Stomach	> 10 times	
34	76	0	2	2	500	0.4	< 0.01	Aug. 7th, 8th	Stomach	> 10 times	
35	65	0	2	2	500	0.4	< 0.01	Aug. 7th	Stomach	> 10 times	
36	92	1	2	3	500	0.4	< 0.01	Aug. 8th	Stomach	10 times	Head CT
37	74	0	22	2	500	0.4	< 0.01	Aug. 8th	Gastric cancer operation		
38	51	1	2	3	500	0.4	< 0.01	Aug. 8th	Gastric ulcer operation		
39	49	0	1	1	500	0.2	< 0.01	Aug. 8th	Stomach	> 10 times	
40	64	0	0	0	500	0	< 0.01	Aug. 7th	Stomach	> 10 times	Barium enema

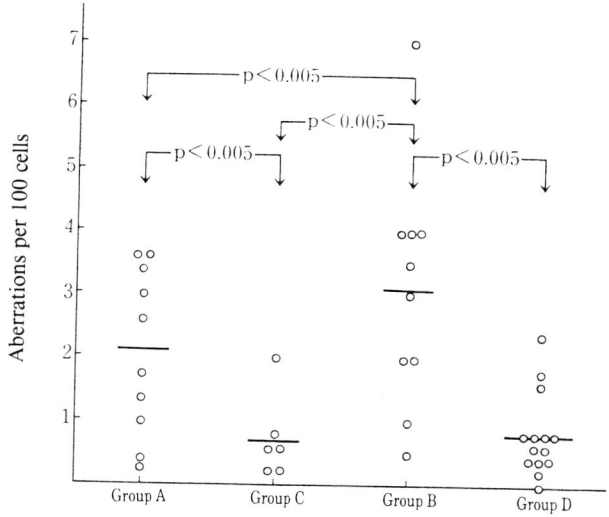

Figure 1 Number of chromosomal aberration in early entrant population

Table 3 Chromosomal aberrations in early entrants

Group	No. of entrants	No. of observed cells	No. of chromosomal aberrations (%)	Significant difference
A	10	5,000	2.1	
B	10	2,000	3.1	
C	6	3,000	0.73	
D	14	7,000	0.83	
Total	40	17,000	1.45	

the same volunteer corps subjects and obtained a maximum total exposure of approximately 0.120 Gy and a minimum figure of approximately 0.035 Gy (the calculation considered external exposure due to fallout, neutron-induced irradiation[12], and internal exposure due to fallout and induced radioactivity). The figures are in approximate agreement with the value of 0.048 Gy obtained from biological dosimetry for exposure to atomic bomb radiation only.

For 135 distally but minimally exposed atomic bomb survivors (estimated dose 0 Gy), Awa and Sawada[13] estimated the medical exposures by considering the type and power of X-ray equipment used (0–0.071 Gy), and found a linear dose-response relationship between the frequency of chromosomal aberrations and bone marrow medical exposure dose. This supports findings suggesting that the contribution of medical exposure is in some cases greater than that of atomic bomb radiation[10]. In other words, it is impossible approximately half a century after the atomic bombing to ignore medical exposure when investigating the effects of atomic bomb radiation.

CONCLUSION

With advances in medicine, the use of X-rays in health management is rapidly increasing. In contrast to the atomic bombing, in which a large amount of radioactivity was released at one time, a future problem to be addressed is how to consider the cumulative dose that the body receives from repeated medical exposure to small amounts of radiation.

The above study concerned subjects who were estimated to have been exposed to large doses of radioactivity. The health effects of the chromosomal aberrations are unclear. That is, although today various types of hemocyte counts exhibit no abnormalities, it cannot be concluded that there is no relationship to future illnesses. It is necessary to perform follow-up studies and also to as far as possible restrict the future medical exposures of these individuals. Although an extremely complex undertaking, it would be worth considering a health management scheme whereby individual records were kept of the date and doses etc. for each medical exposure given to each individual in the country.

Since an analysis of chromosomal aberrations requires observation of a large number of cells, this necessitates both a considerable amount of time and skilled personnel. There is a great need to find easier and more accurate methods of dose estimation (e.g. automation, and the possibility of obtaining measurements from blood serum). For this purpose it is necessary to preserve the precious specimens from those survivors still alive today.

(Nobuo Oguma, Nanao Kamada)

REFERENCES

1. Takeshita K. Dose estimation from residual and fallout radioactivity area survey. *J Radiat Res* 1975; **16** (Suppl): 24–31 .
2. Tough IM, *et al.* X-ray-induced chromosome damage in man. *Lancet* 1960; **2**: 849–51.
3. Sasaki MS, Miyata H. Biological dosimetry in atomic bomb survivors. *Nature* 1968; **220**: 1189–93.
4. Awa AA, *et al.* Chromosome aberration frequency in cultured blood cells in relation to radiation dose of A-bomb survivors. *Lancet* 1971; **2**: 903–5.
5. Oguma N, Kamada N. Chromosome aberrations in the early entrants after A-bomb explosion at Hiroshima. Cooperative medical studies on investigation of the atomic bomb survivors, Ministry of Health and Welfare, 1991; 17–20. (*In Japanese*)
6. Nippon Broadcasting Corporation (NHK), Atomic Bomb Project Team. Hiroshima residual radiation, 1988; 1–241. (*In Japanese*)
7. Moorhead PS, *et al.* Chromosome preparations of leukocytes cultured from human peripheral blood. *Exp Cell Res* 1960; **20**: 613–6.
8. Preston DL, *et al.* Comparison of the dose-response relationships for chromosome aberration frequencies between the T65D and DS86 dosimetries. RERF TR 7–88, 1988.
9. Sawada S, *et al.* Hospital and clinic survey estimates of medical X-ray exposures in Hiroshima and Nagasaki. Part 1. RERF population and the general population. RERF TR 16–79, 1979.
10. Antoku S, *et al.* Hospital and clinic survey estimates of medical X-ray exposures in Hiroshima and Nagasaki. Part 2. Technical exposure factors. RERF TR 6–86, 1986.

11. Yamamoto O, *et al.* Medical X-ray exposure doses as possible contaminants of atomic bomb doses. RERF TR 16–86, 1986.
12. Gritzner ML, Woolson WA. Calculation of doses due to atomic bomb induced soil activation: US-Japan joint reassessment of atomic bomb radiation dosimetry in Hiroshima and Nagasaki. Vol. 2. Hiroshima: Radiation Effects Research Foundation, 1987: 342–51.
13. Awa AA, Sawada S. Chromosome aberration induced by medical X-ray exposures in peripheral lymphocytes of A-bomb survivors. Cooperative medical studies on investigation of the atomic bomb survivors, Ministry of Health and Welfare, 1990; 23–5. (*In Japanese*)

15

Mutation

15.1 SOMATIC CELL MUTATION

INTRODUCTION

Ionizing radiation (such as X-rays and gamma rays), ultraviolet rays and various chemical substances are known to induce somatic cell mutations. Past studies on chromosomal aberrations in the peripheral blood lymphocytes of atomic bomb survivors have proven the persistence of genetic damage (mutations) in their somatic cells[1,2]. Several techniques have recently been established for the quantitative detection of aberrations at specific genetic loci in human blood cells. These have been mainly due to significant advances in the field of immunology and have employed recombinant interleukin-2, monoclonal antibodies which react to specific gene products, and flow cytometry. In contrast to the chromosomal aberration tests for visible abnormalities, these techniques have permitted the detection of gene damage so slight as to be invisible through a microscope. The cancer risk among atomic bomb survivors remains high[3-5], and it is believed that the first step in carcinogenesis is radiation-induced genetic damage that causes somatic cell mutations.

Consequently, the adoption of these new techniques for determining the mutant frequency at specific loci in the somatic cells of atomic bomb survivors (determination of the frequency of DNA damage) is considered extremely valuable in the assessment of the long-term health risks posed by atomic bomb radiation.

Also, even when it is difficult to obtain physical estimates of the radiation dose, it is believed that these methods can provide objective biological estimates.

This chapter summarizes three currently employed techniques and their specific characteristics, and will outline the findings obtained, with particular reference to atomic bomb survivors.

1. T-LYMPHOCYTE HPRT ASSAY[6-8]

This technique employs not flow cytometry but colony formation (Fig. 1a). Since interleukin-2 (T-cell growth factor) has been discovered, peripheral T-cell colony formation has become possible. Then in the same manner that is widely adopted using cultured cells, the frequency of 6-thioguanine resistant lymphocyte colonies gives the mutant frequency in the hypoxanthineguanine phosphoribosyltransferase (HPRT) gene.

Colony formation takes approximately 2 weeks. Approximately 10 ml of blood is required, and it is important to use good quality recombinant human interleukin-2 in order to allow good reproducibility of results. No restrictions are placed on the genetic types of subjects. The HPRT mutant frequency increases significantly with the age of the survivor, rising by 2 mutants per 10^6 lymphocytes for every 10-year increase in age. Also, a significant positive correlation is found between HPRT mutant frequency and the frequency of lymphocytes with chromosomal aberrations[8].

A significant positive correlation exists between the HPRT mutant frequency (Mf) in atomic bomb survivors and DS86 dose estimates (Fig. 2). However, the slope of the linear regression is extremely shallow, e.g. the mean Mf value for a survivor with

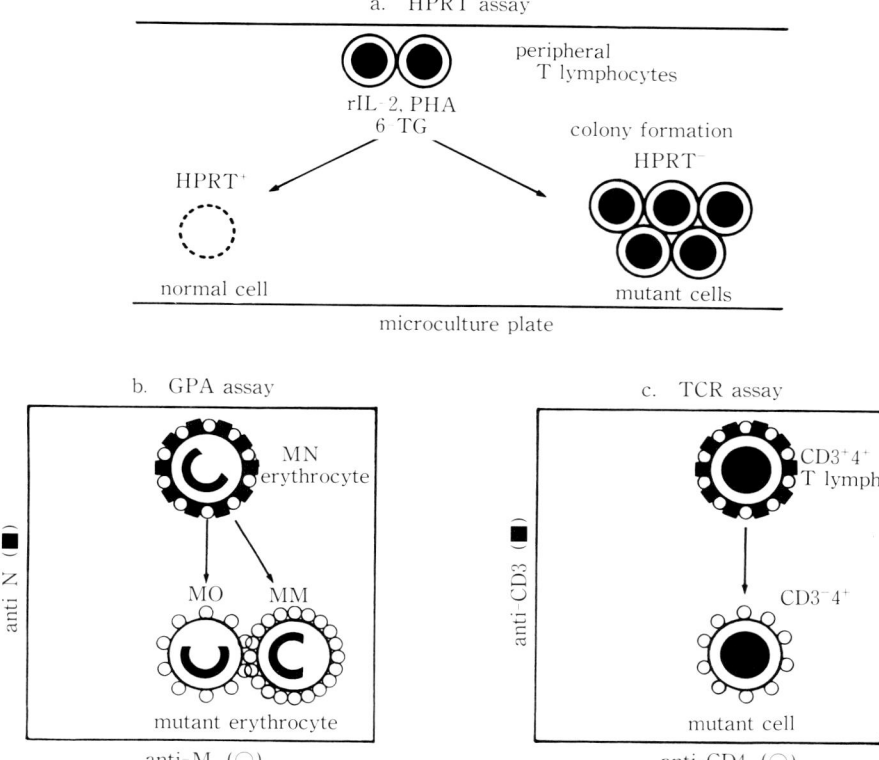

Figure 1 Assays for detecting human somatic mutations

an estimated dose of 3 Gy was only approximately 1.5 times that of the control population.

It is known that HPRT heterozygous females exhibit *in vivo* selection against HPRT-deficient lymphocytes, and the poor correlation of mutant frequency with dose is probably due to the long period that has elapsed since exposure. The HPRT mutant frequency is known to increase in individuals who undergo radiotherapy, but due to the absence of studies on post-therapeutic changes in Mf with respect to time, the rate of mutant cell elimination is unknown, although this author's studies suggest a half-life of 1–2 years.

2. ERYTHROCYTE GLYCOPHORIN A (GPA) ASSAY[8-10] (FIG. 1B)

Erythrocyte glycophorin A (GPA) genes determine MN blood type, with the existence of M and N alleles. The M and N antigens differ in the NH_2 terminals of the 2 amino acids, and thus monoclonal antibodies specific to M and N alleles respectively are produced[12,13]. When these monoclonal antibodies are labeled with two

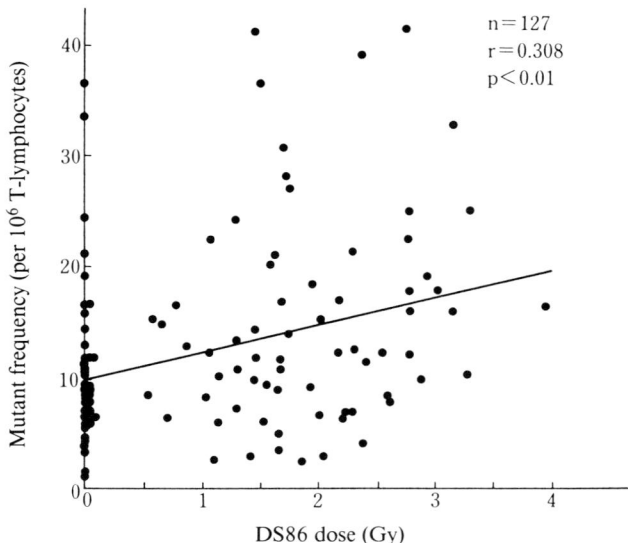

Figure 2   Relationship between mutant frequency and dose (T-lymphocyte HPRT assay; 127 cases)

different fluorescent dyes (red phycoerythrin, PE, and green fluorescein isothiocyanate, FITC), and used to stain fixed human erythrocytes of blood type MN, normal erythrocytes are dyed a mixture of red and green, giving an orange appearance. In contrast, the mutant erythrocytes which lack expression of either M or N alleles (respectively referred to as M0 and N0 mutants) are either red or green, and thus can be automatically determined by flow cytometry.

This procedure permits detection of 4 mutant types (N0, M0, NN, and MM). It is believed that an abundance of either N0 or M0 mutants leads to deletion of M or N alleles, and that NN and MM mutants are probably produced due to somatic recombination of those genes.

The study was performed on individuals of MN blood type, who comprised approximately 50% of the human population. One milliliter of blood was sufficient. The process of subjecting erythrocytes to hypotonic treatment and fixation of the spherical products required several days[9-11].

The frequency of the GPA mutant erythrocytes shows a positive correlation with the age of the survivor, with an average increase of 2×10^{-6} cells per 10 years[8]. It also displays a strong positive correlation with the frequency of lymphocytes with chromosomal aberrations[8]. These correlations are extremely strong in comparison with that observed between HPRT mutant frequency and the frequency of lymphocytes with chromosomal aberrations.

This indicates that the erythrocytes with GPA mutations are different from the cells that possess HPRT mutations, and that the negative *in vivo* selection is not strong. The GPA technique can therefore be employed as a lifetime biological dosimeter for radiation exposure. Figure 3 shows the frequency of GPA mutations in 355 atomic bomb survivors by radiation dose. Since both N0 and M0 GPA mutant

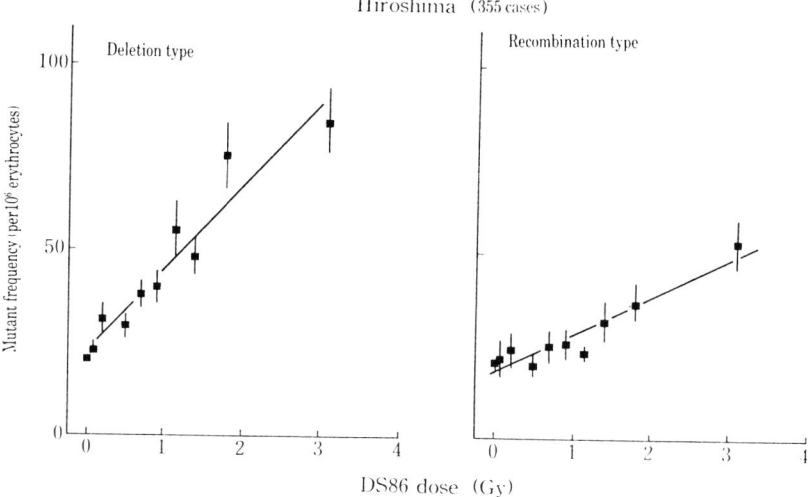

Figure 3   Relationship between mutant frequency in somatic cells and dose (erythrocyte GPA assay; 355 cases)

frequencies exhibit virtually identical strong dose dependencies, the average of the sum of the two indicates the mutant frequency (Mf), which increases by approximately 2.2×10^{-5} per 1 Gy (Fig. 3). The point of interest is that the gradient of this dose-response relationship is derived from cultured human cells, and is virtually the same as that for the HPRT mutant frequency induced by *in vitro* irradiation with X-rays[14]. This also supports the fact that GPA mutant erythrocytes do not undergo negative *in vivo* selection, and suggests they can be adopted as a lifetime biological dosimeter.

3. T-LYMPHOCYTE TCR (T-CELL RECEPTOR) ASSAY[15]

Mature T-cells possess CD3 antigen at the cell surface. This molecule cannot be expressed at the cell surface without formation of a complex with the α-, β, or γ-, δ chain products of the T-cell receptor (TCR). The CD3 antigen itself is a complex derived from various proteins, but since each of these is coded with a pair of genes in the autosomal chromosome, they are not expressed as a phenotype abnormality unless mutations occur in both genes of the pair. In contrast, the α-, β, and γ-, δ chain genes of the T-cell receptor are similar to immunoglobulin genes in B-cells in that expression occurs in only one gene of the pair. Therefore, while TCR α-, β chain genes are autosomal, there is the advantage that functionally they each have the state of being one gene, with a mutation in one gene being expressed directly as a phenotypic abnormality, which can then be detected. As shown in Fig. 1c, by taking advantage of this characteristic, anti-CD3 antibody and anti-CD4 antibody (helper/inducer T-cell markers) are conjugated with different fluorescent dyes. Flow cytometry then allows detection of TCR mutations with a $CD3^-4^+$ phenotypic abnormality.

The TCR mutant frequency (Mf) of healthy individuals increases significantly with age by 3×10^{-6} cells per year[15]. Furthermore, *in vitro* experiments showed a significant dose-dependent increase in TCR mutant frequency upon X-ray irradiation of peripheral blood lymphocytes, with an extremely high gradient of the order of 10^{-3} per Gray. However, a significant dose-response relationship has not to date been observed for the TCR mutant frequency in 342 atomic bomb survivors (Fig. 4), which suggests that the cells with the TCR gene mutations have, in the more than 40 years that have passed since exposure to the bomb, undergone *in vivo* negative selection and have been unable to persist in the long term. Consequently, the TCR technique is not suitable as a lifetime biological dosimeter for radiation exposure, but may be suitable for the detection of recent exposure effects. Indeed, a study on 36 patients who in the past several years underwent radiotherapy (50–60 Gy of external radiation) for gynecological cancers found that the TCR mutant frequency showed a significant short-term increase following radiotherapy, but that this subsequently decreased with time, suggesting a half-life of approximately 2 years. This provides a good explanation for the failure to detect a significant dose-response relationship for survivors more than 40 years after exposure. Furthermore, a TCR mutant frequency study was performed on a population consisting of individuals who were not atomic bomb survivors but who had been recently exposed to radiation, viz. 24 patients recently treated with radioactive iodine-131 (^{131}I) for malignant diseases of the thyroid. The results are shown in Fig. 5, with all the TCR mutant frequencies determined in repeated measurements on the 24 subjects who received multiple administrations of ^{131}I. The ^{131}I dose was calculated on the assumption that the half-life of cells with TCR mutations is approximately 2 years.

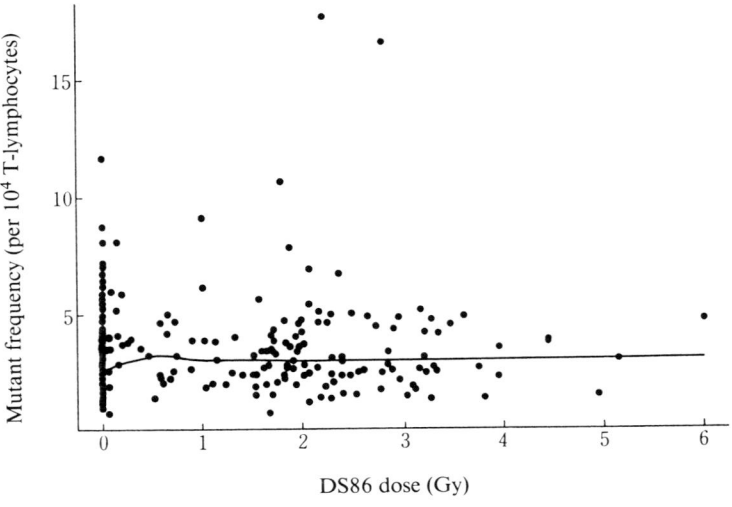

Figure 4 Relationship between mutant frequency and dose (T-lymphocyte TCR assay; 342 cases)

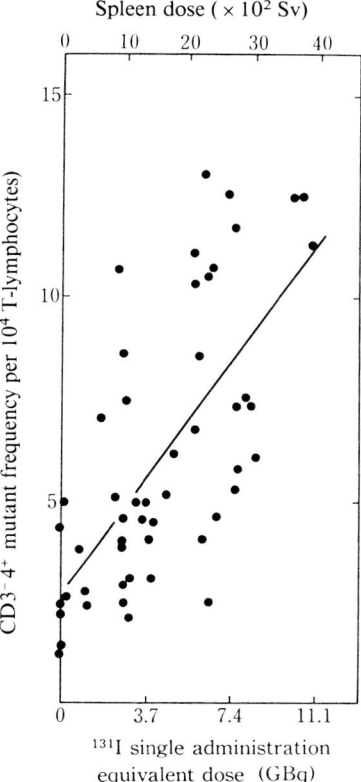

Figure 5   Relationship between mutant frequency and ^{131}I dose among patients undergoing ^{131}I radiotherapy (T-lymphocyte TCR assay)

For example, for a ^{131}I dose of 2 gigabecquerels (GBq) administered 2 years prior to the testing, the dose was taken to be half that (i.e. 1 GBq), and described as a ^{131}I single administration equivalent dose of 1 GBq. The Mf value was found to increase in proportion to the amount of ^{131}I administered, and the gradient of the dose-response curve was almost identical to that obtained during *in vitro* experiments. On the other hand, the Mf value also increased in Thorotrast patients receiving continuous α-ray irradiation[16].

These results show that although there is *in vivo* selection against cells with mutations on TCR genes, an increased Mf can be detected if a long period has not elapsed after exposure (probably within 5–7 years). Therefore, bearing in mind the half-life of these mutants, this could be used as a biological dosimeter. To give an example, measurements of TCR mutant frequency in a fireman approximately 3.5 years after exposure to radiation in the Chernobyl nuclear power plant accident showed an extremely high Mf value of 21.1×10^{-4}, yielding a dose estimate of 3–4 Gy.

The TCR assay has various advantages, e.g. there is no restriction of subjects; the procedure is simple since it is possible to stain the antibodies without cell fixation (approximately 5 hours from collection of specimens to measurement, with measurement requiring 10 minutes); due to the high Mf value (of the order of 10^{-4}) only a small number of cells (i.e. specimen volume) are required to obtain a statistically sufficient number of mutant cells; and every antibody is commercially available.

4. OTHER BIOLOGICAL SOMATIC CELL MUTATION ASSAYS

The chromosomal aberrations in lymphocytes mentioned at the beginning can be broadly classified into stable (Cs) and unstable (Cu) aberrations. Typical Cu-type abnormalities are dicentric aberrations and chromosomal deletions, which are easy to detect in comparison with Cs-type abnormalities such as inversions and reciprocal translocations. On the other hand, they suffer *in vivo* elimination with the passage of time, with a half-life of approximately 1 year. The frequency of Cs-type aberrations is independent of time after exposure and remains approximately constant, but has the disadvantage of demanding skill for detection.

A further technique utilizes lymphocytes and involves determination of the micronucleus frequency. When the acentric segment produced during chromosomal segmentation undergoes nuclear division, it remains at the equatorial plate, and as a result, instead of being incorporated into one of the daughter nuclei, appears in the cytoplasm as a small nucleus. Since the prime cause is the breakage accompanying the Cu-type aberration this also is expected to have a half-life of approximately 1 year. The disadvantage is the existence of rather large individual differences.

5. POST-EXPOSURE DEVELOPMENTS WITH TIME AND APPROPRIATE MONITORING SYSTEMS

When adopting one of the previously mentioned techniques for assessment of the health risks posed by radiation exposure, or to perform biological estimations of dose received, it is important that the chosen technique exploits its special features. For individuals with whole body exposure to high doses ($\geqslant 2$ Gy), various acute symptoms appear (seasickness symptoms, vomiting, fatigue), and the peripheral lymphocyte count decreases drastically within one day. Consequently other methods of health management are necessary for such exposed individuals. Measurements of somatic cell mutant frequencies provide a useful method of monitoring individuals who either suffered no acute symptoms, did not have lymphocyte counts determined, or else were unknowingly exposed to low doses (although later doses are known). In the case of such individuals being exposed to low or moderate doses:

1) *Within several days of exposure*: the simplest measurement should be for frequency of lymphocytes with micronuclei. Unstable (Cu-type) chromosomal aberrations would be easy to detect.

2)   *Within several weeks of exposure*: in tests for chromosomal aberrations such as Cu- and Cs-type abnormalities, culturing is best commenced immediately after exposure, but in testing for somatic cell mutations time is required for mutant phenotypes to be expressed at the surface of the tested cells. At that time, therefore, it is possible to employ the TCR and HPRT methods as well as micronuclei measurements and tests for Cu-type chromosomal aberrations. The time period required for the *in vivo* TCR and HPRT mutant phenotypes to be expressed is not well known, but *in vitro* experiments require 1 week to 10 days, and thus a period of several weeks would probably be appropriate.

3)   *Within several months of exposure*: the GPA technique becomes applicable, since mutant cells formed in nuclear erythroid progenitors within the bone marrow (erythroblasts or less differentiated stem cells) are detected in the peripheries, and since erythrocytes have a life span of 120 days, the maximum number of mutant erythrocytes is observed at 4 months after exposure. By this time it is possible that the value yielded by the HPRT method may have already approached the mutant frequency level of the control population.

4)   *Within 1 to 2 years of exposure*: in each of the techniques based on micronuclear determination, Cu-type chromosomal aberration, and HPRT, the mutant frequency is believed to be considerably reduced, whereas it is thought that the Mf value given by the TCR method will still be above 50%. Detection of mutations by the Cs-type chromosomal aberration and GPA techniques is believed to pose no problem.

5)   *Over 5 years after exposure*: the Mf levels given by the micronucleus determination, Cu-type chromosomal aberration, HPRT and TCR techniques are expected to show virtually no increase, with the only techniques still available being the GPA method and the laborious Cs-type chromosomal aberration test. All the above techniques are summarized in Fig. 6, which indicates the applicability with respect to time for an individual subjected to a low to medium radiation dose of ≤ 2 Gy. In the case of long-term exposure such as occurred due to environmental contamination following the Chernobyl nuclear power plant

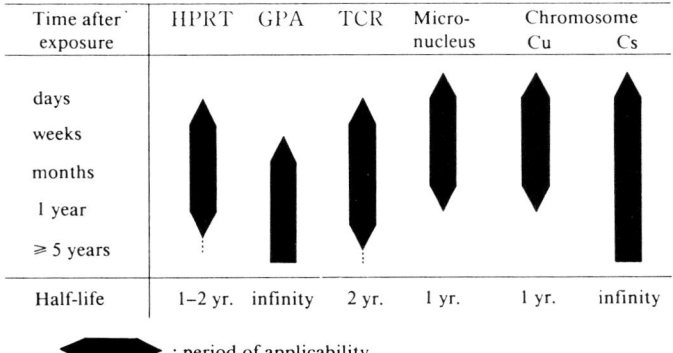

Figure 6   Applicability of somatic mutation assays for biological dosimetry over time for individuals exposed to low to moderate doses of radiation

accident, it is advisable to as far as possible employ biological techniques that utilize long half-lives. The Cs-type chromosomal aberration technique is not feasible for a large population, but it would be possible to adopt the GPA method on a reasonably large scale.

CONCLUSION

The somatic cell mutant frequency data obtained as a result of the long-term medical examinations on the atomic bomb survivors has provided valuable information for the assessment of health risks. On the other hand, dose estimation plays an extremely important role in health risk evaluation, but, as was noted above, earlier physical dose estimations are frequently difficult, and even if they were available they would probably contain a considerable number of errors. Therefore, should biological dose estimation by somatic cell mutant frequency testing prove possible, this would be an extremely significant development.

Besides these mutant frequency measurement methods which can be used with flow cytometry, a method of determining DNA level by means of a polymerase chain reaction is gradually being developed.

It is evident that this field of study holds great promise for the future.

(*Mitoshi Akiyama*)

REFERENCES

1. Awa AA, Sofuni T, Honda T, *et al.* Relationship between the radiation dose and chromosome aberrations in atomic bomb survivors of Hiroshima and Nagasaki. *J Radiat Res* 1978; **19**: 126–40.
2. Awa AA. Radiation-induced chromosome aberrations in A-bomb survivors — a key to biological dosimetry. In: Prentice RL, Thompson DJ, editors. Atomic bomb survivors data: utilization and analysis. Philadelphia: Siam, 1984: 99–111.
3. Darby SC, Nakashima E, Kato H. A parallel analysis of cancer mortality among atomic bomb survivors and patients with ankylosing spondilitis given X-ray therapy. *JNCI* 1985; **75**: 1–21.
4. Preston DI, Kato H, Kopecky KJ, *et al.* Life Span Study report 10. Part 1. Cancer mortality among A-bomb survivors in Hiroshima and Nagasaki 1950–1982. RERF TR 1–86, 1985.
5. Shimizu Y, Kato H, Schull WJ, *et al.* Life Span Study report 11. Part 1. Comparison of risk coefficients for site-specific cancer mortality based on the DS86 and T65DR shielded kerma and organ doses. RERF TR 12–87, 1987.
6. Hakoda M, Akiyama M, Kyoizumi S, *et al.* Increased somatic cell mutant frequency in atomic bomb survivors. *Mutat Res* 1988; **201**: 39–48.
7. Hirai Y, Hakoda M, Kusunoki Y, *et al.* Late effects of A-bomb radiation on bone marrow stem cells. *Nagasaki Med J* 1989; **63**: 120–3. (*In Japanese*)
8. Akiyama M, Kyoizumi S, Hirai Y, *et al.* Studies on chromosome aberrations and HPRT mutations in lymphocytes and GPA mutation in erythrocytes of atomic bomb survivors. In: Medelsohn ML, Albertini RJ, editors. Mutation and the environment, part C. New York: Wiley-Liss, 1990: 69–80.
9. Langlois RG, Bigbee WL, Kyoizumi S, *et al.* Evidence for increased somatic cell mutations at the glycophorin A locus in atomic bomb survivors. *Science* 1987; **236**: 445–8.
10. Akiyama M, Hirai Y, Kyoizumi S, *et al.* Detection of mutant erythrocytes at glycophorin A locus. *Environmental Mutagen Research Communications* 1989; **11**: 47–54. (*In Japanese*).
11. Kyoizumi S, Nakamura N, Hakoda M, *et al.* Detection of somatic mutations at the glycophorin A

locus in erythrocytes of atomic bomb survivors using a single beam flow sorter. *Cancer Res* 1989; **49**: 581–8.

12. Bigbee WL, Vanderlaan M, Fong SSN, *et al.* Monoclonal antibodies specific for the M-and N-forms of human glycophorin A. *Mol Immunol* 1983; **20**: 1353–62.

13. Bigbee WL, Langlois RG, Vanderlaan M, *et al.* Binding specificities of eight monoclonal antibodies to human glycophorin A. Studies with MCM and MkEn (UK) variant human erythrocytes and M- and MNY-type chimpanzee erythrocytes. *J Immunol* 1984; **133**: 3149–55.

14. Nakamura N, Sposto R, Miller RC, *et al.* X-ray-induced mutations in cultured human thyroid cells. *Radiat Res* 1989; **119**: 123–33.

15. Kyoizumi S, Akiyama M, Hirai Y, *et al.* Spontaneous loss and alteration of antigen receptor expression in mature CD4$^+$ T cells. *J Exp Med* 1990; **171**: 1981–99.

16. Umeki S, Kyoizumi S, Kusunoki Y, *et al.* Flow cytometric measurements of somatic cell mutations in Thorotrast patients. *Jpn J Cancer Res* 1991; **82**: 1349–53.

15.2 RADIOSENSITIVITY

INTRODUCTION

In addition to the level of dose, the effect of radiation has long been known to vary with factors such as sex, age, and species of animal etc. Differences in sensitivity are even observed between strains of mice, which is believed due to differences in genetic background. Unlike experimental animals, humans form a heterogenous population, and the importance of such genetic background differences in determining the effect of radiation exposure is not well understood.

If there were some people rather resistant to radiation and others rather sensitive to radiation due to a difference in genetic background, then if they were exposed to a high radiation dose, preferential survival of the resistant population would be expected. In this case, if it is assumed that the relatively resistant population is also resistant to the development of cancer, then the current studies on late effects of the atomic bomb may include certain biases.

In fact, a comparison of individuals suffering an acute post-exposure symptom (severe epilation) with those that did not revealed that the former population was approximately twice as likely to develop leukemia[1]. The population exhibiting the acute symptom was also found to have a higher frequency of chromosomal aberrations in lymphocytes[2]. However, as the DS86 dose estimations used in these studies would contain errors, it is not certain whether individual differences in radiosensitivity actually exist, or simply that this is due to the individuals who exhibited acute symptoms actually being exposed to doses which were on average greater than those received by individuals not displaying the symptoms.

Radiosensitivity studies using blood lymphocytes have recently become possible, whereby evaluations are performed by determining the percentage of cells that survive following *in vitro* irradiation with various doses of X-rays[3-5]. This method primarily involves determining the sensitivity of CD4+ or CD8+ lymphocytes, but no difference in sensitivity was observed between these cells[4]. Therefore although there are differences between individuals regarding the proportion of these cells, this does not lead to a bias in the results of the study.

1. RADIOSENSITIVITY OF LYMPHOCYTES FROM ATOMIC BOMB SURVIVORS

Studies were performed on 113 distally exposed survivors (estimated DS86 dose < 0.005 Gy) and 70 proximally exposed survivors (estimated DS86 dose $\geq$ 1.5 Gy) (Fig. 1). The D_{10} value shown in Fig. 1 represents the X-ray dose required to produce the death of 90% of the lymphocytes (i.e. a survival rate of 10%); it increases with increasing resistance and decreases with a rise in sensitivity. A comparative study on D_{10} distribution failed to reveal a difference between the two populations[6].

Since such studies invariably contain experimental errors, approximately 30 repeat experiments were conducted on one healthy individual[7]. The distribution was found to be quite similar to the D_{10} distribution shown in Fig. 1, indicating that most of the variation in Fig. 1 was due to experimental error. As a consequence, even

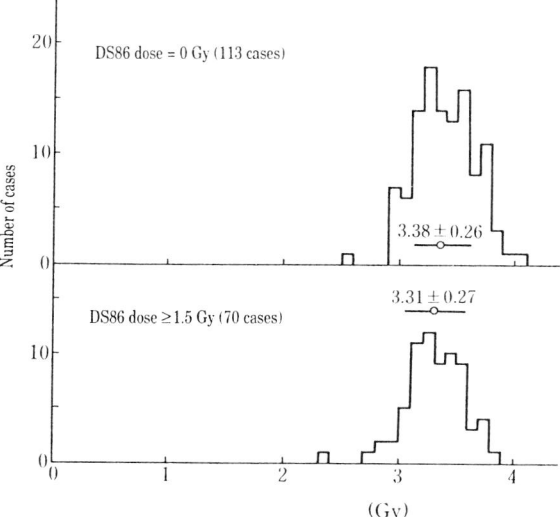

Figure 1   Distribution of lymphocyte radiosensitivity (D_{10} values) between the distally and proximally exposed

if individual variations in lymphocyte radiosensitivity do exist, these are extremely small as far as cell death is concerned.

Furthermore, analysis of the results for the 183 individuals failed to reveal any special sex- or age-specific relationship.

CONCLUSION

A lymphocyte study was conducted on *in vitro* radiosensitivity to X-ray irradiation for 70 heavily exposed survivors and a distally exposed control population (113 individuals). No evidence was found to support the idea that the heavily exposed population included more individuals with a higher resistance to radiation.

(*Nori Nakamura*)

REFERENCES

1. Neriishi K, Stram D, Vaeth M, *et al.* The observed relationship between the occurrence of acute radiation sickness and subsequent cancer mortality among A-bomb survivors in Hiroshima and Nagasaki. *Radiat Res* 1991; **125**: 206–13.
2. Sposto R, Stram D, Awa AA. An investigation of random errors in the DS86 dosimetry using data on chromosome aberrations and severe epilation. RERF TR 7–90, 1990.
3. Nakamura N, Kushiro J, Akiyama M. Improved methods for obtaining colonies of human peripheral blood lymphocytes *in vitro* for radiation dose-survival studies. *Mutat Res* 1990; **234**: 15–22.
4. Nakamura N, Kusunoki Y, Akiyama M. Radiosensitivity of CD4 or CD8 positive human T-lymphocytes by an *in vitro* colony formation assay. *Radiat Res* 1990; **123**: 224–7.

5. Kushiro J, Nakamura N, Kyoizumi S, *et al.* Absence of correlations between radiosensitivities of human T-lymphocytes in G_0 and skin fibroblasts in log phase. *Radiat Res* 1990; **122**: 326–32.
6. Nakamura N, Sposto R, Akiyama M. Dose survival of G_0 lymphocytes irradiated *in vitro*: a test for a possible population bias in the cohort of atomic bomb survivors exposed to high doses. *Radiat Res* 1993; **134**: 316–22.
7. Nakamura N, Sposto R, Kushiro J, *et al.* Is interindividual variation of cellular radiosensitivity real or artificial? *Radiat Res* 1991; **125**: 326–30.

16

Immune Function

16   IMMUNE FUNCTION

INTRODUCTION

The human immune system comprises various types of immunocompetent cells with a variety of functions (Fig. 1). Virtually all foreign antigens and internally produced mutants are recognized as foreign substances by the immunocompetent cells and eliminated. The process of elimination involves a complex and ingenious intercellular network of information transmission, and functional manifestation and suppression. Also, following antigen stimulation a wide range of humoral factors are produced, leading to the differentiation, proliferation, and activation of each immunocompetent cell. On the other hand, the response to certain foreign antigens is governed by immune response genes (in humans, at the gene loci of human lymphocyte antigens, HLA). An individual congenital difference in antigen response has been observed in humans, who belong to a variety of genetic populations.

Consequently, important problems in evaluating human immune response are which population to select and what parameters in the sophisticated systems to adopt. Even with the recent rapid advances in knowledge concerning the immune system and techniques of immunological analysis, this has been a major problem. It is even more difficult to clarify the effects of radiation from the immediate post-bombing destruction of the immune system through to recovery and then the

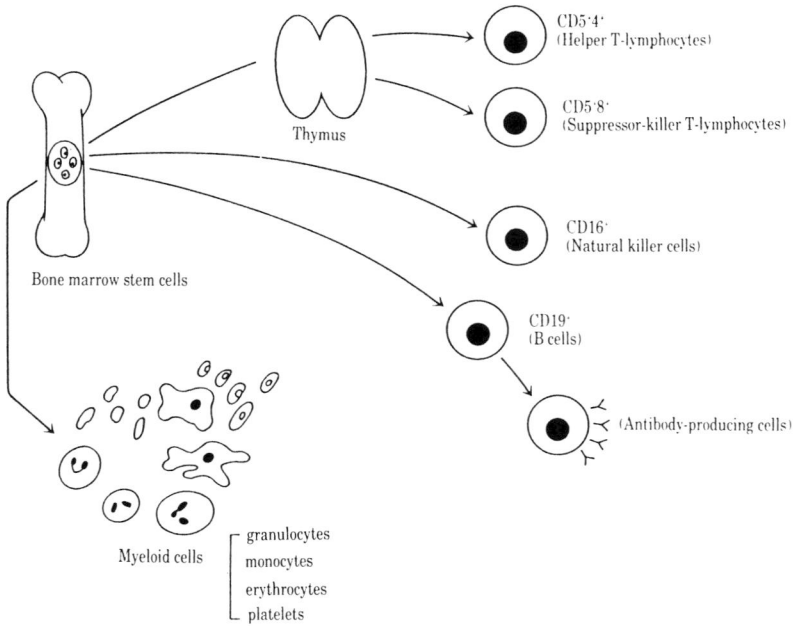

Figure 1   A model for blood cell differentiation

manifestation of late effects. This chapter reviews past results concerning the immunological parameters of atomic bomb survivors, and will, as far as possible, consider the effect of atomic bomb radiation on human immunocompetence from a contemporary immunological standpoint.

1. IMMUNOCOMPETENCE IN THE INITIAL POST-EXPOSURE PERIOD

A. Radiosensitivity of Immunocompetent Cells

The immune system is extremely sensitive to radiation, with a clear difference in radiosensitivity between the cell populations comprising the immune system and cells in the various stages of differentiation. On the other hand, an individual difference in radiosensitivity among human populations has not been clarified to date (for details, please see Chapter 15–2, "Radiosensitivity").

The damage inflicted on the immune system immediately following exposure to the atomic bomb has not been precisely clarified, but knowledge obtained from animal experiments[1,2] permits a certain degree of conjecture. That is, an LD_{50} dose of whole body irradiation first causes a rapid decrease in lymphatic cells, followed by a decrease in myeloid cells. Intrathymus precursor T-cells and mature lymphocytes in peripheral lymph tissue (spleen, and lymph nodes) become necrotic within 1–3 days and the large majority die. Furthermore, the number of circulating lymphocytes in peripheral blood is halved within 24 hours, even with a whole body irradiation dose of 0.5 Gy. Of the lymphocytes, T- and B-cells are both extremely radiosensitive, although resistance is exhibited by some T-cells (approximately 10% of the total, believed to be memory T-cells). Natural killer (NK) cells also display resistance. Mature granulocytes and monocytes show resistance to 10 Gy of irradiation, with the reduction in this cell type observed from 3 days after exposure, at the time the supply of mature cells is inadequate due to damage to the bone marrow's hematopoietic ability. Furthermore, epithelial cells in lymph tissue are highly resistant to radiation.

Hematologic data for the peripheral blood of atomic bomb survivors within 1 week of exposure also reveals a marked reduction in lymphocytes (Table 1)[3], with the number of granulocytes registering a minimum at 4 weeks after exposure[4]. Also, autopsy findings within 2 weeks of exposure revealed atrophy with lymphocyte loss in the spleen, lymph nodes, and thymus, but indicated that the epithelial cells of these organs were relatively unaffected[4].

B. Effect on Immunocompetence

Table 2 summarizes the types of damage to the immune system and their effects on the body's self-defense ability. As previously mentioned, a diverse range of cell types act together in the immune system, which in addition to radiation is greatly affected by burns, trauma, and stress etc. Therefore in the initial period following exposure to the atomic bomb the body's self-defense ability exhibited a general decline without any specific organ hypofunction, with the extent of the decline in an individual survivor believed governed by post-exposure conditions in addition to the radiation dose received.

Table 1   Hematologic data within 1 week of exposure (Kure naval station)[3]

Case number	Erythrocyte count ($\times 10^4$)	Hemoglobin (%)	Color index	Leukocyte count	Basophils	Eosinophils	Myelocytes	Promyelocytes	Neutrophils Stabs	Neutrophils Segs	Neutrophils Total	Lymphocytes	Monocytes	Neutrophil/ Lymphocyte ratio	Status
1.	375	40	0.53	250	0	2	0	4	26	56	86 (215)	8 (20)	4	10.8	
2.	410	42	0.51	400	0	1	0	11	13	53	77 (308)	20 (80)	2	3.9	+
3.	420	50	0.59	150	0	2	0	9	8	66	83 (125)	13 (20)	2	6.4	+
4.	420	45	0.53	400	1	0	0	9	12	62	83 (332)	14 (56)	2	5.9	+
5.	265	32	0.60	400											+
6.	184	23	0.62	340											+
7.	528	43	0.41	150	3	4	0	9	30	34	73 (110)	17 (26)	3	4.3	+
8.	300	49	0.81	4,000	2	3	0	1	8	45	43 (2,160)	36 (1,440)	5	1.5	
9.	405	95	1.17	3,080	1	4	0	0	10	48	58 (1,663)	34 (1,047)	3	1.7	
10.	330	65	0.98	3,800	0	5	0	0	24	44	68 (2,584)	22 (836)	5	3.1	
Normal values	450– 500	90– 100	1.00	6,000– 8,000	0–1	1–5	0	0	3–6	45–55	48–61 (2,880– 4,880)	25–45 (1,500– 3,600)	4–7	1.1– 2.4	

(   ) Actual number

The first characteristic of this period was a decrease in leukocytes (in particular a decrease in neutrophils and monocytes, which registered a minimum at around 30 days after exposure) and an almost identical temporal pattern regarding the development of laryngitis. In addition, excluding the time immediately following exposure, the development of purpura and mortality rate registered a maximum[5] (Fig. 2).

Cause of death was given as sepsis, necrotic pneumonia, and necrotic colitis[4,6–8]. The primary cause of such infectious diseases was the decreased supply of mature neutrophils and monocytes resulting from radiation damage to hematopoietic function. Furthermore, the neutrophils exhibited not only a quantitative decrease but also morphologic abnormalities (nuclear shifts to the left, toxic granule formation, and vacuolation and hypofunction (*in vitro* phagocytosis and peroxidase activity)[9]. Another element believed to contribute to the susceptibility to infection is either a decrease in humoral factors (antibodies, complements[10], etc.) or the fact that the reduction in T-cells results in an inadequate production of factors accelerating the differentiation and activation of neutrophils and monocytes (about which there are no reports).

Table 2   Decrease in the body's self-defense ability in initial period after exposure

Type of damage (and time of manifestation)	Cause	Effect on function
Rapid decrease of lymphocytes (1st day)	Destruction of mature lymphocytes	General decrease
Decrease in humoral factors such as antibodies and complements (immediately after exposure)	• Loss of body fluids by burns and trauma • Decrease in antibody-producing cells (B cells)	Decreased bacteriolysis Decreased phagocytosis by neutrophils, monocytes
Decrease in neutrophils and monocytes (3rd ~ 50th days)	Insufficient supply due to damaged hematopoeitic function	Decreased phagocytosis and bactericidal function
Delayed lymphocyte recovery (after 4th week)	Incomplete differentiation and maturity processes Elimination and non-activation of specific T-lymphocytes due to exposure to bacterial toxins	Delayed recovery from infection Activation of endogenous virus Ease of infection by exogenous viruses Radiation-caused decrease in ability to eliminate mutant cells

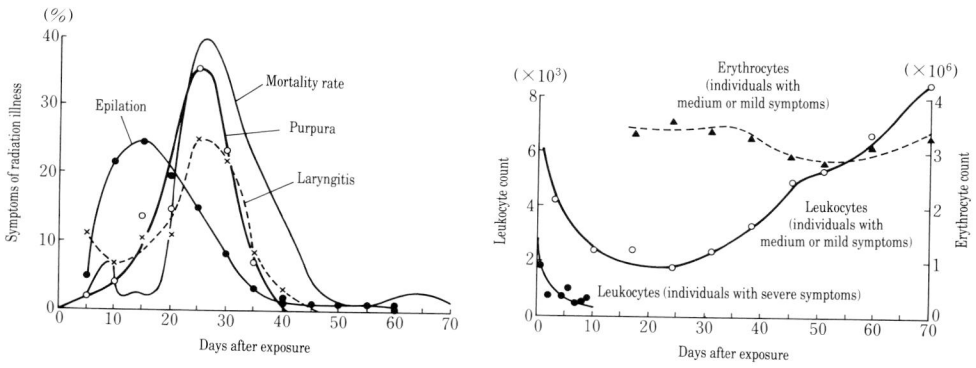

Figure 2   Relationship between post-exposure radiation illness symptoms and changes in blood cells[5]

The second characteristic of this period is that lymphocyte recovery was slower and more moderate than occurred with myeloid cells (granulocytes and monocytes)[4,11-13]. The numbers of monocytes and granulocytes in peripheral blood rapidly recovered after the 5th week following exposure, returning to approximately normal values in the 8th or 9th week. On the other hand, even in the 12th week the number of lymphocytes was of the order of 20% below normal (Table 3). Autopsy findings after the 6th week following exposure showed that whereas almost all cases exhibited bone marrow recovery or hyperplasia, only a few demonstrated formation of lymphatic follicles (the site of antibody production) in the spleen and lymph nodes[4,8]. Autopsy cases were reported to exhibit splenic atrophy even at 14 weeks after exposure[14]. The reasons for the slow recovery of the lymphatic system were

Table 3   Number of peripheral blood cells in Hiroshima and Nagasaki atomic bomb survivors exposed within 1.5 km. of hypocenter[4]

City	Week	Leukocyte count	No. of cases	Lymphocytes	Monocytes	Stabs	Segs	Eosinophils	Basophils
Hiroshima	4	1,000	11	575	55	40	325	10	1
	5	2,435	39	883	104	254	1,093	30	5
	6	3,093	18	1,215	107	244	1,392	100	14
	7	4,113	22	1,152	364	770	1,678	122	16
	8	5,384	13	1,638	276	911	2,309	124	20
	9	7,320	10	2,012	557	247	4,346	236	
	10	6,578	17	1,940	331	590	3,332	292	37
	11	7,048	66	2,048	343	602	3,646	340	25
	12	6,908	91	2,080	369	437	3,594	390	25
Nagasaki	3	3,310	7	1,112	634	611	917	22	56
	4	1,550	12	704	104	145	538	22	14
	5	3,210	6	913	110	424	1,706	70	4
	8	7,230	41	2,060	397	416	3,795	491	48
	9	7,900	137	2,044	509	353	4,331	569	31
	10	7,240	73	2,106	317	102	4,124	559	38
	11	7,940	67	2,487	379	88	4,312	636	30
	12	7,380	26	2,283	376	27	4,017	641	51
Normal value		7,040		2,660	350	154	3,591	252	35

1) degradation of the thymus, which plays an important role in the differentiation of T-cells, due to the aging effect caused at the time of exposure (this will be discussed later); 2) due to the stimulus provided by toxins produced as a result of bacterial infections, receptor-specific T-cells were selectively eliminated or inactivated [a phenomenon recently demonstrated in experiments involving administration of large doses of bacterial toxins to mice[15,16]]; and 3) the genes that code proteins such as T-cell receptors etc., which are necessary for the differentiation and proliferation of lymphocytes, are believed to have undergone considerable mutation following radiation exposure and thus become inactivated (please refer to chapter 15–1, "Somatic Cell Mutations").

The slow recovery of the lymphatic system caused reductions in antigen recognition function, antibody production function, and the ability to activate neutrophils and monocytes, and this inhibited recovery from infection; in particular, depletions in certain T-cell receptors which play a central role in immune response would, if prolonged, mean that certain viruses and mutant cells would not be recognized as foreign substances and would remain in the body. A significant decrease in peripheral blood lymphocytes was observed in atomic bomb survivors until the 1947–48 study[17]. It is unclear whether this decrease was due to a reduction of certain specific types of lymphocyte, but late effects have been observed up to the present day, approximately a half-century after the bombing.

2. LATE EFFECTS

Studies on whether the considerable atomic bomb damage inflicted on the immune system persists in the long term are believed invaluable for clarification of the relationship between radiation exposure and the development of disease (including cancer). Serological and cytobiological analyses have therefore been performed related to various immunological parameters. Finch[18] has already summarized in great detail the results pertaining to atomic bomb survivors up until the 1970s. With the subsequent rapid advances in immunology, the role of immunocompetent cells and their mutual interactions have been clarified. Also, new techniques have been introduced to immunological analysis. This section reviews the literature first pertaining to each of the immunocompetent cells (Table 4), and next with regard to the relationship with disease.

A. T-cells (Table 5)

1. Hypofunction

Between 1974 and 1977 measurements of peripheral lymphocyte response to phyto-hemagglutin (PHA), the mitogen stimulating all T-cells, were conducted on 688 atomic bomb survivors[19]. Atomic bomb survivors exposed to T65D doses of ≥ 2 Gy showed a marked age-related decrease in response relative to the control population (Fig. 3). Also, a 1984–85 study on the response to allogenic antigen (the mixed lymphocyte culture, MLC, response) in 139 survivors revealed a reduced dose-dependent relationship among survivors aged 15 or more at the time of bombing (ATB) (Fig. 4)[20]. These studies investigated the ability of mature *in vivo* T-cells to respond and proliferate in the presence of foreign antigens, and found that the function decreased with increasing dose and age ATB. A 1983–86 study on 1,328 survivors also found an age-related decrease in the number of mature peripheral blood T-cells (Fig. 5)[21].

On the other hand, no decreases in the number and function of these T-cells were observed in young survivors. However, the question remains of how to explain such age-related radiation effects on T-cells. The authors surmise that this was not a direct effect of radiation, but that the post-exposure recovery of mature T-cells became increasingly impaired with advancing age due to an age-related involution of the thymus (Fig. 6). That is, as previously mentioned, mature peripheral lymphocytes exhibit extreme sensitivity to radiation, and many die. Later, mature T-cells differentiate from bone marrow stem cells via the thymus and are supplied to the peripheral regions; however, thymic involution had begun 1 year after birth (Fig. 7)[37], and consequently the efficiency of differentiation and maturity of thymic T-cells had already declined substantially with increasing age by the time of the bombing. This hypothesis is well supported by the work of Hirokawa and Sado[38], who compared T-cell regeneration in newborn and mature mice following bone marrow transplantation.

Table 4   Studies on late effects related to immunocompetence

Type of cell etc.		Study period	Radiation effect	Reference
Bone marrow cells				
	Number of cells	1947–59	Absent	22
	Granulocyte bacterolysis	1959	Absent	23
	Neutrophil phagocytosis	1962	Absent	24
	Granulocyte migration	1977	Absent	25
	Whole blood bactericidal activity	1978–79	Absent	26
Lymphocytes				
	Spleen index	1963–70	Absent	27
	Number of lymphocytes	1958–72	Absent	28
T-cells				
	PHA response	1974–77	Decreased in aging survivors	19
	MLC response	1984–85	Decreased in aging survivors	20
	IL2 production	1983–86	Absent	29
	Number of cells	1983–86	Decreased in aging survivors	21
B-cells				
	Number of cells	1983–86	Absent	21
Natural killer cells				
	NK activity	1983–86	Absent	29
	Interferon production (including T-cells)	1983–86	Absent	29
	Number of cells	1983–86	Absent	21
Humoral factors				
	Immunoglobulin levels	1968–69	Absent	30
		1970–71	Absent	31
		1987–89	Increased IgA in females Increased IgM in aging survivors	32
Autoantibodies				
	Antiparietal antibody	1971–72	Absent	33
	Antinuclear antibody	1987–89	Absent	32
	Antithyroglobulin antibody	1987–89	Absent	32
	Antithyroid microsome antibody	1987–89	Absent	32
	Rheumatoid factor (RF)	1987–89	Increased	32
Immune complex (IC)		1983–86	Absent	29
Anti-influenza virus				
Antibody production		1961	Decreased	34
Anti-EB virus antibody		1983	Increased anti-EA antibody levels	35
		1988–89	Increased anti-EA antibody levels	36
Interferon		1983–86	Absent	29

2. *Increase in Mutant T-cells*

Many T-cells have to date been found to possess radiation-induced chromosomal aberrations, with the number related to received dose (approximately 15% at 2 Gy)[39] (please refer to Chapter 14–1a, "Chromosomal Aberrations in Peripheral Blood Lymphocytes"). Research on the frequency of T-cells with mutations in specific genes has been performed since 1984. Such mutant T-cells exhibit incomplete or abnormal function, and it is possible that the increase may result in decreased T-cell function in

Table 5   Late effects on T-lymphocytes

Type of cell	Late radiation effects	Change in functional ability	Reference
Normal cells Repertoire imbalance	Decrease in aging survivors (present) ?	Decrease —	19–21
Mutants	Chromosomal aberrations (increase) HPRT deficiency (increase) T-cell receptor loss (unchanged) HLA antigen loss (unchanged)	? ? Decrease Decrease or abnormality	39 40 41, 42 43, 44

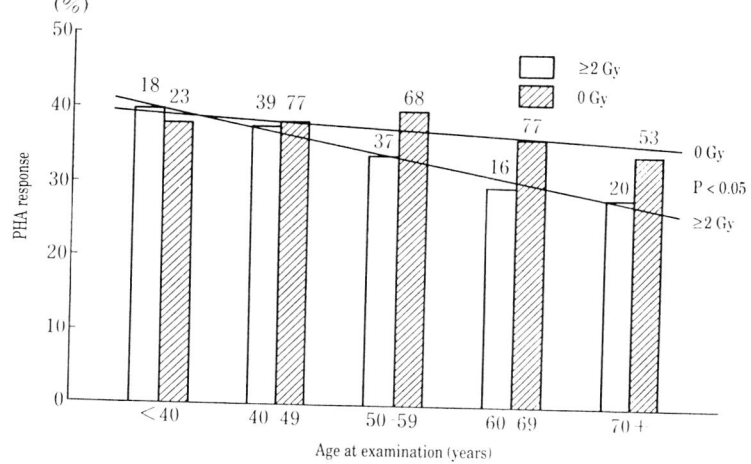

Figure 3   Phytohemagglutinin (PHA) response of peripheral blood lymphocytes in atomic bomb survivors, 1974–77[19]

the atomic bomb survivors. However, today a dose-related increase in mutant cells has been detected only with hypoxanthine guanine phosphoribosyl transferase (HPRT), a nucleic acid metabolic enzyme[40]; no increase was observed in either T-cell receptors (which have a substantial effect on function)[41,42] or human lymphocyte antigens (HLA)[43,44]. (For details, please refer to Chapter 15–1, "Somatic Cell Mutations"). It is surmised that the *in vivo* selection against many of such mutants had already been completed during the initial period following exposure. In addition, it is believed that even among the cells that caused chromosome aberrations, only those that possess abnormalities unrelated to function may exhibit long-term persistence.

B. B-Lymphocytes and Humoral Immunity

The B-cells of atomic bomb survivors were measured at the same time as the numbers of mature peripheral blood T-cells[21]. Although the number of B-cells displayed an age-related decrease, the effect of radiation was not statistically signifi-

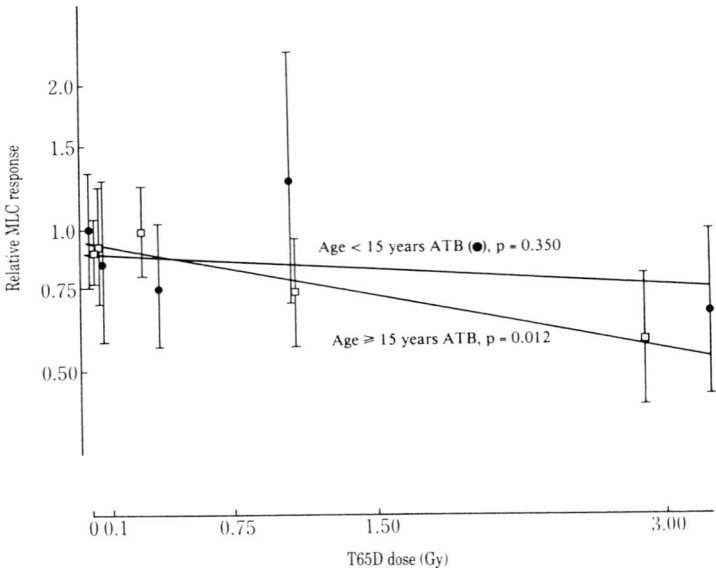

Figure 4   Mixed lymphocyte culture (MLC) response of peripheral blood lymphocytes by dose, 1984–85[20]

cant. However, as with T-cells, there was a decrease in heavily exposed survivors (Fig. 8), and studies are continuing.

Two past studies (1968–69 and 1970–71) on serum immunoglobulin (antibody) levels failed to demonstrate a significant atomic bomb radiation effect[30,31]. However, a further study on 2,061 survivors in 1987–89 showed that, while small, increases were observed in the immunoglobulin A (IgA) antibody levels in female survivors and in immunoglobulin M (IgM) levels in aging survivors[32]. These results show that radiation has no direct effect on B-cell lineage, and may indicate chronic stimulation by some antigen.

C. Natural Killer Cells and Natural Immunity

Natural killer (NK) cells are lymphocytes that differ from T- and B-cells in that they kill certain cancer cells and viral infection cells without being sensitized by antigens. The measurement of the numbers and function of NK cells is believed extremely important for clarifying the role of the immune system in the development of cancer in atomic bomb survivors. A 1982–86 study on 1,314 survivors found that the results concerning the number and function of NK cells were the exact opposite of T- and B-cells, showing a significant increase with age but no relationship with radiation[21,29]. In addition, measurements were simultaneously conducted on the activity in serum and lymphocyte culture supernatant of interferon, a protein exhibiting an anti-cancer and anti-virus effect which is produced primarily by NK and T cells, but no radiation effect was observed[29].

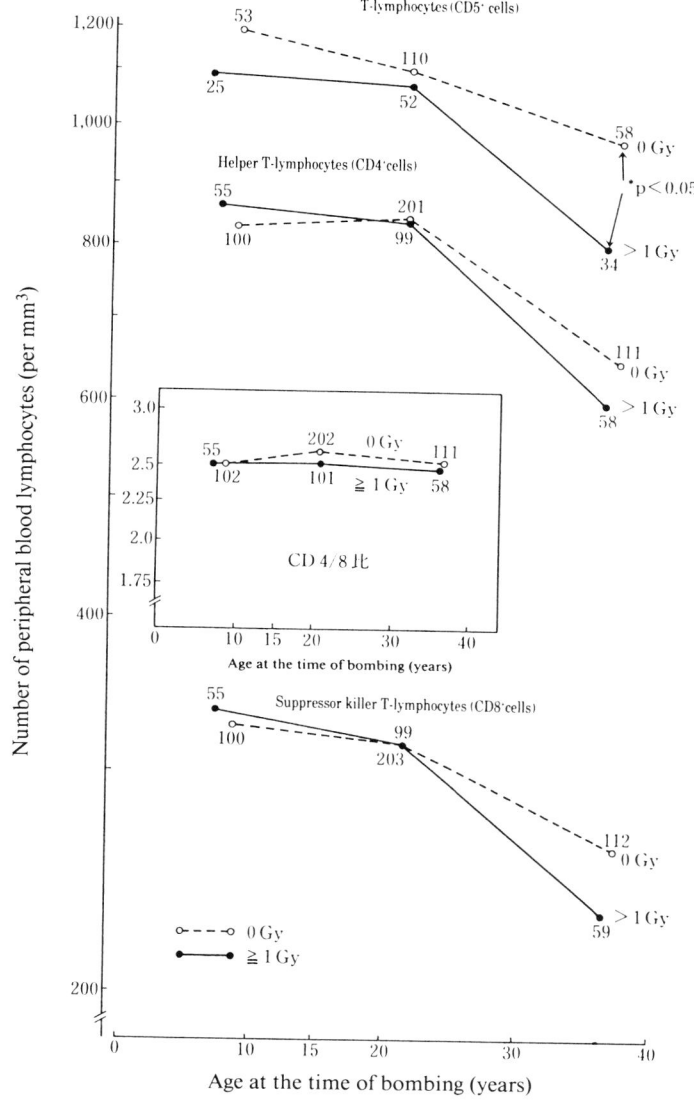

Figure 5 Number of peripheral blood T-lymphocytes, 1983–86[21]

D. Myeloid Cells

The many studies on peripheral blood neutrophil function regarding phagocytosis, migration and bactericidal activity have all failed to show radiation effects[22–26]. In addition, no difference between the exposed and non-exposed populations has been observed since the previously-mentioned recovery in the relatively early period following the bombing[22]. Functional studies have not been performed on other

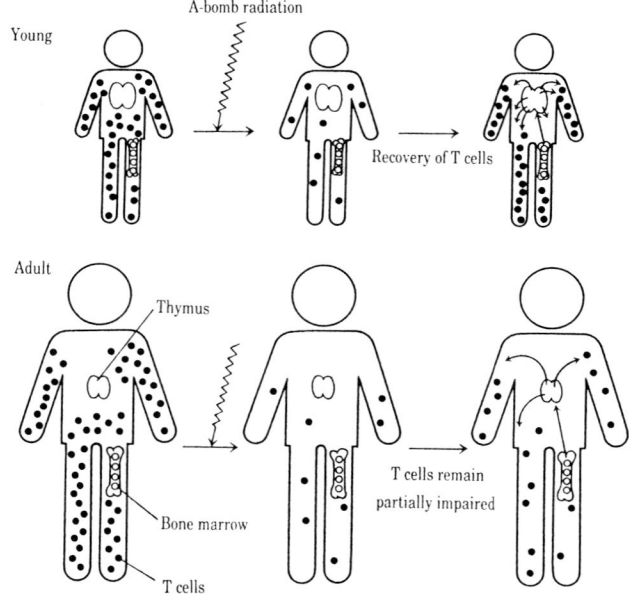

Figure 6   A hypothesis for age-dependent effects on T-cell development

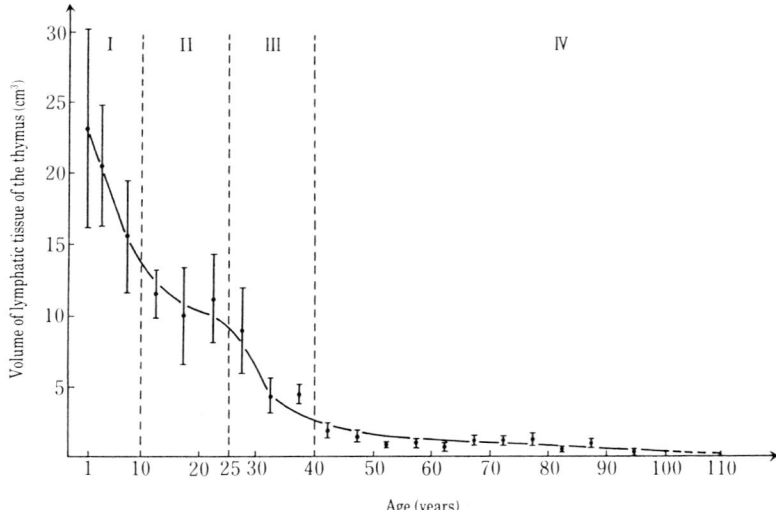

Figure 7   Age-dependent changes in lymphatic tissue of the human thymus

granulocytes (eosinophils and basophils) or monocytes, but quantitative changes have not been observed. It is thought that radiation probably exerts no late effects on these myeloid cell populations.

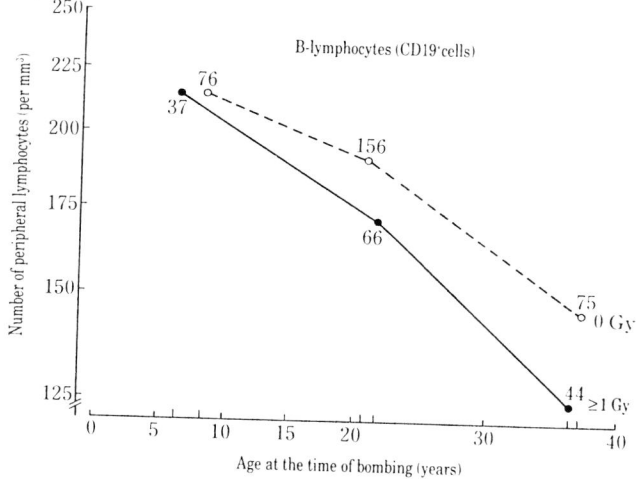

Figure 8   Number of peripheral blood B-lymphocytes, 1983–86[21]

E. Immunity to Infection

The results of infection studies to date are shown in Table 6. No reports have as yet demonstrated a significantly high prevalence of infectious diseases among atomic bomb survivors. However, results suggestive of a high proportion of urinary tract infections among the exposed population have been reported[49,50]. Also, a few observations indicated decreased immunocompetence with respect to viruses. In 1961 prenatally exposed atomic bomb survivors were inoculated with Asia-type influenza virus vaccine; the results of anti-viral antibody measurements revealed that proximally exposed survivors exhibited a significant decrease in antibody production with respect to mutant strains of certain influenza viruses[34], and that heavily exposed survivors displayed an increased positive rate for serum hepatitis B virus antigen (HBs antigen)[46] and an increased level of antibody (the anti-EA

Table 6   Studies on late effects related to infectious diseases

Subject of study	Study period	Radiation effect	Reference
Frequency of positive hepatitis-related antigen findings	1971	Absent	45
	1972	Absent	46
Frequency of positive HBs antigen findings	1975 ~ 77	Present (increase)	47
	1975 ~ 77	Absent	47
Prevalence of tuberculosis	1954 ~ 60	Absent	48
	1958 ~ 60	Absent	49
Frequency of urinary tract infection	1962 ~ 63	Suggested (increase)	50
	1969	Suggested (increase)	51

antibody) produced upon activation of the EB virus[35,36]. These findings show that the infecting viruses are not adequately controlled by the body's immune system. The primary cause of such decreased response with respect to infection might be the inactivation or elimination of specific T-cells as a result of a general decrease in T-cell function (impairment of mature T-cell recovery in aging survivors) or due to exposure to bacterial toxins in the initial period following the bombing.

F. Autoimmunity

It was predicted that a high rate of development of autoimmune diseases might be observed in atomic bomb survivors as a result of radiation-induced changes in the antigenecity of autologous cells or decreased suppressor T-cell function. However, no relationship was observed between atomic bomb radiation and the prevalence of typical autoimmune diseases such as rheumatoid arthritis[52,53], Hashimoto's disease[54], systemic lupus erytematosus[55], and scleroderma[55], etc. Although an age-dependent increase has been observed, recent studies on the positive rate of various autoantibodies[32] and immune complex levels[29] have, with the exception of rheumatic factors, revealed no effect due to atomic bomb radiation. It has been surmised that the increased rheumatoid factor positive rate is primarily related not to autoimmunity but to chronic antigen stimulus related to increased levels of IgA and IgM[32].

G. Tumor Immunity

The high cancer mortality rate among atomic bomb survivors is well known, but it has not been adequately clarified as to whether the immune system in some way affects the development and progress of cancer. Also, there is no good method of evaluating immune response function to tumors, and at the present time the only way is to consider overall immunocompetence. However, in murine systems in which tumor-specific immune responses were induced, the previous irradiation was found to decrease the tumor suppression response[56]. Also, from the fact that late effects on T-cell lineage were observed in atomic bomb survivors[19-21], it would appear that if a radiation-related decrease did occur in anti-tumor immunity, then this would probably be due not to non-specific natural immunity but to tumor-specific immunity (and in particular to T-cells).

CONCLUSION

With regard to the results yielded to date by atomic bomb survivor immunocompetence studies, firstly the decreased T-cell function in aging survivors was found to be in good agreement with animal experiments using aging mice[57]. The thymus is believed to participate in this process, but it has also been suggested that something independent of the thymus is involved in the T-cell differentiation process [58-60], possibly that extrathymically differentiated T-cells display a function different from normal. It is also surmised that such cells increase in aging atomic bomb survivors since extrathymic differentiation occurs to a greater extent at the time of post-exposure T-cell recovery. This necessitates further and more sophisticated detection of T-cell subpopulations and analysis of clone levels.

On the other hand, no clear late effects have been observed among young atomic bomb survivors. Animal experiments have also been reported to show contradictory results regarding the existence of late radiation effects among the young, suggesting the possibility of variations depending on the rearing environment. That is, radiation effects are not observed in an environment lacking pathogens[2], but are seen under normal conditions[61]. As mentioned earlier in the book, the atomic bomb survivors in Hiroshima and Nagasaki not only sustained direct injury from radiation but also suffered greatly from burns, trauma, and pathogenic infections arising from the poor sanitary conditions. This was possibly not only a matter of life and death at the time for the survivors, but also had later effects on the immune system. It is hoped that future research will consider such viewpoints, including the suggested decrease in anti-viral immunocompetence among atomic bomb survivors. Specifically, did immunogenetic differences contribute to post-exposure deaths resulting from infectious diseases? In other words, do the survivors still alive today tend to possess certain HLA types? Also, do the T-cells of atomic bomb survivors exhibit some kind of response to those agents such as bacterial toxins (the so-called "super antigens") that exert a great effect on the formation of the repertoire of T-cells (the range of possible responses of T-cells to antigens)? And so on. This may possibly yield valuable data concerning not only the various infectious and inflammatory diseases occurring in atomic bomb survivors, but also regarding the development of autoimmune diseases and the advancement of tumors.

The second point is the increase in mutant cells (including chromosomal aberrations) that directly reflect the effect of radiation. It is necessary to both develop new methods of mutant cell detection and to investigate mutant cell functions.

Finally, with the aging of the atomic bomb survivors there is today some anxiety concerning the reduction in the study population, and it is important to accumulate under favorable conditions as much data as possible in preparation for the time when exemplary immunological techniques of analysis have been developed. The development of analytical methods for procuring immunological information using old pathologic tissue is also desirable.

(Mitoshi Akiyama, Youichiro Kusunoki)

REFERENCES

1. Anderson RE, Warner NL. Ionizing radiation and the immune response. In: Dixon FJ, Kunkel HG, editors. *Advances in immunology.* Academic Press, 1976; **24**: 215–335.
2. Sado T, Kamisaku H, Ikarashi Y, *et al.* Immediate and long-term effects of radiation on the immune system of specific-pathogen free mice. *Int J Radiat Biol* 1988; **53**: 177–87.
3. Sassa K, Nakao Y, Kobayashi G, *et al.* Hematological study of A-bomb radiation sickness. In: *Genshibakudan saigai chousa Houkokushu* [Collection of the reports on the investigation of the atomic bomb casualties] Vol. 1. Tokyo: Japan Society for the Promotion of Science, 1953: 649–62. (*In Japanese*)

4. Oughtersen AW, Warren S. Hematology of atomic bomb injuries, pathology of atomic bomb injuries. In: *Medical effects of the atomic bomb in Japan*. Natl Nuclear Energy Ser Div. McGraw-Hill, 1956; **III**: 191–430.

5. Ohkita T. Acute effects. *J Radiat Res* 1975; **16** (Suppl): 49–6.

6. Sassa K. Clinic of the atomic bomb radiation sickness. In: *Genshibakudan saigai chousa Houkokushu* [Collection of the reports on the investigation of the atomic bomb casualties] Vol. 2. Tokyo: Japan Society for the Promotion of Science, 1953: 50–70. (*In Japanese*)

7. Medical investigation report on A-bomb casualty of Hiroshima by Army Medical School, Provisional Tokyo No. 1 Army Hospital. In: *Genshibakudan saigai chousa Houkokushu* [Collection of the reports on the investigation of the atomic bomb casualties] Vol. 1. Tokyo: Japan Society for the Promotion of Science, 1953: 285–412. (*In Japanese*)

8. Amano S. Pathological study of A-bomb patients. In: Japanese textbook of hematology. Part 3. Japanese Society of Hematology. Tokyo: Maruzen, 1964: 630–59. (*In Japanese*)

9. Mashita S, Kikuchi T, Funaoka S, *et al.* Study of A-bomb injuries in Hiroshima (clinical report). In: *Genshibakudan saigai chousa Houkokushu* [Collection of the reports on the investigation of the atomic bomb casualties] Vol. 2. Tokyo: Japan Society for the Promotion of Science, 1953: 769–803. (*In Japanese*)

10. Kimura K, Azuma N, Goto M, *et al.* Bacteriological study of serum in A-bomb patients. In: *Genshibakudan saigai chousa Houkokushu* [Collection of the reports on the investigation of the atomic bomb casualties] Vol. 2. Tokyo: Japan Society for the Promotion of Science, 1953: 806–10. (*In Japanese*)

11. Kure Naval Station. Investigation concerning A-bomb in Hiroshima city (medical aspects). In: *Genshibakudan saigai chousa Houkokushu* [Collection of the reports on the investigation of the atomic bomb casualties] Vol. 1. Tokyo: Japan Society for the Promotion of Science, 1953: 423–36. (*In Japanese*)

12. Kikuchi T, Kimoto S. Clinical phase of A-bomb sickness. In: *Genshibakudan saigai chousa Houkokushu* [Collection of the reports on the investigation of the atomic bomb casualties] Vol. 2. Tokyo: Japan Society for the Promotion of Science, 1953: 1580–642. (*In Japanese*)

13. Wakisaki K. Clinical study of A-bomb patients. In: Japanese textbook of hematology. Part 3. Japanese Society of Hematology. Tokyo: Maruzen, 1964: 600–29. (*In Japanese*)

14. Tamagawa C. Autopsy records on 19 cases of A-bomb sickness in Hiroshima city. In: *Genshibakudan saigai chousa Houkokushu* [Collection of the reports on the investigation of the atomic bomb casualties] Vol. 2. Tokyo: Japan Society for the Promotion of Science, 1953: 1497–561. (*In Japanese*)

15. Kawabe Y, Ochi A. Selective anergy of Vβ8$^+$, CD4$^+$ T cells in staphylococcus entero-toxin B-primed mice. *J Exp Med* 1990; **172**: 1065–70.

16. Rellahan BL, Jones LA, Kruisbeek AM, *et al. In vivo* induction of anergy in peripheral Vβ8$^+$ T cells by staphylococcal enterotoxin B. *J Exp Med* 1990; **172**: 1091–100.

17. Snell FM, Neel JV, Ishibashi K. Hematologic studies in Hiroshima and a control city two years after the atomic bombing. ABCC TR 27–59, 1959.

18. Finch SC. A review of immunological and infectious disease studies at ABCC-RERF. RERF TR 22–79, 1979.

19. Akiyama M, Yamakido M, Kobuke K, *et al.* Peripheral lymphocyte response to PHA and T cell population among atomic bomb survivors. *Radiat Res* 1983; **93**: 572–80.

20. Akiyama M, Zhou OL, Kusunoki Y, *et al.* Age and dose related alteration of *in vitro* mixed lymphocyte culture response of blood lymphocytes from A-bomb survivors. *Radiat Res* 1989; **117**: 26–34.

21. Kusunoki Y, Akiyama M, Kyoizumi S, *et al.* Age-related alteration in the composition of immuno-competent blood cells in atomic bomb survivors. *Int J Radiat Biol* 1988; **53**: 189–98.

22. Blaisdell RK, Akamoto K. Review of ABCC hematologic studies 1947–59. ABCC TR 25–66, 1966.

23. Hollingsworth JW, Hamilton HB. Blood bactericidal activity, Hiroshima. ABCC TR 14–60, 1960.

24. Barreras RF, Finch SC. Peripheral blood leukocyte phagocytosis and respiratory response to certain micromolecular substances in the ABCC-JNIH Adult Health Study. Hiroshima ABCC TR 8–74, 1974.

25. Pinkston JA, Finch SC, Hamilton HB, *et al.* Granulocyte random migration and chemotaxis in atomic bomb survivors, Hiroshima and Nagasaki. Unpublished data.

26. Sasagawa S, Yoshimoto Y, Toyota E, *et al.* Whole-blood phagocytic and bactericidal activities of atomic bomb survivors, Hiroshima and Nagasaki. *Radiat Res* 1990; **123**: 275–84.

27. Doughty WE, Anderson RE, Yamamoto T, *et al.* Spleen index in atomic bomb survivors. *Arch Pathol* 1973; **96**: 395–98.

28. Oesterle SN, Norman JE Jr. Long term observation on absolute lymphocyte counts in the Adult Health Study sample, Hiroshima and Nagasaki. *J Hiroshima Med Ass* 1981; **34**: 570–78.

29. Bloom ET, Akiyama M, Korn EL, *et al.* Immunological responses of aging Japanese A-bomb survivors. *Radiat Res* 1988; **116**: 343–55.

30. Hall CB, Hall WJ, Ashley FW, *et al.* Serum immunoglobulin levels in atomic bomb survivors in Hiroshima, Japan. *Am J Epidemiol* 1973; **98**: 423–9.

31. King RA, Milton RC, Hamilton HB. Serum immunoglobulin levels in the ABCC-JNIH Adult Health Study, Hiroshima-Nagasaki. ABCC TR 14–73, 1973.

32. Fujiwara S, Carter RL, Akiyama M, *et al.* Autoantibodies and immunoglobulins in A-bomb survivors. *Radiation Res* 1994; **139**: 89–95.

33. Akiyama M, Okawa T, Otake M, *et al.* Stomach cancer screening in the Adult Health Study population, 1971–72, Hiroshima. RERF TR 7–77, 1977.

34. Kanamitsu M, Morita K, Finch SC, *et al.* Serologic response of atomic bomb survivors following Asian influenza vaccination. *Jpn J Med Sci Biol* 1966; **19**: 73–84.

36. Ozaki K, Kyoizumi S, Mizuno S, *et al.* Late effects of A-bomb radiation on human immune response. VI. Anti-EB virus antibody titer in sera of A-bomb survivors. *J Hiroshima Med Ass* 1990; **43**: 523–4. (*In Japanese*)

37. Steinmann GG. Changes in the human thymus during aging. *Current Topics in Pathol* 1986; **75**: 43–88.

38. Hirokawa K, Sado T. Radiation effects on regeneration and T-cell-inducing function of the thymus. *Cell Immunol* 1984; **84**: 372–9.

39. Awa AA. Review of thirty years study of Hiroshima and Nagasaki atomic bomb survivors. II. Biological effects. G. Chromosome aberrations in somatic cells. *J Radiat Res* 1975; **16** (Suppl): 122–31.

40. Hakoda M, Akiyama M, Kyoizumi S, *et al.* Increased somatic cell mutant frequency in atomic bomb survivors. *Mutat Res* 1988; **201**: 39–48.

41. Kyoizumi S, Akiyama M, Hirai Y, *et al.* Spontaneous loss and alteration of antigen receptor expression in mature CD4[+] T cells. *J Exp Med* 1990; **171**: 1981–99.

42. Kyoizumi S, Umeki S, Akiyama M, *et al.* Frequency of mutant T lymphocytes defective in the expression of the T-cell antigen receptor gene among radiation-exposed people. *Mutation Res* 1992; **265**: 173–180.

43. Kushiro J. Detection of somatic mutation at HLA-A locus in human peripheral blood T-lymphocytes. *Med J Hiroshima Univ* 1990; **38**: 865–891.

44. Kushiro J, Hirai Y, Kusunoki Y, *et al.* Development of a flow-cytometric HLA-A locus mutation assay for human peripheral blood lymphocytes. *Mutation Res* 1992; **272**: 17–29.

45. Belsky IL, Okochi K, Ishimaru T, *et al.* Hepatitis associated antigen and antibody in A-bomb survivors and nonexposed subjects in Hiroshima and Nagasaki. *Radiat Res* 1972; **52**: 528–35.

46. McGregor DH, Belsky JL, Ishimaru T, *et al.* Postmortem hepatitis associated antigen in blood and liver histology among Japanese. ABCC TR 18–72, 1972.

47. Kato H, Mayumi M, Nishioka K, *et al.* The relationship of HBs antigen and antibody to atomic bomb radiation in the Adult Health Study sample, 1975–77. RERF TR 13–80, 1980.

48. Komatsu T, Onishi S. Tuberculosis and A-bomb exposure, a study of shipyard workers. *J Hiroshima Med Ass* **15**: 59–66 (ABCC TR 15–61, 1962).

49. Turner RW, Hollingsworth DR. Tuberculosis in Hiroshima. *Yale J Biol Med* **36**: 165–82 (ABCC TR 13–63, 1963).

50. Freedman LR, Phair JP, Seki M, *et al.* The epidemiology of tract infections in Hiroshima. *Yale U Biol Med* 1965; **37**: 262–82 (ABCC TR 21–64, 1964).

51. Sawada H, Otake M, Omori Y, *et al.* Long-term follow-up of urinary tract infection in women, Hiroshima. ABCC TR 31–72, 1972.

52. Wood JW, Kato H, Johnson KG, *et al.* Rheumatoid arthritis in Hiroshima and Nagasaki, Japan: prevalence, incidence, and clinical characteristics. *Arthritis Rheum* 1967; **10**: 21–31.

53. Kato H, Duff IF, Russell WJ, *et al.* Rheumatoid arthritis and gout in Hiroshima and Nagasaki, Japan: a prevalence and incidence study. *J Chronic Dis* 1971; **23**: 659–79.

54. Asano M, Norman JE Jr, Kato H, *et al.* Autopsy studies of Hashimoto's thyroiditis in Hiroshima and Nagasaki (1954–74): relation to atomic bomb radiation. *J Radiat Res* 1978; **19**: 306–18.

55. Sasaki S, Fujiwara S, Akiba S, *et al.* Incidence of systemic lupus erythematosus and progressive systemic sclerosis among a fixed population. Report of Intractable Disease Research Team. Tokyo: Ministry of Health and Welfare, 1990: 136–8.

56. Norimura T, Tsuchiya T. Long-term effect of whole-body X-irradiation on cell-mediated immune reaction in mice. *J Radiat Res* 1989; **30**: 226–37.

57. Peterson WJ, Perkins EH, Makinodan T. Recovery of immune competence following sublethal X-irradiation of young and old mice: a model for studying age-related loss of immunologic homeostasis. *Radiat Res* 1982; **89**: 53–64.

58. MacDonald HR, Lees RK, Bron C, *et al.* T cell antigen receptor expression in athymic (nu/nu) mice. Evidence for an oligoclonal β-chain repertoire. *J Exp Med* 1987; **166**: 195–209.

59. Ohteki T, Seki S, Abo T, *et al.* Liver is a possible site for the proliferation of abnormal CD3$^+$4$^-$8$^-$ double negative lymphocytes in autoimmune MRL *lpr/lpr* mice. *J Exp Med* 1990; **172**: 7–12.

60. Bandeira A, Itohara S, Bonneville M, *et al.* Extrathymic origin of intestinal intraepithelial lymphocytes bearing T-cell antigen receptor γδ. *Proc Natl Acad Sci USA* 1991; **88**: 43–7.

61. Yuhas JM. Immunosuppression as a co-factor in radiation carcinogenesis. In: Okada ES, Imamura M, Terashima T, Yamaguchi H, editors. *Radiation Research*. Japanese Association for Radiat Res 1979: 736–42.

17

Effects on Growth
and Development

17 EFFECTS ON GROWTH AND DEVELOPMENT

INTRODUCTION

Measurements of height, body weight, sitting height, chest circumference, and head size etc. were performed as indices of the growth of atomic bomb survivors, and it was found that infantile exposure generally resulted in growth retardation. However, it is possible that besides radiation these indices were affected by factors such as chronic illness and stress due to disruption of everyday life, not to mention nutrition. Consequently, care is needed in the interpretation of results. For example, prior to 1965, estimates of individual dose were restricted to an extremely small number of survivors, and it was not possible to analyze radiation effects with respect to dose. Early studies were conducted, e.g. a study first comparing children in Hiroshima and Kure, and then children in Nagasaki and Sasebo[1], and other studies contrasting proximally exposed survivors (exposed within 2 km) with the distally exposed (the control population)[2,3]; however, it is extremely difficult to interpret the extent to which radiation was the cause of the differences in results[3]. Close to the hypocenter, this is because besides the effect of radiation, there was also great confusion in daily life (houses destroyed by fire, and families broken up, etc.). Although these are also undoubtedly effects of the atomic bomb, this section summarizes the effects due to radiation. The discussion will therefore be restricted to relationships with received dose, and will not describe reports[1-4] which appeared prior to establishment of the T65D system of dosimetry.

Regarding dose estimations, in 1986 the DS86 system was proposed as a revision of the previous T65D system, and has been used to evaluate various risks including cancer development (for details, please refer to Chapter 20, "Dose Estimations"). Unfortunately, however, since reevaluations of growth and development studies using DS86 doses have not yet been performed, the following discussion employs only T65D data (should DS86 reassessments be conducted, it is very likely that the doses would be revised downward).

1. CHILDHOOD EXPOSURE

The height and body weight data for Hiroshima survivors exposed to the atomic bomb at under 18 years of age is summarized in Fig. 1[5].

The effects of radiation on growth are believed to be more severe among growing children, and therefore this discussion will first consider 3 populations classified according to age at the time of bombing (ATB), i.e. 0–5 years, 6–11 years, and 12–17 years. Estimates were performed in 1966–68, and thus even those aged 0 ATB had attained adulthood; consequently heights would not increase further. It can be seen from the diagram that for both the 0–5 and 6–11 year old populations, no constant tendency regarding height or body weight is observed between group A (those not present in the city ATB, but who entered later), group B (individuals with an estimated dose of 0–0.09 Gy), and group C (estimated dose of 0.10–0.99 Gy).

Age at the time of bombing (years)

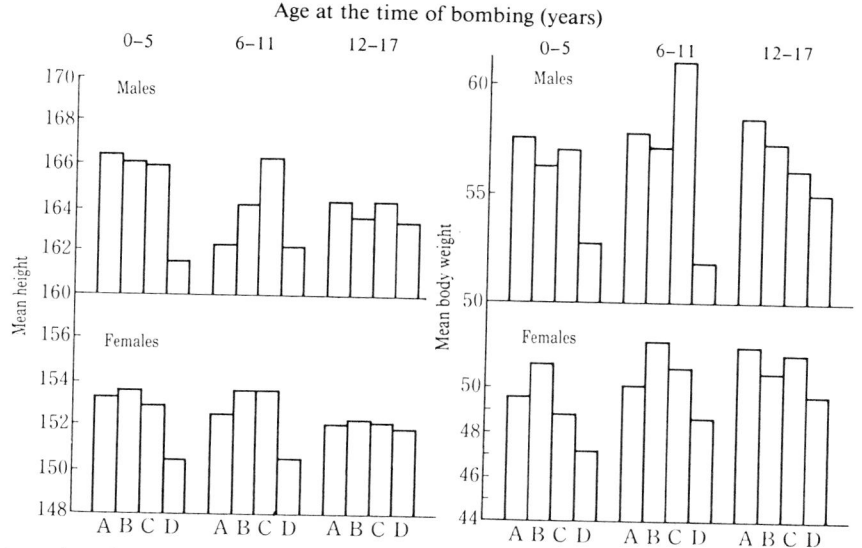

Group A consists of persons not in Hiroshima at the time of the bombing (ATB). Groups B, C, and D were respectively exposed to 0–0.9 Gy, 0.10–0.99 Gy and ≥ 1.0 Gy (T65D doses). A radiation effect was observed in group D subjects in the populations aged 0–5 ATB and 6–11 ATB, but no clear effect was observed among subjects aged 12–17 ATB.

Figure 1   Height and weight of young Hiroshima survivors based on measurements conducted in 1966–68

However, in group D (estimated dose of ≥ 1 Gy) both males and females exhibit a reduced mean height and body weight in comparison with groups A, B, and C in the same age population. The effect of radiation on height and weight for subjects in the 12–17 years ATB population, however, is not as marked as in the populations aged 11 or less.

A similar survey on Nagasaki survivors found that females exhibited very similar results to those observed in Hiroshima, but that males were somewhat different. Ishimaru et al[6] analyzed the radiation effects on height in survivors aged under 10 ATB, and found that for these subjects also there was no clear radiation effect on Nagasaki males. The reason is unknown, but may be related to either a difference between the cities in the method of dose estimation resulting from the different forms of radiation, or caused by inter-city environmental differences. However, as will be mentioned later, studies on the prenatally exposed found that in common with other post-natal populations, the heights of the heavily exposed Nagasaki males were small.

With respect to developmental indices, it is possible that the age at menarche in females was delayed as a result of radiation exposure, but no reports confirming this have as yet appeared.

To summarize, the effect of radiation on growth is believed to increase with decreasing age ATB, although a statistical analysis on subjects aged under 10 ATB indicated that the relationship with age ATB is not significant[6]. It therefore cannot be said with certainty that the effects do increase with decreasing age, and it is hoped that future analyses will be performed using DS86 dose estimates.

2. PRENATAL EXPOSURE

As mentioned at the beginning, studies on growth and development used only T65D data. No prenatal dose estimations were performed until the work by Kerr[7] in 1979; consequently, unless otherwise stated, the figures in the following discussion refer to the maternal kerma dose (the estimated fetal dose was postulated to be approximately half the maternal kerma dose[7]).

Figure 2 shows the height measurements obtained at 10 and 17 years of age in one study on prenatally exposed survivors. No clear difference was observed between group A (distally exposed controls) and group B (exposed to 0.01–0.99 Gy), but a clear effect was seen in group C ($\geq$ 1 Gy)[8]. Although not shown in the diagram, similar results were obtained for Nagasaki. Also, Ishimaru et al[9] analyzed prenatally exposed survivors at the age of 18 using T65D fetal dose estimates, and similarly found a clear effect (the $\geq$ 0.5 Gy population in this study was approximately equivalent to group C in Fig. 2). The first appearance of this difference in height was not after the start of puberty but seems to have been continuous from childhood. From Fig. 2, which compares heights at ages 10 and 17, it can be seen that the difference between groups A and C was already distinct by age 10. The diagram indicates no radiation effect for females aged 10, but this is probably due to the limited size of the sample group (group C consisted of only 13 subjects). Although not shown in the diagram, this is supported by a radiation effect being detected among Nagasaki males and females at both age 10 and age 17[8]. On the other hand, growth measurements between the ages of 10 and 17 show no clear radiation effect (Fig. 3). This also is believed to indicate pre-puberty growth retardation in cases of prenatal exposure.

No direct comparative study has been conducted between childhood and prenatal exposure, but a comparison of the results from two studies by Ishimaru et al[6,9] shows that the effect of radiation on height is greater in the case of the prenatally exposed.

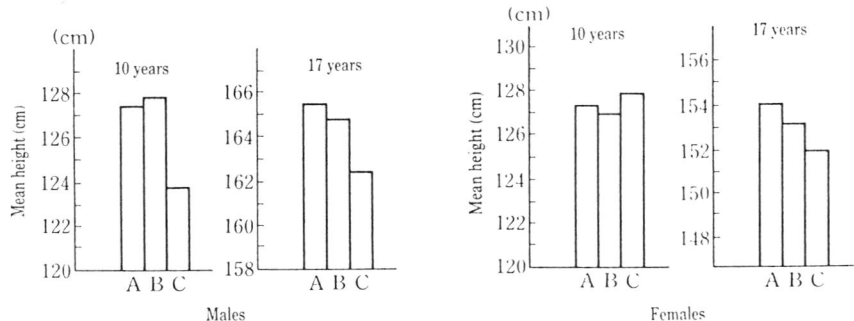

Populations A, B, and C were respectively exposed to 0 Gy, 0.01–0.99 Gy, and $\geq$ 1 Gy (maternal T65D kerma doses). A marked effect can be seen in population C.[8]

Figure 2   Heights of prenatally exposed Hiroshima survivors at ages 10 and 17

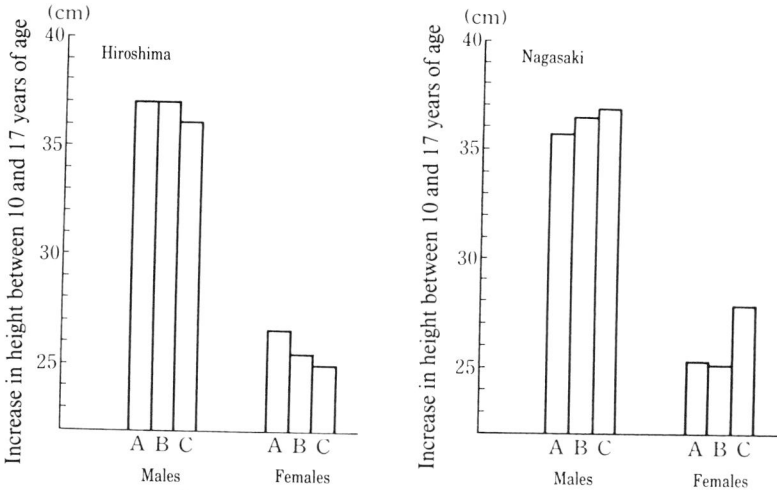

Populations A, B, and C were respectively exposed to 0 Gy, 0.01–0.99 Gy, and ⩾ 1 Gy (maternal T65D kerma doses)[8]

Figure 3   Height increases in prenatally exposed Hiroshima and Nagasaki survivors between ages 10 and 17

This is consistent with the fetus containing a greater number of cells undergoing cell cycle progression and being more sensitive to radiation.

With regard to indices other than height, it has been reported that a radiation effect has been observed on body weight and head size, but not on chest circumference[9]. However, the number of prenatally exposed survivors was small from the outset, not to mention the fact that the totals of prenatally exposed (both male and female) receiving an estimated dose of ⩾ 0.25 Gy amounted to only 45 in Hiroshima and 30 in Nagasaki. With such low numbers, even if an effect were actually present, it might not be possible to detect a statistically significant difference. The actual values for the population estimated to have been prenatally exposed to ⩾ 0.50 Gy show a reduced mean chest circumference relative to the lightly exposed populations for both Hiroshima and Nagasaki, and for both males and females[9].

To summarize, in comparison with other children, children prenatally exposed to a large dose of radiation already had small bodies and small heads by age 10, with similar smallness also observed at age 17. However, between the ages of 10 and 17 there appeared to be no clear difference in growth rate.

Regarding radiosensitivity and the stage of fetal development at the time of exposure, the effect on height was unrelated to developmental stage, whereas there appears to have been a large effect on head size in survivors exposed during the first trimester of pregnancy[8]. This coincides with the radiosensitive period of brain cells, with the reduction in head size believed probably due to the death of cells (please refer to Chapter 13, "Prenatal Exposure").

Another study on prenatal survivors used epiphyseal closure as a measure of development[10]. When bone grows, the epiphysis becomes separated from the main body of bone by cartilage, with bone growth occurring from the cartilage. The epiphysis later undergoes fusion with the main body of bone, becoming part of a large bone (a process known as "epiphyseal closure") (Fig. 4). The epiphyseal center appears at ages 0–6, and undergoes closure at ages 13–21, with the time period said to vary as the result of illness, nutrition, and radiation exposure etc. Based on regular annual X-ray photographs of the left hand conducted between the ages of 9 and 21, the epiphyseal fusion period was investigated at 21 locations, including the wrist.

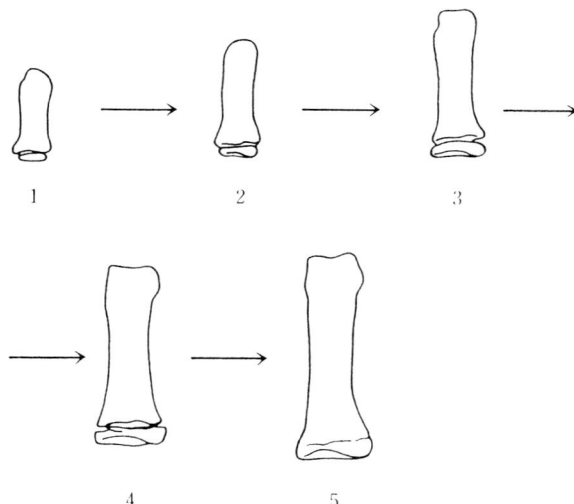

Figure 4   Epiphyseal fusion accompanying bone growth[10]

The average age at epiphyseal fusion for all sites was a little under 17 for males and over 15 for females, with the process thus occurring approximately 1.5 years earlier in females. Radiation appears to reduce this difference between the sexes. That is, the age at which the process occurred in males was reduced on average by 1 month among males exposed to $\geqslant 0.40$ Gy, and by 3.6 months among those receiving $\geqslant 1$ Gy; conversely, the process was delayed in females by an average of 1.4 months for those exposed to $\geqslant 0.40$ Gy, and by an average of 3.5 months for those receiving $\geqslant 1$ Gy. However, due to the small size of the $\geqslant 1$ Gy population (35 subjects), a statistically significant radiation effect was not detected.

No report has appeared concerning the use of the age at menarche among prenatally exposed females as an index of later growth and maturity.

3. CHILDREN OF THE ATOMIC BOMB SURVIVORS

Five studies[11-15] have been performed on the children of atomic bomb survivors between the ages of 6 and 17 with respect to height, body weight, sitting height, and chest circumference, but all have failed to detect an atomic bomb radiation effect.

CONCLUSION

Various possible biological explanations exist for radiation-caused growth distur-bance, but there is little hard evidence. Bones are known to be weakened by localized application of high doses of radiation during radiotherapy. Consequently, with regard to bone formation, it is possible that bone growth deteriorates due to a reduction in the number of bone cells themselves. On the other hand, whole body irradiation causes continual fatigue, and it is well known that many atomic bomb survivors suffered long-term fatigue and general malaise. However, the reasons for this are virtually unexplained. It might be that the combination of a changed systemic hormonal environment, decreased immunocompetence, and slow atrophy due to gradual tissue destruction etc. leads to long-term systemic disturbances in metabolic processes. In the case of prenatal exposure, the finding that growth retardation already exists at age 10 is believed to infer that systemic development is retarded by radiation exposure. On the other hand, studies on epiphyseal fusion suggest that radiation exposure acts to reduce the difference between the sexes. A reduced hormonal environment related to secondary sex characteristics has been suggested, but there are no actual measurements concerning this. Reduced heights have also been observed among children in the Marshall Islands who were exposed to radioactive fallout as a result of atmospheric nuclear tests, but in this case thyroid dysfunction is suspected to have been caused by the ingestion of radioactive iodine[16,17]. With respect to the Hiroshima and Nagasaki atomic bomb survivors, the extent of the effect of fallout is unclear, but as the incidence of thyroid tumors is strongly dependent on the DS86 doses (the doses due to external irradiation), it appears that the fallout effect was small. A study has been performed on the thyroid stimulating hormone (TSH) level in blood in Hiroshima survivors, but this was based on T65D doses[18], and it is thus hoped that the data will be reanalyzed using DS86 values.

(*Nori Nakamura, Mitoshi Akiyama*)

REFERENCES

1. Greulich WN, Crismon CS, Turner ML. The physical growth and development of children who survived the atomic bombings of Hiroshima or Nagasaki. *J Pediatr* 1953; **43**: 121–45.
2. Reynolds EL. Growth and development of Hiroshima children exposed to the atomic bomb. Three-year study (1951–53). ABCC TR 20–59, 1959.
3. Nehemias JV. Multivariate analysis and the IBM 704 computer applied to ABCC data on growth of surviving Hiroshima children. *Health Phys* 1962; **8**: 165–86.
4. Burrow GN, Hamilton HB, Hrubec Z. Study of adolescents exposed *in utero*. Clinical and laboratory data, Nagasaki 1958–59. *JAMA* 1965; **192**: 357–64.
5. Belsky JL, Blot WJ. Adult stature in relation to childhood exposure to the atomic bombs of Hiroshima and Nagasaki. ABCC TR 35–71, 1971.
6. Ishimaru T, Amano T, Kawamoto S. Relationship of stature to gamma and neutron exposure among atomic bomb survivors aged less than 10 at the time of the bomb, Hiroshima and Nagasaki. ABCC TR 18–81, 1981.
7. Kerr GD. Organ dose estimates for Japanese atomic bomb survivors. *Health Phys* 1979; **37**: 487–508.

8. Conner RJ, Kawamoto S, Omori Y. Growth and development age 10 to age 17 of children exposed *in utero* to the atomic bomb, Hiroshima and Nagasaki. ABCC TR 5–71, 1971.

9. Ishimaru T, Nakashima E, Kawamoto S. Relationship of height, body weight, head circumference at age 18 to gamma and neutron doses among *in utero* exposed children, Hiroshima and Nagasaki. RERF TR 19–84, 1984.

10. Russell WJ, Keehn RJ, Iino Y, *et al.* Bone maturation in children exposed *in utero* to the atomic bomb. ABCC TR 1–72, 1972.

11. Furusho T, Otake M. A search for genetic effects of atomic bomb radiation on the growth and development of the F_1 generation. 1. Stature of 15- to 17-year-old senior high school students in Hiroshima. RERF TR 4–78, 1978.

12. Furusho T, Otake M. A search for genetic effects of atomic bomb radiation on the growth and development of the F_1 generation. 2. Body weight, sitting height, and chest circumference of 15- to 17-year-old senior high school students in Hiroshima. RERF TR 5–78, 1978.

13. Furusho T, Otake M. A search for genetic effects of atomic bomb radiation on the growth and development of the F_1 generation. 3. Stature of 12- to 14-year-old junior high school students in Hiroshima. RERF TR 14–79, 1979.

14. Furusho T, Otake M. A search for genetic effects of atomic bomb radiation on the growth and development of the F_1 generation. 4. Body weight, sitting height, and chest circumference of 12- to 14-year-old junior high school students in Hiroshima. RERF TR 1–80, 1980.

15. Furusho T, Otake M. A search for genetic effects of atomic bomb radiation on the growth and development of the F_1 generation. 5. Stature of 6- to 11-year-old elementary school pupils in Hiroshima. RERF TR 9–85, 1985.

16. Sutow WW, Conard RA, Griffith KM. Growth status of children exposed to fallout radiation on the Marshall Islands. *Pediatrics* 1965; **36**: 721–31.

17. Robbins J, Rall JE, Conard RA. Late effects of radioactive iodine in fallout. *Ann Intern Med* 1967; **66**: 1214–42.

18. Ito C, Kato M, Mito K, *et al.* Study on the effect of atomic bomb radiation on thyroid function. *Hiroshima J Med Sci* 1987; **36**: 13–24.

18

Aging and Life Span

18.1 AGING

INTRODUCTION

The hypothesis that ionizing radiation accelerates the aging process derives from the results of diverse animal experiments performed since the 1930s[1-6]. That is, several reports showed that the life span of animals undergoing irradiation was reduced relative to the controls, with the effects of radiation believed to have either accelerated natural senescence or the aging process[3]. However, this argument has frequently been opposed on the basis that the senescence brought about by radiation may be different to the natural process[4-6]; in addition, many researchers reject the hypothesis maintaining that radiation-induced life shortening is merely the result of an increased number of tumors. The point of contention in the debate is whether or not the reduction in life span is specific. In order to demonstrate that it is non-specific, it is necessary to show that the irradiated population exhibits the same spectrum of illnesses that accompany aging at an earlier age than in the control population. Also, the same observations found with natural aging should also be manifested at the histologic and cytologic levels. Many researchers believe that observations of the vascular system etc. show that the aging process is not specific, and the debate has not yet reached a conclusion[7,8]. The question of specificity also poses a great problem epidemiologically, but this will be examined in detail in another section.

This chapter reviews the main results of the numerous clinical, pathological, and basic medical studies conducted in order to determine whether non-specific aging in the atomic bomb survivors was accelerated by radiation.

1. PATHOLOGICAL STUDIES

Various pathological studies have been performed on the atomic bomb survivors, with those pertaining to radiation and aging presented in Table 1. Although numerous age-related changes have been reported, the only one found to be radiogenic was tubular sclerosis of the testis. Jordan et al[13] studied 349 autopsy cases and detected age-related changes regarding tubular sclerosis and interstitial cell hypoplasia, but found that only the former was related to distance from the hypocenter. The hexamine : collagen ratio in skin and the aorta suggested an association with radiation[12].

Table 1 Pathological Studies

Study	Ref.	Chronological age correlation	Radiation effect
Heart muscle lipofuscin	9	↑ thru age 80	None
Papillary muscle fibrosis (focal)	10	↑ with age	None
Aorta extensibility	11	↓ with age	None
Hexamine: collagen ratio of skin and aorta	12	↓ with age	Suggested
Testicular changes	13	TS* ↑ with age	Positive
Giant hepatic nuclei	14	↑ with age	None
Neurofibrillary tangle, senile plaque or granulovascular degeneration	15	↑ with age	None

*TS: tubular sclerosis

A series of studies involving cardiac tissue found correlations between age and focal cardiac myocytolysis, papillary muscle fibrosis, and small vessel sclerosis, but failed to demonstrate a relationship with radiation[9,10].

2. PHYSIOLOGICAL STUDIES

Although there are individual differences, it is well known that the physiological functions of the whole body begin to decline when an individual matures. Consequently, it is believed that these physiological indices are a good tool in aging studies. Table 2 shows the main physiological tests performed on atomic bomb survivors.

Although forced vital capacity, an important index of lung function, exhibited a linear decrease with age[16], no relationship was found with radiation.

Both systolic and diastolic blood pressure increase with age[18-20], but this is more marked in the case of systolic pressure; as the aging process advances, the diastolic pressure begins to decrease, resulting in the elderly being liable to exhibit systolic hypertension. The same tendencies are observed among atomic bomb survivors, but again no difference is found with respect to radiation dose. Furthermore, the blood pressure response to cold stimulus is the same. The occurrence of arteriosclerosis is important in aging studies since it is believed to be an aging phenomenon of the blood vessels, and attempts have been made to detect it clinically[23-26]. These have

Table 2   Functional and physical tests

Tests or measurement	Ref.	Chronological age correlation	Radiation effect
Forced vital capacity	16	↓ with age	None
Grip strength	16	↓ with age	in > 1.00 Gy population
Visual acuity	16	↓ with age	Not consistent
Vibration sense	16	↓ with age	Not consistent
Hearing	16	↓ with age	in 0.50 ~ 0.99 Gy population
Amplitude of visual accommodation	16	↓ with age	Not consistent
Light extinction	16	↓ with age	Not consistent
Skin elasticity	16	↓ with age	Not consistent
Physiological age	16, 17	↑ with chronologic age	None
Systolic blood pressure	18, 19, 20	↑ with age	None
Diastolic blood pressure	19, 20	↑ with age until 60–69	None
Cold pressor test	21	Systolic pressure ↑ with age	None
Cardiac performance	22	Not consistent	None
Aortic arch diameter	23	↑ with age*	None
Cardio thoracic ratio	23	↑ with age*	None
Transverse thoracic diameter	23	↑ with age	None
Electrocardiogram	24, 25	"Aging index" ↑ with age	None
PWV**	26	↑ with age	None
Achilles tendon reflex	27	Reflex time ↑ with age	None
Hair graying	28	↑ with age	None

*Longitudinal study
**PWV: Pulse wave velocity

mainly involved X-ray studies of aortic shadows and pulse transmission velocity, but in each case radiation was found to have no effect.

Certain electrocardiographic changes increase with age, and from these Yano and Ueda[24] selected seven age-related categories as aging parameters, but failed to show a relationship with radiation.

Physiological tests on hearing, visual acuity, and grip strength etc. all demonstrated age-related changes, and it is believed that consideration of these variables allows determination of an individual's aging status. Hollingworth et al[18] first used this concept in an attempt to define the so-called "physiological age" using strongly age-related physiological parameters. Based on the same concept, Belsky et al[16] later carried out physiological tests on the Adult Health Study sample under six categories i.e. grip strength, hearing ability, vibratory perception, amplitude of visual accommo-dation, skin elasticity, and visual reaction time. A linear multiple regression analysis of the scores for the age at the time of testing permitted establishment of aging parameters. No relationship was observed between these parameters and radiation. Furthermore, while there was naturally a significant relationship between each test score and age, certain results also demonstrated a relationship with radiation, e.g. the grip strength in the ≥ 1 Gy population was low in comparison with the 0–0.09 Gy population, and hearing ability in the 0.50–0.99 Gy population was poorer than in the control population. However, since no consistent pattern of differences was observed, it is believed that the results offer no support at all to the hypothesis that radiation accelerates the aging process. Over 15 years have passed since these studies were performed, and a follow-up study is currently under way, according to which individu-als deemed physiologically older than their chronological age based on these aging indices were found to exhibit a higher mortality rate than individuals of the same chronological age who were classified as physiologically younger.

Almost all aging studies using these physiological test scores employed the so-called cross-sectional study format. That is, tests are performed on a fixed cohort over a given time period, and the relationship with aging investigated by the difference in test scores between various age groups. The technique is relatively simple, but it is possible that differences exist in the various background factors among the different age populations, thereby introducing the so-called cohort effect. In order to avoid this, it is necessary to perform a longitudinal study over a period of years examining changes with age in the same individual. Fortunately, in the case of the atomic bomb survivors long-term data has been accumulated for the same individuals, thus permitting the future application of such studies.

3. CLINICAL STUDIES

Various clinical studies have been conducted on atomic bomb survivors, e.g. using blood samples; the main findings are presented in Table 3. Although many of the results show a significant relationship with age, there is no consistency with respect to radiation. For example, impaired glucose tolerance increases with age, but a radiation effect is observed only among the young populations[31].

Table 3   Laboratory tests (1)

Tests	Ref.	Chronological age correlation	Radiation effect
Blood sedimentation rate	29, 30	↑ with age	Positive
Glucose tolerance test	31, 32	↑ with age in borderline type	Positive only in younger survivors
α, β-globulin	33	↑ with age	Positive
Serum immunoglobulin	34	↑ with age	None
Total leukocyte count	29	↓ with age	None
Lymphocyte cytotoxicity	35	↑ with age	None
Serum anti-EB titers	36	↑ with age	Equivocal
PHA response	37	↓ with age	Positive
Number of T-cells	38	↓ with age	Positive at age > 30 years ATB
Con A-induced suppressor T-lymphocytes	38	↓ with age	Equivocal
Helper/inducer T cells	38, 39	↓ with age, especially at ages < 75	None
B-cells and monocytes	38, 39	↑ with age, especially at ages < 75	None
Natural killer cell activity	40	↑ with age	None

*PHA: phytohemagglutinin
ATB: at the time of bombing

Laboratory tests (2)

Stomatic mutation			
T-lymphocyte HPRT*	41	↑ with age	Weak positive
Erythrocyte GPA*	42	↑ with age	None
T-lymphocyte TCR*	43	↑ with age	Positive
Chromosome aneuploidy	44	↑ with age	None

*PHA : phytohemagglutinin
*HPRT: hypoxanthine guanine phosphoribosyl transferase
TCR :T-cell receptor
GPA : glycophorin-A
ATB : at the time of bombing

On the other hand, blood sedimentation rates and serum α- and β-globulin levels increase with age, and furthermore exhibit a radiation effect[29,30].

Several immunological studies have been performed on the Adult Health Study sample. $CD3^- 4^+ (8^-)$ T-cells (atypical T-cells) in peripheral blood exhibited an age-dependent increase which is believed to be related to an age-dependent decrease in T-cell function[38]. B-cells exhibited a similar decrease in function with age, although no radiation effect was found[38,39]. On the other hand, both the numbers and activities of natural killer (NK) cells increased with age, although no relationship with radiation was observed[40].

Somatic cell mutation studies[41–43] began with the objective of estimating the biological doses in order to evaluate the radiation doses received by atomic bomb survivors. In each case, the spontaneous mutation rate increased with age, with the mutation rates of T-lymphocyte hypoxanthine guanine phosphoribosyl transferase (HPRT) and erythrocyte glycophorin-A (GPA) demonstrating a suggested radiation-related increase.

Long-term cytogenetic studies on atomic bomb survivors have yielded numerous important findings, particularly from studies on lymphocyte chromosomes. One such finding involved aneuploid cells; studies of aneuploidy (the loss or gain of a certain chromosome within a cell due to mitotic errors) showed a tendency for an increased loss with advancing age of X chromosomes in females and Y chromosomes in males. However, no radiation-related effects were observed.

4. DISEASE

Investigations concerning the development of diseases that increase with age are another valuable technique in aging studies. The main diseases investigated among the atomic bomb survivors are shown in Table 4. Most of these involve some tissue degeneration, and each exhibits a positive correlation with age. However, no consistent relationship with radiation has been observed.

Both stroke and ischemic heart disease are primarily arteriosclerotic lesions which increase with age, and are very strongly related to the aging process. In cardiovascular studies on the Adult Health Study sample, investigations have been performed on the relationship between incidence and radiation exposure using diagnoses of these diseases made according to standardized diagnostic criteria based on clinical data and autopsy findings etc. Although discussion of the detailed results will be deferred until another section, this study revealed an association with radiation for Hiroshima females only[45]. The study period was subsequently extended and an even more detailed analysis is currently under way.

Several cataract studies have also been conducted[48], showing a clear age-related increase in prevalence and a relationship with radiation exposure. However, since it is well-known that radiogenic cataracts (so-called atomic bomb cataracts) demonstrate a weak relationship with age, care is needed when interpreting these results.

Epidemiological studies on these diseases obviously require long-term longitudinal study to avoid the previously mentioned cohort effect. Furthermore, in order to investigate whether radiation causes an increase in age-related disease it is necessary to consider many other confounding factors, such as the roles of blood pressure, cholesterol, and smoking etc. in the development of ischemic heart disease.

Table 4   Tissue changes or diseases

Disorder	Ref.	Chronological age correlation	Radiation effect
Hypertension	19	↑ with age	None
Stroke	45	↑ with age	Significant in Hiroshima women
Coronary heart disease	29, 45, 46	↑ with age	Significant in Hiroshima women
Diabetes mellitus	47	↑ with age	None
Lenticular opacities	48	↑ with age	Good
Rheumatoid arthritis	49	↑ with age	None
Thoracic vertebral fracture	50	↑ with age, only for females	None
Senile dementia	51	↑ with age	None

CONCLUSION

A considerable amount of data concerning the atomic bomb survivors has been accumulated from various fields with respect to the question of whether radiation accelerates the aging process. The incidence of arteriosclerosis-related disease, changes in immunocompetence, and some pathological and physiological tests have shown an association between radiation and age-related changes, although at the present time the overall results concerning the relationship between atomic bomb exposure and the aging process appear to be inconsistent or negative. However, in order to allow definite conclusions to be drawn, it is hoped that analyses based on longitudinal studies will proceed, and furthermore that studies will be conducted that employ the molecular biology techniques which have advanced rapidly during recent years.

(Hideo Sasaki)

REFERENCES

1. Russ S, Scott GM. Biological effects of gamma irradiation. *Br J Radiol.* 1939; **12**: 440–1.
2. Walburg HE Jr. Radiation-induced life shortening and premature aging. *Adv Radiat Biol* 1975; **5**: 145–79.
3. Comfort A. Natural aging and the effects of radiation. *Radiat Res* 1959; **1** (Suppl): 216–34.
4. Upton AC. Ionizing radiation and the aging process. A review. *J Gerontol* 1957; **12**: 306–13.
5. Upton AC, Kimball AW, Furth J, *et al.* Some delayed effects of atomic radiation in mice. *Cancer Res* 1960; **20**: 1–60.
6. Lindop PJ. Radiation and life span. *Sci Basis Med Annu Rev* London, 1965; 91–109.
7. Casarett GW. Similarities and contrasts between radiation and time pathology. *Adv Gerontol Res* 1964; **1**: 109–63.
8. Cutler RG. Cross linkage hypothesis of aging: DNA adducts in chromatin as a primary aging process. In: Smith KC, editor. Aging, carcinogenesis and radiation biology. New York: Plenum Press, 1976: 443–92.
9. Anderson RE, Yamamoto T, Ishida K, *et al.* Aging in Hiroshima and Nagasaki atomic bomb survivors: accumulation of cardiac lipofuscin. *Am J Geriat Soc* 1971; **19**: 193–8.
10. Steer A, Danzig MD, Robertson TL, *et al.* Focal and diffuse papillary muscle fibrosis and small vessel sclerosis of the heart. ABCC TR 15–75, 1975.
11. Nishimura ET, Matsuoka M, Ishii G, *et al.* Effects of age upon the extensibility of isolated aortic segments of the Japanese. ABCC TR 6–60, 1960.
12. Anderson RE. Aging in Hiroshima atomic bomb survivors. *Arch Pathol* 1965; **79**: 1–6.
13. Jordan SW, Hasegawa CM, Keehn RJ. Testicular changes in atomic bomb survivors. *Arch Pathol* 1965; **82**: 542–54.
14. Anderson RE. Longevity in human irradiated populations with particular reference to the atomic bomb survivors. ABCC TR 9–72, 1972.
15. Wollmann RL, Mitsuyama Y, Webber LS. A morphologic study of central nervous system aging, Hiroshima 1961–72. ABCC TR 22–75, 1975.
16. Belsky JL, Moriyama IM, Fujita S, *et al.* Aging studies in atomic bomb survivors. RERF TR 11–78, 1978.
17. Okajima S, Miyajima J, Ichimaru M, *et al.* Effects of radiation on aging in atomic bomb survivors. *Nagasaki Med J* 1979; **55**: 716–21. (*In Japanese*)
18. Hollingworth JW, Hashizume A, Jablon S. Correlation between tests of aging, Hiroshima. An attempt to define "physiologic age". *Yale J Biol Med* 1965; **38**: 11–26.
19. Yano K, Ueda S. Cardiovascular studies, Hiroshima 1958–60. Report 3. Cardiovascular disease in relation to exposure to ionizing radiation. ABCC TR 22–62, 1962.

20. Dock DS, Fukushima K. A longitudinal study of arterial blood pressure in the Japanese, 1958–1972. *J Chron Dis* 1978; **31**: 669–89.

21. Sasaki T, Sweedler DR, Okamoto A. Cold pressor test on atomic survivors, Nagasaki. ABCC TR 3–64, 1964.

22. Sasaki H, Yamada M, Sawada H, *et al.* Study of cardiac performance of A-bomb survivors (using the mechano-cardiogram). *Nagasaki Med J* 1984; **59**: 554–9. (*In Japanese*)

23. Mihara F, Fukuya T, Nakata H, *et al.* Manifestations of aging on serial chest radiography: a longitudinal observation. RERF TR 3–86, 1986.

24. Yano K, Ueda S. Cardiovascular studies, Hiroshima 1958–60. Report 2. Electrocardiographic findings related to aging. ABCC TR 20–62, 1962.

25. Miyanishi M, Yoshida M, Furonaka H, *et al.* Cardiovascular changes in atomic bomb survivors in term of aging with special reference to electrocardiographic findings. *Hiroshima J Med Sci* 1971; **24**: 1183–95. (*In Japanese*)

26. Takayama S, Ito Y, Okazaki K, *et al.* Study on arteriosclerosis among atomic bomb survivors (second report). *Hiroshima J Med Sci* 1990; **43**: 502–5. (*In Japanese*)

27. Omori Y, Ashley FW, Belsky JL. Achilles tendon reflex and aging in atomic bomb survivors, Hiroshima. *J Chron Dis* 1972; **25**: 111–20.

28. Hollingworth JW, Ishii G, Conard RA. Skin aging and hair graying, Hiroshima. *Geriatrics* 1961; **16**: 27–36.

29. Belsky JL, Tachikawa K, Jablon S. ABCC-JNIH Adult Health Study. Report 5. Results of the first five examination cycles, Hiroshima and Nagasaki M958–68. ABCC TR 9–71, 1971.

30. Yamada M, Neriishi K, Fujiwara S, *et al.* Erythrocyte sedimentation rate in Adult Health Study participants. *Hiroshima J Med Sci* 1986; **39**: 446–51. (*In Japanese*)

31. Bizzozero OJ Jr, Omori Y, Archer PG, *et al.* The relation of oral glucose tolerance to age and sex in the Japanese, Hiroshima. ABCC TR 21–67, 1967.

32. Kawate R, Naito Y, Noka K, *et al.* Aging and metabolism in the atomic bomb survivors. *Hiroshima J Med Sci* 1971; **24**: 1196–204. (*In Japanese*)

33. Neriishi K, Matsuo T, Ishimaru T, *et al.* Radiation exposure and serum protein, globulin fraction. *Nagasaki Med J* 1986; **61**: 449–54. (*In Japanese*)

34. Hall CB, Hall WJ, Ashley FW, *et al.* Serum immunoglobulin levels in atomic bomb survivors, Hiroshima. *Am J Epidemiol* 1973; **98**: 423–9.

35. Caplan RA, Odoroff CL, Ozaki K, *et al.* Lymphocyte cytotoxicity of colchicine in Hiroshima atomic bomb survivors. RERF TR 9–78, 1978.

36. Ozaki K, Kyoizumi S, Mizuno S, *et al.* Late effects of A-bomb radiation on human immune response. VI Anti-EB virus antibody titer in sera of A-bomb survivors. *Hiroshima J Med Sci* 1990; **43**: 523–4. (*In Japanese*)

37. Yamakido M, Akiyama M, Dock DS, *et al.* T and B cells and PHA response of peripheral lymphocytes among atomic bomb survivors. *Radiat Res* 1983; **93**: 572–80.

38. Kusunoki Y, Akiyama M, Kyoizumi S, *et al.* Age-related alteration in the composition of immuno-competent blood cells in atomic bomb survivors. *Int J Radiat Biol* 1988; **53**: 189–98.

39. Fujiwara S, Akiyama M, Kobuke K, *et al.* Analysis of peripheral blood lymphocytes of atomic bomb survivors using monoclonal antibodies. *J Radiat Res* 1986; **27**: 255–66.

40. Akiyama M, Kusunoki Y, Bloom ET, *et al.* Immunological responses of A-bomb survivors. *Radiat Res* 1988; **116**: 343–55.

41. Hakoda M, Akiyama M, Kyoizumi S, *et al.* Increased somatic cell mutant frequency in atomic bomb survivors. *Mutat Res* 1988; **201**: 39–48.

42. Kyoizumi S, Nakamura N, Hakoda M, *et al.* Detection of somatic mutations at the glycophorin-A locus in erythrocytes of atomic bomb survivors using a single beam flow sorter. *Cancer Res* 1989; **49**: 581–8.

43. Kyoizumi S, Akiyama M, Hirai Y, *et al.* Spontaneous loss and alteration of antigen receptor expression in mature CD4 T cells. RERF TR 22–89, 1989.

44. Awa AA, Sofuni T, Honda T. Chromosome aneuploidy and radiation in a human population. In the ninth NIRS symposium on carcinogenesis and genetic disorders — toward risk estimates of radiation. NIRS-M-27: 212–8, 1977.

45. Kodama K, Shimizu Y, Sawada H, *et al.* Incidence of stroke and coronary heart disease in the Adult Health Study sample, 1958–78. RERF TR 22–84, 1984.

46. Johnson KG, Yano K, Kato H. Coronary heart disease in Hiroshima, Japan: a report of a 6 year period of surveillance, 1958–64. *Am J Public Health* 1968; **58**: 1355–67.

47. Brodsky JB, Moore DF, Kawate R. Diabetes, glycosuria, and proteinuria in a Japanese cohort followed for 20 years. RERF TR 11–85, 1985.

48. Choshi K, Takaku 1, Mishima H, *et al.* Ophthalmologic changes related to radiation exposure and age in the Adult Health Study sample, Hiroshima and Nagasaki. RERF TR 8–82, 1982.

49. Kato H, Duff IF, Russel WJ, *et al.* Rheumatoid arthritis and gout in Hiroshima and Nagasaki, Japan. A prevalence and incidence study. *J Chron Dis* 1971; **23**: 659–79.

50. Fujiwara S, Mizuno S, Ochi Y, *et al.* Incidence of thoracic vertebral fracture among Adult Health Study participants, Hiroshima and Nagasaki, 1958–86. RERF TR 12–89, 1989.

51. Akahoshi M, Matsuo T, Kodama K, *et al.* Occurrence of dementia in Adult Health Study population. *Hiroshima J Med Sci* 1990; **43**: 548–50. (*In Japanese*)

18.2 LIFE SPAN

INTRODUCTION

Life shortening (or an increased mortality rate) was one late effect of exposure to the atomic bomb. Animal experiments have shown that radiation increases the mortality rate from leukemia and other cancers, but although an increased non-cancer mortality rate is observed following exposure to high doses (several dozen Grays), such an increase is not observed with low or medium doses[1].

As mentioned in Chapter 1.1, the atomic bomb survivors exhibited an increased cancer mortality rate[2]. No clear evidence, however, existed regarding an increased non-malignant disease mortality rate, although recent observations have suggested such an increase among survivors exposed to doses greater than 2 Gy[3].

Since the contribution of cancer in life-shortening is clear, this chapter focuses on the results obtained in the Life Span Study at the Radiation Effects Research Foundation (RERF), with particular reference to the effects on life span of radiation-related non-cancer diseases. In other words, the chapter will examine whether an increased mortality rate from non-malignant disease is observed among atomic bomb survivors; cancer mortality is also discussed from the viewpoint of life span.

1. MORTALITY RATES FROM NON-MALIGNANT DISEASE

Of the 120,000 subjects in the RERF Life Span Study sample (90,000 atomic bomb survivors plus 30,000 non-exposed), DS86 dose estimates were available for a total of 75,991 of the 90,000 exposed persons. The number of deaths occurring in this population during the period 1950–85 totaled 28,737; of these, 27,147 died from disease, 1,515 from all extrinsic causes such as accidents and suicide etc., and 75 from unknown causes. Among the 27,147 disease deaths, 23% (6,224 cases) died due to neoplasm and 77% (20,923 cases) from other diseases (Table 1).

Table 1   Number of deaths by cause of death during 1950–85 among the 75, 991 subjects in the RERF cohort[3]

Cause of death	No. of deaths	
All causes	28,737	
Extrinsic factors	1,515	
Unknown causes	75	
All disease	27,147	
Neoplasm	6,224	
Malignant neoplasm	5,936	
Neoplasm of benign and unspecified nature	288	
All disease except neoplasm	20,923	(100%)
Infectious disease	1,413	(7)
Diseases of blood and hematopoietic organs	146	(1)
Circulatory disease	11,164	(53)
Stroke	6,202	(29)
Circulatory disease except stroke	4,962	(24)
Respiratory tract disease	2,036	(10)
Digetsive tract disease	2,149	(10)
Other diseases	4,015	(19)

Of the 6,224 neoplasm deaths, the large majority (5,936) were due to malignant neoplasm (cancer), with only the remaining 288 dying from "neoplasms of benign or unspecified nature" (although most of these are believed to have actually had cancer). Cancer mortality among atomic bomb survivors has been discussed in an earlier chapter. Of the 20,923 non-neoplasm deaths, 53% (11,164 cases) died from circulatory disease.

This discussion of non-malignant diseases will exclude from the disease totals not only malignant neoplasm but all other neoplasm and blood disease (146 cases) (many of the cases in which the cause of death was recorded as a hematologic disorder had leukemia or other malignant neoplasm).

Consideration of the 20,777 deaths from non-malignant disease reveals that the dose-response relationship for the sex and age totals over the period 1950–85 increased at doses greater than 2 Gy, with the dose-response curve being not linear but having a threshold value (i.e. no increase from the baseline value is observed until a certain minimum (threshold) dose is received) (Fig. 1). Examination by age at the time of bombing (ATB) and observation period shows that among the young ATB population the mortality rate from non-malignant disease has recently been increasing among the heavily exposed (Fig. 2).

Scrutiny of the dose-response relationship by disease for the population aged < 40 ATB in the period 1965–85 reveals no evidence of a dose-related trend in mortality

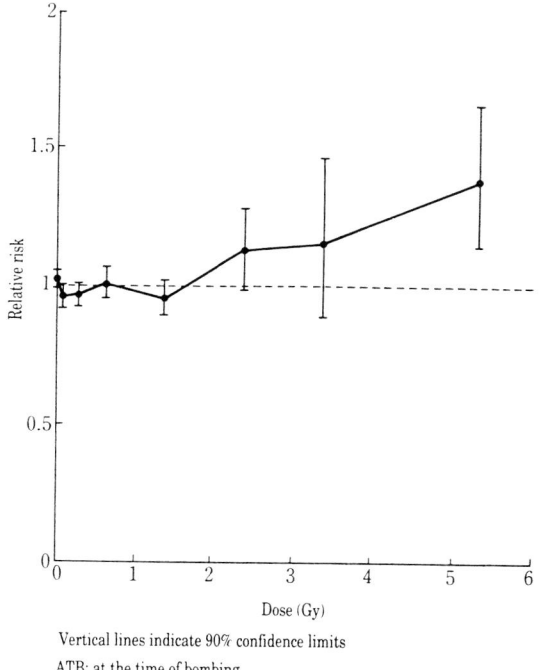

Vertical lines indicate 90% confidence limits

ATB: at the time of bombing

Figure 1   Dose-response curve for mortality rates from non-malignant disease (all ages ATB, 1950–85)[3]

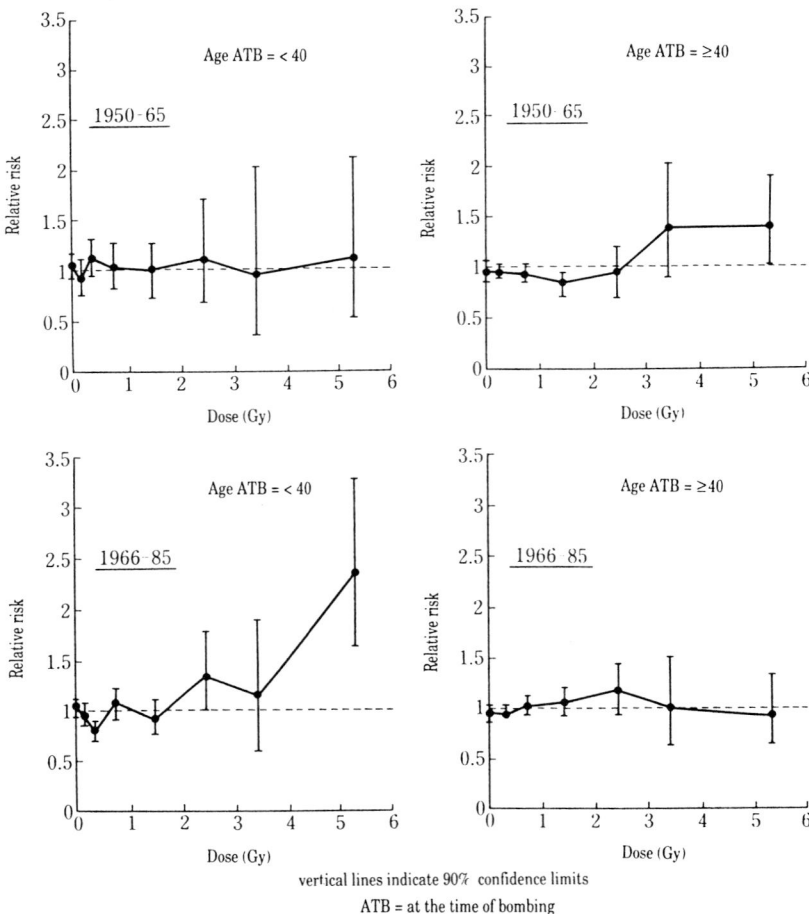

vertical lines indicate 90% confidence limits

ATB = at the time of bombing

Figure 2   Dose-response curve for mortality rates from non-malignant disease by age at the time of bombing (ATB) and observation period[3]

rates for infectious disease and respiratory tract disease; however, high mortality rates are observed among the heavily exposed for all circulatory disease, stroke, circulatory disease other than stroke, and digestive tract disease (Fig. 3).

Compared with a relative cancer risk of 1.78 among subjects exposed to 2 Gy, the risk of non-malignant disease is a low 1.06 (Table 2). The excess number of deaths per Gray per 10,000 person years is respectively 10.0 and 1.18, and thus the number of excess deaths due to non-malignant disease is small despite the background rate being high in comparison with cancer deaths.

Since these mortality study findings are based on death certificates, a problem arises regarding the accuracy of the listed cause of death. In particular, the high mortality rate from non-malignant disease among the heavily exposed may arise due to the misclassification of cases of radiation-induced cancer. In order to resolve this

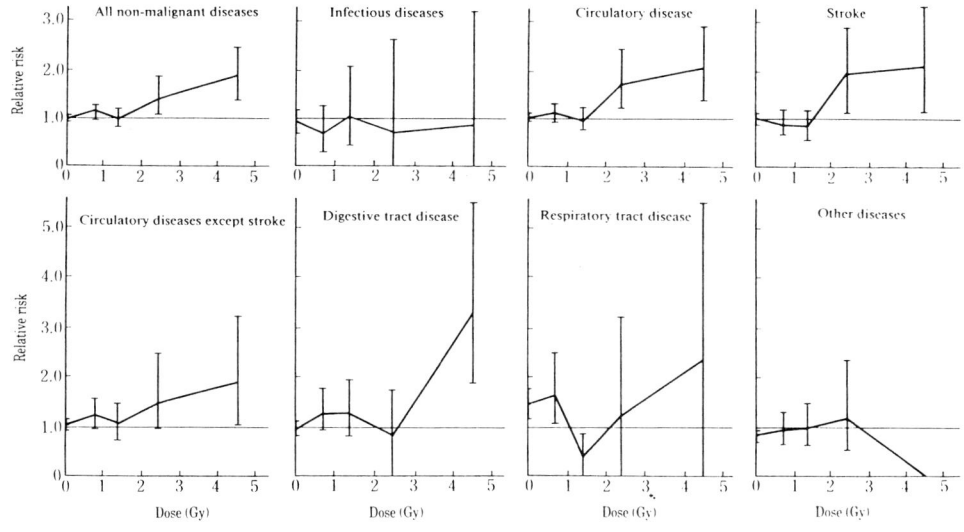

Vertical lines indicate 90% confidence limits
ATB: at the time of bombing

Figure 3   Dose-response curve for mortality rates of specific non-malignant diseases (Age < 40 ATB, 1966–85)[3]

Table 2   Comparison of risks from cancer and non-malignant disease[3]

		Relative risk at 2 Gy	Excess deaths per Gy per 10,000 person years
Non-malignant diseases	Total	1.06 (1.02, 1.09)	1.18 (0.51, 1.19)
	Age under 40 ATB Observation period 1966–85	1.19 (1.10, 1.29)	1.69 (0.90, 2.62)
Cancer	Total	1.78 (1.64, 1.92)	10.00 (8.36, 11.8)

( ) 90% confidence limit
ATB = at the time of bombing

N.B. Estimates are based on the linear risk model for cancer, and the linear risk model with a threshold value (1.4 Gy) for non-malignant diseases

problem, a study was performed on the relationship between radiation dose and the adjusted non-cancer mortality rate, which was calculated using a correction factor determined from a comparison of the causes of death listed in the death certificates and the autopsy findings. However, a high mortality rate was still observed among the heavily exposed population.

That is, although it has until now been believed that no association exists between radiation and non-malignant disease, the young ATB population has begun to reach the age at which non-malignant adult diseases such as circulatory disease frequently appear, and recently a radiation effect has been suggested among the heavily exposed population (≥ 2 Gy). In order to confirm these observations, in addition to the mortality studies it is necessary to perform incidence studies such as those on RERF's Adult Health Study sample.

There are virtually no other studies with which these findings can be compared. At the present time, the only study to find an increased mortality rate from non-malignant disease is a mortality study on American radiologists[4]; no such increase was observed among British radiologists[5]. Patients in Britain who underwent radiotherapy for ankylosing spondylitis showed increases in mortality rate of both cancer and non-malignant disease[6]; however, the increased from non-malignant disease is likely to be associated with ankylosing spondylitis itself, so the relationship with radiotherapy is not clear.

2. LIFE SHORTENING

The relationship between mortality rate and age is known to generally obey Gompertz's Law, which states that the logarithm of the mortality rate is proportional to age, i.e. the age-specific death rate is linear[7]. The radiation-related life shortening is suggested by an upward but parallel shift of the straight Gompertz function. Figure 4 shows the Gompertz function for atomic bomb survivors exposed to 0 Gy and ≥ 2 Gy with regard to mortality rates for all disease, cancer, and non-malignant diseases. In each of these disease classifications the line for the ≥ 2 Gy population is shifted to a higher position than the corresponding line for the 0 Gy population, with the shift for cancer being the most marked. Even the line for non-malignant diseases is elevated, although by only a small amount relative to that for cancer. As mentioned previously, the mortality rate from non-malignant disease is marked among those exposed while young; consequently, an examination by age ATB shows a clear reduction in life span among the < 40 years ATB population (Fig. 5).

Another index of life shortening is the difference in average life expectancy between the exposed and non-exposed populations (which at 0 years is equivalent to

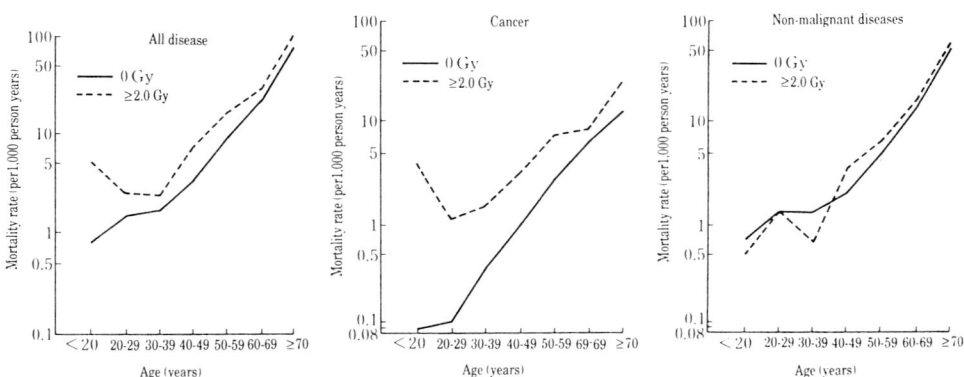

Figure 4   Age-specific mortality rates per 1,000 person years by radiation dose (Gompertz's function)[3] (for all diseases, cancer, and non-malignant diseases)

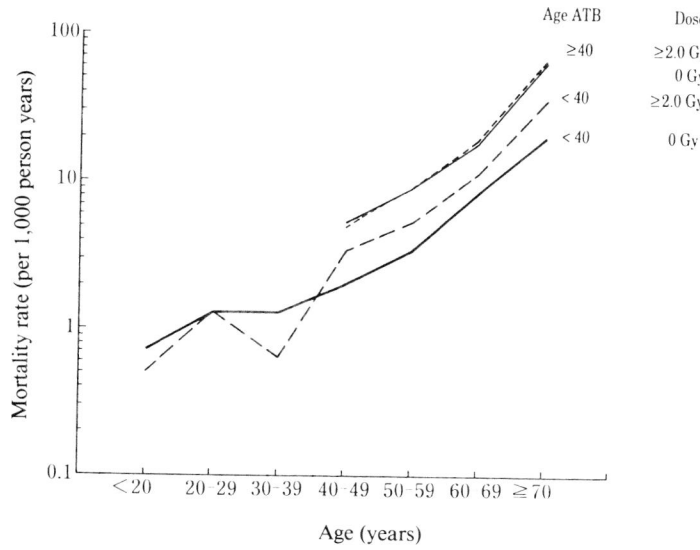

Figure 5 Age-specific mortality rates per 1,000 person years by radiation dose, and age at the time of bombing (ATB), (Gompertz's function)[3] (for non-malignant diseases)

the difference in life span). It is not possible to calculate the life expectancy for the RERF Life Span Study sample since approximately 60% of the subjects are still alive. Therefore calculations of life expectancy were performed using the risk coefficient in the Life Span Study sample and the stationary population in the 1985 Japanese "life table" ["life table" is a summarizing technique used to describe the pattern of mortality and survival in a population]. No increase in non-malignant disease mortality rate was observed in the < 2 Gy population, so for the ≥ 2 Gy population (with an average dose of 3.3 Gy) calculations were performed separately for cancer and non-cancer diseases. The life shortening at 0 years for males was approximately 3 years for cancer and approximately 0.4 years for non-malignant diseases (Table 3).

Estimated life expectancy can be expected to vary greatly with the age-sex composition of the population selected, mortality rates in the background population, and average radiation dose received. Consequently, the afore-mentioned esti-

Table 3 Life shortening (in years) among survivors exposed to ≥ 2 Gy (average dose = 3.3 Gy)[3]

		Age ATB							
		0	10	20	30	40	50	60	70
Non-malignant diseases	Males	0.42	0.42	0.42	0.40	0.37	0.30	0.21	0.06
	Females	0.32	0.31	0.31	0.30	0.28	0.25	0.18	0.05
Cancer	Males	2.91	2.90	2.87	2.79	2.55	1.92	1.03	0.17
	Females	2.17	2.16	2.12	1.99	1.71	1.27	0.68	0.12

ATB = at the time of bombing

mated life span reduction in years is merely a calculated value. However, the relative difference in magnitude of life shortening between cancer and non-malignant disease cases in this group does not change significantly.

Supplementary note: Comments on the "selection effect" argument by Stewart and Kneale[8].

As shown in Fig. 2, the dose-response relationship for the pre-1965 mortality rate from non-malignant disease shows that the mortality rate among the ≥ 40 years ATB population tends to decrease with received dose at doses of ≤ 2 Gy. As asserted by Stewart and Kneale[8], this is in part due to the RERF Life Span Study sample being comprised of survivors alive 5 years after exposure to the atomic bomb, causing the population to be biased toward individuals with a strong resistance to radiation, and possibly resulting in the so-called "healthy worker effect" which is observed in general epidemiological studies (the effect whereby healthy individuals are selected as subjects).

However, even if such a bias is postulated, then as shown in Fig. 2 such an effect is restricted to the initial period following exposure (until approximately 1965), and so when considered with the fact that the development of radiation-induced cancer (except for leukemia) requires a minimum latency period of 10–15 years, it is believed that there is almost no effect on the estimated risk of radiation-induced cancer in this population. Thus it does not follow that the cancer risk in the RERF Life Span Study is underestimated, as suggested by Stewart and Kneale.

In passing, it might be added that the radiogenic cancer risk coefficient estimated from the Life Span Study is approximately the same as the risk coefficient estimated from a medically irradiated population. For details, the reader is referred to reference 3.

(Yukiko Shimizu, Hiroo Kato)

REFERENCES

1. United Nations Scientific Committee on the Effects of Atomic Radiation. 1982 Report Annex K: Radiation-induced life shortening. New York: United Nations, 1982: 655–727.
2. Shimizu Y, Kato H, Schull WJ. Studies of the mortality of A-bomb survivors. Report 9. Mortality, 1950–85: Part 2. Cancer mortality based on the recently revised doses (DS86). *Radiat Res* 1990; **121**: 120–41.
3. Shimizu Y, Kato H, Schull WJ, *et al.* Studies of the mortality of A-bomb survivors. 9. Mortality, 1950–85: Part 3. Non-cancer mortality based on the revised dose (DS86). *Radiat Res* 1992; **130**: 249–66. (RERF TR 2-91, 1991)
4. Matanoski GM, Selster R, Sartwell PE, *et al.* The current mortality rates of radiologists and other physician specialists: specific causes of death. *Am J Epidemiol* 1975; **101**: 199–210.
5. Court Brown WM, Doll R. Expectation of life and mortality from cancer among British radiologists. *Brit Med J* 1958; **2**: 181–7.
6. Darby SC, Doll R, Gill SK, *et al.* Long term mortality after a single treatment course with X-rays in patients treated for ankylosing spondylitis. *Br J Cancer* 1987; **55**: 179–90.
7. Last JM, editor. A dictionary of epidemiology. New York: Oxford University Press, 1988: 53–4.
8. Stewart AM, Kneale GW. Non-cancer effects of exposure to A-bomb radiation. *J Epid Comm Health* 1984; **38**: 108–12.

19

Genetic Effects

19.1 GENETIC EFFECTS

1) ABORTIONS, STILLBIRTHS, AND MALFORMATIONS

INTRODUCTION

Radiation exposure exerts a genetic effect on the following generations by inflicting injury to the gonadal germ cells (sperm, ova, and their precursor cells), with the degree of injury varying according to the received dose. Should the damage be great, with the death of the germ cells or the loss of their mitotic and proliferative ability, then sterility results and adverse genetic effects are not manifested. However, if germ cells undergo mutation while retaining their reproductive ability, it is possible for genetic effects to appear, with mutations occurring in genes and chromosomes. The former occur in the bases constituting DNA in a certain part of the gene, and the latter cause changes in the genetic information due to abnormalities in the numbers and structures of the chromosomes. Stable chromosomal aberrations are transmitted to daughter cells via mitosis, but in many instances cells with severe chromosomal abnormalities die in the early generations of mitosis, resulting in no genetic succession. In contrast, gene mutations are transmitted at every mitotic division, and in the case of germ cells it is possible for the mutation to be transmitted to descendants. The fact that radiation induces mutations has been known since 1927 when Muller[1] experimentally induced mutations by irradiating fruit flies (*Drosophila*) with X-rays and observed a visible phenotype. Based on such historical knowledge, long-term studies were performed on the human genetic effects of the atomic bombings in Hiroshima and Nagasaki. This chapter reviews the background to those studies and summarizes the findings.

1. EARLY GENETIC STUDIES

In order to comprehend the genetic effects of the atomic bombing, Japanese and American researchers began studies 2–3 years after the bombing in order to investigate questions such as 1) whether or not there was an increase in fetal abortions and stillbirths in the offspring of exposed parents; 2) whether malformations increased in their fetuses and newborns; and 3) whether there was a change in the sex ratio of offspring.

2. STILLBIRTHS AND MALFORMATIONS

Studies were performed in order to determine the rate of increase in fetal deaths and malformations in the next generation (i.e. to estimate the increased injurious effect caused when a human population is exposed to a fixed quantity of radiation). Before making comparisons with controls, it is first necessary to know:

(1) the frequency of genetic abnormalities among a non-exposed human population (in Hiroshima, Nagasaki, or an average Japanese population);

(2)   the expected abnormality rate due to spontaneous mutations which would be repeated among that population (the constant long-term frequency of genetic abnormality and disease evident to date in human beings). Japanese family registers had previously been accurate, but such documents were difficult to obtain in the postwar confusion. It was believed that valid subjects for the studies would be populations such as those on outlying islands who at one time were totally isolated, but today it is difficult to obtain a suitable cohort due to population migrations. Recently results have appeared such as those published by Stevenson[2] on Northern Ireland:

(1)   The frequencies of traits at the time of birth which are maintained due to spontaneous mutations which repeat the frequency governed by a single gene are:

Autosomal dominant trait	Approx. 0.96%
Autosomal recessive character	Approx. 0.13%
Sex-linked recessive character	Approx. 0.04%

(2)   Genetic forms which show family accumulations at the time of birth (polygenes, primarily including congenital abnormalities), approximately 0.98%.

(3)   Abnormalities governed by single recessive genes with mutation dependence, approximately 0.09%

(4)   Abnormalities governed by polygenes whose genetic form is not adequately clear, estimated at approximately 1.48%.

According to this, those in which frequency was maintained due to natural mutations belong to type (1) and thus account for approximately 1.1% of the total at the time of birth. It is believed that the genetic effect of mutations caused by radiation exposure increases in frequency, and therefore, for example, if the number of abnormalities increased at the same rate as the natural mutations, then the number of autosomal dominant and sex-linked recessive genetic abnormalities appearing in the offspring would be of the order of 1%, while the number of abnormalities due to autosomal recessive genes (whose effects appear slowly) would be 0.13%. The possibility cannot be discounted that these will increase in the grandchildren of the atomic bomb survivors (the F_2 generation).

Therefore even in non-exposed human populations, it is not easy to elucidate genetic information. However, in animal experiments using mice etc., Russell[3] reported radiation-caused changes in specific genetic loci with ensuing trait abnormalities in the next generation. Based on these experimental findings and data concerning human cohorts, a United Nations Scientific Committee report[4] determined the genetic risk posed to humans by radiation exposure (Table 1). Three years after the atomic explosion, Neel and Schull[5] commenced a study on congenital malformation and infantile deaths etc. occurring in Hiroshima and Nagasaki. In the 1948–53 study, subjects were classified into 5 populations according to the distances from the hypocenter of each parent and the radiation-caused acute symptoms. The doses received by these populations were estimated as 0, 0.005–0.10, 0.50–1.00,

Table 1   Estimated effect of 0.01 Gy per generation of low-dose, low-dose rate radiation on a population of one million individuals born alive[4]

Disease classification	Current incidence	First generation (F_1)
Autosomal dominant and X-linked diseases	10,000	20
Recessive diseases	1,100	relatively slight
Chromosomal diseases	6,000	40
Congenital anomalies, anomalies expressed later, constitutional and degenerative diseases	90,100	5
Total	107,200	65
Percentage of current incidence		0.06

1.00–1.50, and 2.00–3.00 Gy. The study considered 15,410 survivors with pregnancy records, and 55,870 non-exposed controls with similar records, giving a total study population in Hiroshima and Nagasaki of 71,280. Categories examined by the study included stillbirths, neonatal deaths, infant mortality within 9 months of birth, malformations observed at birth and at 9 months, and the sex ratio of the offspring. Retrospective calculations on this sample size showed that none of the categories displayed a significant statistical difference between the exposed populations and controls.

On the other hand, Hayashi et al[6] autopsied 887 fetuses and newborns in Nagasaki between September 1949 and December 1953, and found a significant difference in the malformation rate between the non-exposed controls (11.0%) and offspring born to atomic bomb survivors (18.5%). However, no specific genetic malformations were found among the exposed population.

3. SEX RATIO STUDIES

Kaplan[7] studied the sex ratio among children born to women who had undergone X-ray treatment for sterility, and found that at birth the sex ratio (i.e. the percentage of boys in the total number of children) was considerably lower than in the general population. Tanaka and Ohkura[8] compared 326 male X-ray technologists with 750 male pharmacist controls of approximately the same age, and found an increase in stillbirths and sex ratio in the offspring. Maternal exposure was found to lead to a reduction in the sex ratio and an increased mortality rate among male children due to fatal sex-linked recessive mutations; paternal exposure led to an increased sex ratio and increased mortality among female children due to fatal sex-linked dominant mutations. These results were consistent with the hypothesis of sex-linked mutations. The proposition that exposure of either one or both parents to radiation may produce a change in the sex ratio of the offspring in this way underlies the suggestion that rather than the radiation causing physical functional damage to exposed females, the effects are due to a radiation-caused genetic effect. Behind the sex ratio changes is the fact that the fatal abnormalities in the male or female children may be inherent, leaving open the question of whether this is related to fetal death.

Although Neel and Schull[5] found a tendency for a sex ratio change in their first study (1948–53), in 1968 Schull et al[9] reported less evidence for this in a follow-up study conducted on 47,624 children born in Hiroshima and Nagasaki in the period 1956–62. In 1966 Tabuchi et al[10] performed a similar study at Hiroshima University's Department of Obstetrics and Gynecology, but reached no definite conclusion.

4. STUDIES OF QUANTIFIABLE CHARACTERISTICS IN THE OFFSPRING OF ATOMIC BOMB SURVIVORS

When genetic mutations are caused by radiation, rather than the radiation producing base substitution in DNA ("point mutation"), damage more frequently occurs to various genetic loci. Generally damage to multiple genetic loci leads easily to cell death, and it is known that changes in quantifiable characteristics originating from inherited polygenes with multiple genetic damage are more difficult to demonstrate than similar changes arising from point mutations consistent with mendelism. Examples of quantifiable characteristics are intellectual development, height, body weight, several malformations, and various adult illnesses etc., which are governed by hereditary and environmental factors. Furusho[11] adopted height as an index of quantifiable characteristics in a study of the effects on the offspring of parental exposure. The analysis was based on a 1965 survey on the physical development of approximately 200,000 elementary, junior high, and senior high school students in Hiroshima and Nagasaki. However, no significant difference was found between comparable populations consisting of the offspring of exposed parents and non-exposed controls.

5. LATER STUDIES ON CHILD MALFORMATION

As a means to investigate the genetic effects of atomic bomb radiation, Satow and Hori[12] have continued to perform autopsies on fetal and newborn deaths arising from spontaneous or artificial abortions in the offspring of atomic bomb survivors (the F_1 generation) and also in the following generation (the F_2 generation). Data was collected at obstetric and gynecological hospitals in Hiroshima, commencing in 1963 for the F_1 generation (i.e. the children of atomic bomb survivors) and in 1971 for the F_2 generation (i.e. the grandchildren of atomic bomb survivors). An analysis was performed on 652 F_1 subjects and 115 F_2 subjects for whom data was available, with the control population consisting of approximately 8,000 fetuses who underwent artificial abortion under approximately identical conditions and for whom autopsy results showed no evidence of abnormalities. The autopsy findings were classified into 3 categories: a normal population, who exhibited no abnormalities; an abnormal population, who exhibited pathological symptoms such as hemorrhaging and inflammation; and a malformation population, who exhibited either single or complicated malformations (Table 2). One of the aims of these studies was to investigate whether the limited autopsy population displayed

Table 2   Comparison of autopsy findings for controls and the F_1 and F_2 populations

Autopsy findings	Artificial abortions			Spontaneous abortions		
	Controls	F_1	F_2	Controls	F_1	F_2
Normal	2,871 (64.0)*	63 (78.8)**	32 (100)	594 (18.4)	74 (22.0)	14 (14.0)
Pathological	1,367 (30.5)	14 (17.5)**	0	1,743 (54.1)*	167 (49.7)*	40 (40.0)**
Anomalies	248 (5.5)	3 (3.7)*	0	885 (27.5)	95 (28.3)	46 (46.0)**
Total	4,486 (100%)	80 (100)	32 (100)	3,222 (100%)	336 (100)	100 (100)

*$p < 0.05$ **$p < 0.01$

In the artificial abortion population, normal findings were predominant in the controls and F_1 generation. In the spontaneous abortion population, pathological findings were predominant in the controls, and in the F_1 and F_2 generations.

increases in accordance with Mendel's Laws with respect to disorders such as autosomal dominant hereditary chondrodystrophy, polycystic kidney, or autosomal recessive hereditary osteogenesis imperfecta etc. Another objective was to determine whether the exposed population exhibited a high rate of multifactorial inheritance abnormalities (which account for the vast majority of malformations), i.e. abnormalities arising from interactions between polygenes and various environmental factors. However, for each organ no particular difference in malformations was seen between the F_1 and F_2 generations of the control and exposed populations. Furthermore, no significant differences were observed in the differences in genetic effect caused by exposure of sperm or ova, which were classified according to whether exposure was of the father only, the mother only, or both parents, and according to distance from the hypocenter (within 2 km, or further than 2 km). (Tables 3 and 4).

CONCLUSION

Early studies, which were restricted to indices such as dominant lethal effects and malformation etc. among the offspring of atomic bomb survivors, and even later studies that covered 40 years following exposure, revealed no positive evidence of genetic effects being produced by atomic bomb radiation. Analogical radiation-induced genetic effects observed in experimental animals such as mice and frogs are difficult to demonstrate in humans due to the limited number of subjects studied; another reason is that in humans the numbers of pregnancies and offspring are small, and the harmful genetic mutations produced were selected from spontaneous abortions occurring in early pregnancy, thus making it difficult to systematically collect data. Also, as the number of marriages with close relatives has decreased in recent years, and the pattern of human marriage has been essentially heterogeneous, the opportunities of detecting the recessive hereditary character which is exhibited in homogeneity have been low, and are related to social conditions. However, the various above factors are certainly not a basis for asserting that atomic bomb

Table 3 Relationship between malformations and distance from the hypocenter among natural births in the F_1 population ('D' indicates dominant gene abnormality)

Distance from hypocenter Person exposed	< 2 km	2 ~ 4 km	Early entrants	Unknown
Paternal exposure Maternal exposure Both parents exposed	2 9 4	3 7 1	3	9 28 8
No. of subjects	15	11	3	45
♀/♂	7/8	6/5	2/1	23/22

Malformation	Anencephalia 6
	Accessory spleen, 4
	  lien accessorius
	Abnormal lobation 3
	  of right lung
	Patent ductus 3
	  arteriosus
	Cleft lip & cleft 2
	  palate
	Ventricular septal 2
	  defect
	Meningocele 1
	Chondrodystrophy 1 D
	Abnormal lobation 1
	  of both lungs
	Transposition of 1
	  the great arteries
	Probe patency 1
	  (of foramen ovale)
	Agenesis of both 1
	  kidneys
	Nephrocystosis 1
	Meckel's 1
	  diverticulum
	Cecum mobile 1
	Single umbilical 1
	  artery
		Anencephalia 1
		Accessory spleen, 3
		  lien accessorius
		Abnormal lobation 1
		  of the right lung
		Tetralogy of Fallot 2
		Cleft lip & cleft 1
		  palate
		Ventricular septal 1
		  defect
		Abnormal arch 1
		  of aorta
		Chondrodystrophy, 1 D
		  chondralloplasia
		Abnormal lobation 1
		  of both lungs
		Female 1
		  pseudohermaphroditism
		Transposition of 1
		  the great arteries
		Horoprosencephaly 1
		Hydrocephaly 1
		Left heart syndrome 1
		
		Abnormal lobation 1
		  of left lung
		Diaphragmatic hernia 1
		Cecum mobile 1
		Abdominal fissure 1
		Megalocystis 1
		Horseshoe kidney 1
		Anal atresia 1
		Duplex uterus, 1
		  uterus duplex
		Hydrometer 1
		Male pseudoher- 1
		  maphroditism
		Clubfoot 1
		Pschyotia 1
		Erythroblastosis 1
		Trisomy E syndrome 1
			Anencephalia 1
			
			Abnormal lobation 1
			  of right lung
			Tetralogy of Fallot 1
			Cleft lip & cleft 1
			  palate
			Facial cleft, 1
			  prosoposchisis
			Meningocele 1
			Clubfoot 1
			
			Meckel's 1
			  diverticulum
			
			Megalocytosis 1
			
			Hydroureter 1
				Anencephalia 6
				Accessory spleen, 9
				  lien accessprius
				Abnormal lobation 9
				  of the right lung
				Hypoplasia of the 2
				  aorta
				Patent ductus 2
				  arteriosus
				Cleft lip & cleft 6
				  palate
				Unilateral cleft 3
				  lip and cleft palate
				Ventricular septal 7
				  defect
				Atrial septal defect 1
				Coarctation of the 1
				  aorta
				Meningocele 1
				Microcephaly 1
				Micrognathia 1
				Abnormal lobation 4
				  of both lungs
				Heterotaxis, 1
				  visceral inversion
				Hydrocephaly 1
				Syndactylia 2
				Spina bifida 2
				Agenesis of right 1
				  kidney
				Agenesis of both 2
				  kidneys
				Left heart syndrome 1
				Abnormal lobation 1
				  of left lung
				Meckel's 3
				  diverticulum
				Cecum mobile 1
				Diaphragmatic 4
				  hernia
				Omphaocele 1
				Megalocytosis 1
				Pelvic kidney 1
				Bicornate uterus, 1
				  uterus bicornis
				Anal atresia 4
				Hydronephrosis 2
				Polycystic kidney 1 D
				Acystia 1
				Clubfoot 1
				Agenesis of the 3
				  bilateral internal ear
				Tracheoesophageal 1
				  fistual
				Double ureter 1

Total no. of malformations	30	32	11	91
No. of malformations per individual	30/15 = 2.0	32/11 = 2.9	11/3 = 3.7	91/45 = 2.0

Table 4   Relationship between malformations and distance from the hypocenter among natural births in the F_2 population. ('D' and 'R' respectively indicate dominant and recessive gene abnormalities)

Distance from hypocenter / Person exposed	< 2 km		2 ~4 km		Early entrants		Unknown	
	No. of cases	Malformation	No. of cases	Malformation	No. of cases	Malformation	No. of cases	Malformation
Paternal grandfather	1	Anencephalia 1 Transposition 1 of the great arteries	1	Diaphragmatic 1 hernia	1	Anencephalia 1	1	Hydronephrosis 1
Paternal grandmother	1	Meningocele 1 Polydactylia 1			2	Acardius ancepts, 1 acephacardia Artrial septal 1 defect Patent ductus 1 arteriosus	2	Ancencephalia 1 Manus valga 1
Both paternal grandparents	1	Transposition 1 of the great arteries Polycystic 1 D kidney	1	Anal atresia 1 Agenesis of 1 the left kidney Tetralogy of 1 Fallot Partial visceral 1 inversion			1	Diaphragmatic 1 hernia Hydronephrosis 1
Maternal grandfather	1	Anencephalia 1 Hydroureter 1					4	Otocleisis 1 Hydronephrosis 1 Anencephalia 1
Maternal grandmother			1	Osteogenesis 1 R imperfecta Inguinal hernia 1	1	Horoprosen- 1 cephaly Esophageal 1 atresia Cleft lip 1 Atrial septal 1 defect		Hydroureter 1 Ventricular septal 1 defect Patent ductus 1 arteriosus Clubfoot 1 Spina bifida 1 Hypoplasia of 1 the lungs Meningocele 1
Both maternal grandparents			2	Polycystic 1 D kidney Spina bifida 1 Phocomelia, 1 phocomely Polydactylia 1 Microphthalmia 1				
No. of malformations	4	8	5	12	4	8	9	16
♀/♂	3/1		2/3		2/2		3/6	
No. of malformations per individual		8/4 = 2		12/5 = 2.4		8/4 = 2		1/9 = 1.7

radiation had no genetic effect on humans. The number of the F_1 generation born in 1946–1980 is estimated at approximately 60,000 in Hiroshima and approximately 40,000 in Nagasaki, with the F_2 generation already having been given birth to by this generation. It is therefore necessary to perform long-term studies in order to determine whether or not any visible or inherent mutations are produced in these or subsequent generations.

(*Yukio Satow*)

REFERENCES

1. Muller HJ. Artificial transmission of the gene. *Science* 1927; **66**: 84.
2. Stevenson AC. Some data, estimates and reflections on congenital and hereditary anomalies in the population of Northern Ireland. United Nations document. New York: United Nations, 1985.
3. Russell WL. The effect of radiation dose rate and fractionation on mutation in mice. In: Sobels FH, editor. Repair from genetic radiation damage. New York: Pergamon Press, 1963: 205.
4. United Nations Scientific Committee on the Effects of Atomic Radiation (UNSCEAR). Ionizing Radiation. Levels and effects. New York: United Nations, 1972.
5. Neel JV, Schull EJ. The effect of exposure to the atomic bombs of pregnancy termination in Hiroshima and Nagasaki. National Academy of Science-National Research Council, USA, 1956: 491.
6. Hayashi I, Okamoto N, *et al.* Atomic bomb and morphogenesis *in utero. J Clin Obst Gynec* 1955; **9**: 923. (*In Japanese*).
7. Kaplan I. The treatment of female sterility with X-rays to the ovaries and the pituitary. *Can Med Ass J* 1957; **76**: 43–6.
8. Tanaka K, Ohkura K. Evidence for genetic effects of radiation in offspring of radiological technicians. *Jpn J Hum Genet* 1958; **3**: 135–45.
9. Schull WJ, Neel JV. Radiation and the sex ratio in man. *Science* 1958; **128**: 343–8.
10. Tabuchi A, Nakayama S, *et al.* Summary report on disorders noted among A-bomb exposed women. *Hiroshima J Med Sci* 1966; **15**: 1.
11. Furusho T. On the sex ratio of the descendants of the A-bomb survivors. *J Hiroshima Med Ass* 1982; **35**: 301–306. (*In Japanese*).
12. Satow Y, *et al.* Autopsy findings of the first and second filial generation of atomic bomb survivors. *Proc Hiroshima Univ RINMB* 1992; **33**: 189–96. (*In Japanese*).

19.2 CHROMOSOME STUDIES ON THE OFFSPRING OF ATOMIC BOMB SURVIVORS

INTRODUCTION

Attempts to clarify the genetic damage caused by atomic bomb radiation commenced immediately after the Second World War, and have continued to the present day. These include cytogenetic investigations on the offspring of atomic bomb survivors which were initiated at the Atomic Bomb Casualty Commission (ABCC) in 1967 and used the frequency of chromosomal aberrations as an index. Following an organizational reorganization, these studies were continued by the ABCC's successor, the Radiation Effects Research Foundation (RERF), and completed in 1985.

The scientific objectives of this study were the evaluation of the type and frequency of radiation-induced chromosomal changes in the children of exposed individuals. Details regarding chromosomal abnormalities are presented in Chapter 14, "Chromosomal Aberrations"; this section focuses on radiation-induced chromosome injury (breakage, and various accompanying morphological abnormalities) in the cell nuclei of living bodies, and the relationship between radiation dose and the frequency of induced chromosomal aberrations. In addition to the long-term persistence of certain chromosomal aberrations induced in stem cells, the possibility that clones of abnormal cells may be produced is particularly noteworthy. If this should occur in the germ cells it is clear that the genetic risk will increase. That is, if it is hypothesized that chromosomal aberrations are induced in spermatogonial cells, which form the basis of spermatogenesis, then within the limits of possible fertilization with the sperm carrying radiation-induced chromosomal damage, individuals with chromosomal aberrations will increase in frequency in the next generation. This section reviews and attempts to evaluate the cytogenetic studies.

1. CYTOGENETIC STUDY

A. Subjects

The subjects were the proximally and distally exposed populations established by Neel *et al*[1] from the Mortality Study sample of the offspring of atomic bomb survivors. In the following discussion the proximally exposed population will be referred to simply as the exposed population; and since the distally exposed population was established in order for comparisons with the proximally exposed population, it will be referred to as the control population.

The exposed population consisted of the offspring of atomic bomb survivors for whom either one or both parents had been exposed within 2,000 m of the hypocenter, and who had received an estimated T65D dose of $\geqslant 0.01$ Gy. The control population was comprised of offspring whose parents were both exposed at a distance greater than 2,500 m from the hypocenter (with an estimated T65D dose of $\leqslant 0.005$ Gy), and children whose parents were not in the city at the time of bombing. The populations were sex- and age-matched as much as possible. Most of the subjects were born between May 1st, 1946 and December 31st, 1958; however, the latter half of the study was expanded to include offspring born between 1959 and 1972, although these accounted for only approximately 10% of the total.

Of the initial population approximately 5% died, and 35% moved away from the two cities, thus rendering study impossible. Of the remainder, approximately 75% agreed to participate in the study, thus making 45% of the original population available for study. The subjects themselves or the parents of subjects gave consent prior to commencement of the study. In many cases, the subjects came to RERF, at which time they were given an oral questionnaire concerning their health; blood specimens were then taken. For those who wished, various clinical tests were performed in addition to the main medical examination. When necessary, blood samples for various tests were taken during home visits.

The number of subjects thus amounted to 16,298 (Table 1), of whom 9,828 were in Hiroshima (4,716 exposed, and 5,112 controls) and 6,470 in Nagasaki (3,606 exposed; 2,864 controls). By sex, there were 7,596 males and 8,702 females, i.e. females slightly outnumbered males. This is believed to be related to the rather higher percentage of males leaving the cities.

The average age at the time of examination was 24 years for both the exposed and control populations, with the minimum age set at 12 years (the time of entry into

Table 1 Cytogenetic findings

Chromosome aberrations		Exposed	Controls
Number of examines	Males	3,914	3,682
	Females	4,408	4,294
	Total	8,322	7,976
A. Sex chromosome abnormalities			
Males	XYY	3 (0.77)	5 (1.36)
	XXY	7 (1.79)	9 (2.44)
	Mosaicism	1 (0.26)	—
	Others	1 (0.26)	2 (0.54)
Females	XXX	5 (1.13)	—
	Mosaicism	2 (0.45)	3 (0.70)
	Others	—	1 (0.23)
B. Autosomal structural rearrangements			
Reciprocal translocations (balanced)		7 (0.84)	13 (1.63)
D/D, D/G translocations (balanced)		10 (1.20)	6 (0.75)
Inversions (balanced)		1 (0.12)	6 (0.75)
Others (including unbalanced)		5 (0.60)	2 (0.25)
C. Autosomal trisomy			
21 trisomy		1 (0.12)	—
Total aberrations	43 (5.17)	51 (6.39)	

( ) Figures in parentheses indicate frequency per 1,000 examinees. However, the percentages for sex chromsome abnormalities apply only to the affected sex.

junior high school). If parents so desired, blood samples for various tests were taken from children in the early grades of elementary school. Ages ranged from 12 to 38 years. The number of offspring per couple in the exposed population was 1.4, and 1.2 in the control population. Although this difference is not statistically significant, if considered together with the rather higher cooperation rate evident among the exposed population, it is consistent with the tendency for the atomic bomb survivors and their offspring to display a greater concern about health.

B. Cytogenetic Methods

Blood samples (1–2 ml) from the subjects were collected, treated with heparin, and cultured for 48 hours according to the conventional blood culture method[2]. (For details, please see Chapter 14, "Chromosomal Aberrations").

For each case, chromosomal analysis was conducted directly under the microscope on 10 metaphase cells, and the presence or absence of aberrations ascertained. Three of these cells were photographed and karyotypic analyses performed. When the number of cells observed was less than 10, the results were deemed ineligible. The rate of successful cultures for Hiroshima and Nagasaki combined was 99.9%.

When any chromosomal abnormalities were suspected, the number of cells observed was increased to 100 and analysis performed according to the conventional staining technique. In the case of mosaicism, the number of cells observed was, if necessary, increased up to 200. Besides these routine procedures, G-, Q- and C-banding methods were introduced to accurately identify the types of anomaly, and the aberrant chromosome (and chromosomal region) concerned. The method of determination and description of the abnormalities were performed according to the International System for Human Cytogenetic Nomenclature (ISCN)[3].

When an individual with a chromosomal aberration was identified, a detailed family study was performed to determine the origin of the abnormality and whether it was inherited. When an identical aberration was found in either of the parents, it was deemed an inherited trait; when the abnormality (structural chromosomal abnormalities in particular) was found to be absent in both parents, the abnormality was judged a chromosomal mutant.

Anomalies are usually classified into two categories, i.e. numerical abnormalities (aneuploidy and trisomy) and structural abnormalities. In this discussion, however, they are divided into three categories: sex chromosome abnormalities, autosomal (structural) abnormalities, and autosomal trisomy.

2. RESULTS OF CYTOGENETIC TESTS: TYPE AND FREQUENCY OF CHROMOSOMAL ABNORMALITIES

It has been experimentally confirmed that radiation can induce numerical abnormalities (both aneuploidy and polyploidy) as well as structural rearrangements in human chromosomes. Prior to a discussion of the effects of radiation, an outline of the types and frequencies of chromosomal aberrations occurring in the general human population will be presented, along with a review of current knowledge concerning the rate of spontaneous formation of chromosomal abnormalities in the prenatal population. Comparison of the results with those for the offspring of atomic bomb survivors thus permits an objective assessment of the genetic effects of radiation.

A. Chromosomal Abnormalities in the Neonatal Population

Since the latter half of the 1960s attempts have been made worldwide (especially in Western Europe) to estimate the genetic risk in the general human population using the frequency of individuals displaying chromosomal abnormalities. Analysis of the genetic risk of chromosomal aberrations requires the monitoring of all pregnancies across an entire specific region, the registration of data pertaining to spontaneous abortions, stillbirths and live births, and the procurement of blood specimens from all live neonates. In particular, blood is obtained from the umbilical cord at the time of parturition, and from the frequency of chromosomal aberrations in each study cohort it is possible to estimate the genetic load.

The results of chromosomal studies on neonates in various parts of the world have been described in detail in a United Nations Scientific Committee report[5]. In addition, a further report by Kuroki[6] covers data concerning the Japanese. Estimates of the genetic risk due to chromosomal abnormalities are discussed below.

Out of 10,000 recognized pregnancies it is estimated that 1,450 undergo spontaneous abortion and another 100 are stillborn, resulting in 8,450 live births. Chromosomal studies to date suggest that chromosomal abnormalities cause 50% of spontaneous abortions and 5.7% of stillbirths, i.e. 725 of the 1,450 spontaneous abortions and 6 of the 100 stillbirths are the characterized by chromosomal anomalies. Consequently, individuals with chromosomal aberrations are lost due to spontaneous abortions and stillbirths in 731 out of 10,000 pregnancies (7.31%). On the other hand, neonatal studies show that chromosomal aberrations are present in 0.63% of newborns, and it is thus estimated that chromosomal aberrations exist in 53 of the 8,450 live births. Summarizing the above results, it is estimated that out of a total of 10,000 pregnancies, chromosomal aberrations are present in 784, but only 7% (53/784) of these are present in neonates. That is, 93% of chromosomal aberrations are eliminated during the prenatal period.

As is evident from the above results, 0.63% of neonates possess chromosomal anomalies which, depending on the type of aberration, affect the postnatal mortality rate. In many cases of sex chromosome aneuploidy (e.g. Klinefelter's syndrome, 47, XXY) the neonates can survive, and even with structural chromosomal rearrangements, abnormalities of balanced type (i.e. when there is neither loss nor gain of chromosomal material, and therefore no loss or gain of genes) would lead to no manifestation of phenotypic changes, and thus no change in viability.

Since autosomal numerical abnormalities (mostly trisomy) accompany phenotypic abnormalities, their viability is noticeably inferior. One exceptional chromosomal anomaly is 21 trisomy, known as Down's syndrome, which occurs at a frequency of 0.95 per 1,000 births. Since this congenital abnormality, which manifests mild mental retardation and characteristic facial features, is susceptible to infectious diseases etc., the viability used to be conspicuously low, but due to recent advances in medical treatment the mortality rate has markedly declined. The incidence of this disease shows a strong correlation with an increase in maternal age. Although extremely infrequent, some newborns exhibit other autosomal trisomies (such as 13 trisomy or 18 trisomy). Since all of these are accompanied by serious malformations, the mortality rates are high.

To summarize the results of neonatal studies, chromosomal anomalies are the primary cause of genetic damage, with half of all spontaneous abortions attributed to chromosomal aberrations (and numerical abnormalities in chromosomes in particular). As pregnancy progresses, the genetic risk due to chromosomal aberrations gradually decreases.

As previously mentioned, 0.63% of neonates possess chromosomal aberrations. Two-thirds of these are chromosome aneuploidy, and arise from either an excess of a sex chromosome, such as XXY, XYY and XXX, or from autosomal trisomies such as Down's syndrome. In each case spontaneous chromosomal mutations are caused in the germ cells of one of the parents. In the case of sex chromosome abnormality, due to inactivation of one of the two X chromosomes there may be no effects upon viability, although various congenital abnormalities are observed. Due to poor differentiation of the germ cells, in many cases no viable offspring could be produced. As an exception, XXX females are known to be normal, and since their reproductive function is also normal they produce descendants (most being normal descendants). Similarly, XYY males are believed able to survive and leave descendants. Also, in cases of mosaicism (e.g. 46, XX/47, XXX, etc.) produced from various combinations of sex chromosomes, the viability varies depending on the distribution of cells with normal genotypes.

Due to its hazardous genetic make-up, autosomal trisomy has a low viability, and no offspring can be produced. An exception is the case of 21 trisomy (Down's syndrome), since with the extension of life span that leads to sexual maturity of the proband, there is a possibility of producing offspring. This now poses a serious problem.

If autosomal structural rearrangements are of balanced type, the phenotype is normal; however, in the case of an unbalanced type (such as the deletion or duplication of chromosomes or chromosomal regions) the manifestation of a harmful character results in a high mortality rate that would cause reduced viability and reproductive ability. Over 80% of structural rearrangements are transmitted to the offspring from either carrier parent. Family studies have clarified that in the natural population around 20% of new abnormalities with structural rearrangements arise from spontaneous germ-line mutations.

B. Chromosomal Abnormalities in the Offspring of Atomic Bomb Survivors

As previously mentioned, chromosomal abnormalities identified in the children of atomic bomb survivors are classified into the following three categories: sex chromosome anomalies (including aneuploidy, mosaicism, inverted Y chromosomes and structural rearrangements of X chromosomes), autosomal structural rearrangements (reciprocal translocation, Robertsonian translocation, inversion, supernumerary marker chromosomes, etc.) and autosomal trisomies (Table 1).

1. Sex Chromosome Abnormalities

The chromosomal abnormalities in this category are mainly XYY and XXY (Klinefelter's syndrome) in males, and XXX in females, including mosaicism with normal cells (46, XX, or 46, XY). Except for mosaicism, Turner's syndrome (45, X) was not detected in this study. In these numerical alterations the genotypic effect is small because of genetic inactivation of the X chromosomes. Due to infertility, the abnormality in the proband is not inherited in the following generation. Aneuploidy is classified as spontaneous mutation produced from the nondisjunction of chromosomes at meiotic division. On the other hand, mosaicism does not belong to the same category since it is believed to be caused by nondisjunction occurring at post-zygotic cell divisions. Nondisjunction is sometimes related to the age of the parent, but in this study the age of the parents at the time of birth was of the same order in both the exposed and control populations, and thus parental age is not believed to exert an effect.

Inversion of the Y chromosome (a structural abnormality of the sex chromosomes) was confirmed in 2 cases, but in both of these cases the father was the carrier of the abnormality, and it was judged to be inherited. Observed abnormalities included a case of mosaicism in a female exhibiting one ring X chromosome, a case with deletion of a long X arm, and an XX male.

The frequency of sex chromosome abnormalities in the exposed population was 0.23%, while in the control population it was rather high at 0.30%. Neonatal studies yielded a figure of 0.22–0.24%, the same as in the exposed population. A detailed investigation of individual abnormalities showed a biased distribution in abnormality by type and sex, but this is due to the limited size of the study population. No significant difference was found between the two populations with respect to the frequency of sex chromosome abnormalities.

2. Autosomal Structural Rearrangements

Structural rearrangements are those abnormalities in which a chromosome has a different configuration from the original due to breakage and recombination. The structural rearrangement whereby breakages also occur in different chromosomes followed by the exchange of two segments between the two chromosomes is termed translocation (or reciprocal translocation). If the same phenomenon occurs within the same chromosome, the structural rearrangement is known as inversion. The centromeres of two acrocentric chromosomes may fuse and form a new aberrant chromosome. Since in the case of humans the abnormality is produced between D group and G group chromosomes it is called either a D/D type or a D/G type (or G/G type) translocation, and is also known as a Robertsonian translocation. When chromosome 21 in the G group is involved, this often leads to translocation-type

Down's syndrome (trisomy 21 due to translocation). In many cases, one of the parents is a carrier of the abnormality.

Structural rearrangements are the most reliable indicator for evaluation of genetic risk because they can in theory be induced by ionizing radiation (with the rate of induction proportional to the dose received) and since family study shows whether the observed rearrangement is due to germ-line mutation of the exposed parent or whether it is inherited from the carrier parent. Furthermore, neonatal studies estimate that balanced translocation and structural rearrangements occur in approximately 2 out of 1,000 live births. Also, since new mutations occur in 20% of these, the rate becomes 1 in 2,500. As can be seen from Table 1, the majority of structural rearrangements are balanced translocations and inversions. The family study revealed 1 case of new mutation in each of the exposed and control populations. Due either to a refusal to cooperate or to absence of family members, the family study did not cover all abnormal cases. However, due to recognition of the same abnormality in siblings, one of the parents was in some cases presumed to be the carrier of the anomaly. The results showed no difference between the two populations with respect to the frequency of spontaneous mutations involving balanced structural rearrangements.

A minute marker chromosome was present in the majority of other structural rearrangements (including unbalanced types); no abnormalities were observed in either phenotype or infertility. The origin of these excess chromosomes is unknown, but may be caused by deletion of a short arm of the D or G group chromosome, including the satellite. Cases of deletion of a short arm of chromosome 18 and an iso-chromosome formed by two long arms of chromosome 18 were identified among children with exposed fathers. There was, however, no evidence of a causative relationship between these structural rearrangements and paternal exposure. From the fact that they were in the form of mosaicism, it is likely that chromosomal rearrangement and subsequent nondisjunction occur following zygote formation.

The study failed to detect any case of unbalanced-type translocation. As previously mentioned, the study commenced 22 years after the bombing, and it is presumed that children possessing unbalanced rearrangements must have been born before the start of the study. Although there seem to be considerable differences in individual viability related to the severity of unbalanced rearrangements, their viability should be extremely low; for example, even if the anomaly had been present, there is a strong likelihood that death would have occurred before the time of the study.

3. Autosomal Trisomy

This category is represented by 21 trisomy Down's syndrome. Although only 1 case was observed among the exposed population in this study, the expected rate in the population studied was 1 case per 1,000 births[7]. Uchida and Curtis[8] indicated the possibility of an increase in Down's syndrome due to diagnostic X-ray irradiation of the mother. However, this was disputed by Schull and Neel[7] on the basis of epidemiological observations on the atomic bomb survivors. Down's syndrome can be diagnosed with certainty even without making use of the chromosome study. However, when monitoring Down's syndrome patients, the study needs to take into consideration all information relating to a range of genetic and socioeconomic factors, and maternal age in particular.

CONCLUSION

Although an attempt was made to assess the genetic effects of atomic bomb radiation through the cytogenetic analysis of the offspring of atomic bomb survivors, the results failed to provide any evidence of increased genetic damage. However, this does not preclude the possibility that radiation exposure causes an increased genetic risk, since it is necessary to consider various confounding factors, e.g. 1) the possibility that various mechanisms may lead to genetic damage being eliminated; 2) the possibility that the study population was too small to adequately evaluate the risk; and 3) the fact that the chromosomal analysis method itself was of limited sensitivity with regard to the identification of radiation-induced abnormalities. Therefore, the conclusion currently reached is that exposure to atomic bomb radiation may have produced an increased level of genetic damage, but as yet this can not be quantitatively proven.

By combining the results of the untoward pregnancy outcome study, the mortality study (including cancer mortality), the chromosome study (aneuploid anomalies in particular), and the protein variant study, Neel et al[9] attempted to estimate the genetic doubling dose of atomic bomb radiation. A calculation taking the relative biological effectiveness (RBE) of neutrons to be 20 yielded a doubling dose value of 1.7–2.2 sieverts, but experimental observations showed that this is greater than the doubling dose in mice, thus indicating that the radiosensitivity of humans might be less than that of mice.

Attempts to assess the genetic risk of radiation have been described in reports such as those published by a United Nations Scientific Committee[5] and by BEIR-V[10], with predictions that the increased risk of chromosomal aberrations is not necessarily large. The genetic effect of radiation on humans is currently inadequately understood, and it is hoped that as the human genome project develops it will be possible to evaluate the rate of spontaneous mutations at the DNA level.

(Akio Awa)

REFERENCES

1. Neel JV, Kato H, Schull WJ. Mortality in children of atomic bomb survivors and controls. *Genetics* 1974; **76**: 433–53.
2. Awa AA, Sofuni T, Honda T, *et al.* Relationship between the radiation dose and chromosome aberrations in atomic bomb survivors of Hiroshima and Nagasaki. *J Radiat Res* 1978; **19**: 126–40.
3. ISCN (1985): An International System for Human Cytogenetic Nomenclature. Harnden DG and Klinger HP, Editors Published in collaboration with Cytogenet Cell Genet (Karger, Basel 1985); also in Birth Defects: Original Article Series, Vol. 21, No. 1 (March of Dimes Birth Defects Foundation, New York 1985).
4. Awa AA, Honda T, Neriishi S, *et al.* Cytogenetic study of the offspring of atomic bomb survivors, Hiroshima and Nagasaki. RERF TR 21–88, 1988.

5. United Nations Scientific Committee on the Effects of Atomic Radiation. Ionizing radiation: sources and biological effects. Report to the General Assembly, Thirty-seventh Session. New York: United Nations, 1982; Suppl No. 40 (A/37/45).

6. Kuroki Y. Genetic load of chromosome abnormalities — prevalence, selection and estimates of detriment. In: Ishihara T, Tobari I, editors. The new developments in chromosome studies — with special reference to human chromosomes. *Proceedings of the 18th National Institute of Radiological Sciences (NIRS) Symposium*; 1986 Dec. 10–11; Chiba, Japan. Chiba: National Institute of Radiological Sciences, 1987: 31–40. (*In Japanese*)

7. Schull WJ, Neel JV. Maternal radiation and mongolism. *Lancet* 1962; **1**: 537–8.

8. Uchida IA, Curtis EJ. A possible association between maternal radiation and mongolism. *Lancet* 1961; **2**: 848–50.

9. Neel JV, Schull WJ, Awa AA, *et al.* The children of parents exposed to atomic bombs: estimates of the genetic doubling dose of radiation for humans. *Am J Hum Genet* 1990; **46**: 1053–72.

10. Committee on the Biological Effects of Ionizing Radiation. Commission on Life Science. Health effects of exposure to low levels of ionizing radiation (BEIR-V). National Academy of Sciences-National Research Council. Washington, DC: National Academy Press, 1990.

19.3 CANCER INCIDENCE AND MORTALITY RATES AMONG THE OFFSPRING OF ATOMIC BOMB SURVIVORS

INTRODUCTION

Radiation has been used in genetic research to create mutations in experimental animals since radiogenic damage to the genetic materials of germ cells is inherited by the following generation. It is therefore important to comprehend the degree to which radiation affects the health of humans genetically.

Genetic studies require consideration of the effects on several generations, and thus epidemiological studies are of little practical significance in this field. For example, even if it is considered that the genetic effects persist until the 5th generation and that humans have a reproductive period of 30 years, the total time period involved amounts to 150 years. It is not possible to imagine what changes may occur in our future living environment, but at least there is little genetic effect on humans at the dose levels usually employed. This degree of genetic effect will probably be obscured by the health effects accompanying the long-term changes in the living environment occurring over 150 years.

This section summarizes the results of studies on cancer incidence and mortality rates in the offspring of atomic bomb survivors, taking into consideration the direct effects observable in the first generation.

1. THE OFFSPRING OF ATOMIC BOMB SURVIVORS

The Radiation Effects Research Foundation (RERF) has continued to perform follow-up mortality studies on children who were conceived after the dropping of the atomic bombs (thus born after April 1946) and for whom at least one parent was a survivor of either the Hiroshima or Nagasaki atomic bombs; the number of subjects studied (including controls) was approximately 72,000 (Table 1). The mortality study sample initially consisted of approximately 50,000 subjects born between May 1946 and December 1958, but later this was expanded to include children born during the period 1959–84[1]. The sampling procedure employed for determining the cohort will not be discussed in detail here. The 0 sievert (Sv) population, for whom the conjoint parental atomic bomb radiation dose to the gonads (ovaries and testes) can be ignored, consisted of 41,069 subjects; the number in the population exposed to a significant dose of ⩾ 0.01 Sv was 31,159, with a mean gonadal dose of 0.435 Sv.

The death of the subjects was confirmed by means of family registers, and causes of death ascertained from death certificates[1]; for subjects holding Japanese citizenship the confirmation rate was 99%, but since the first program for ascertaining causes of death was conducted retrospectively in the 1960s, the causes of death could not be determined for approximately 380 individuals who had been born during the period 1946–58 (including approximately 250 subjects in the 0 Sv population). However, the number who died of unknown causes (approximately 90% of whom died before reaching the age of one) is unrelated to the parental radiation dose.

Table 1   Offspring of atomic bomb survivors

Total subjects		72,228
Year of birth	May 1946–1958	50,529
	Jan. 1959–1984	21,699
City	Hiroshima	44,852
	Nagasaki	27,376
Sex	Males	37,044
	Females	35,184
Gonadal dose	0 Sv	41,069 [377]
	≥ 0.01 Sv	31,159 [4,265]
		(0.435 Sv)

[ ]: No. of individuals for whom tentative doses were used.
( ): Average dose of ≥ 0.01 Sv

The medical records of cancer cases were reinvestigated using the causes of death listed in the death certificates and the tumor registries supervised by the medical associations in Hiroshima and Nagasaki[2]. In the case of fatal cancer it was possible to confirm data both for the whole period and also for the whole of Japan. For non-fatal cancer, data was restricted to cases manifested after establishment of the tumor registries in 1958, and moreover was limited to cases within the tumor registry areas. However, it is believed that the frequency of tumors which were overlooked (due to migration) did not correlate with parental radiation doses. In particular, many cancers in subjects aged under 20 proved fatal, and since only a small percentage moved away from the areas covered by the tumor registries, the number for whom documents are missing is probably small.

2. GENETIC EFFECTS OF ATOMIC BOMB RADIATION

Rather than beginning with somatic cell damage, systematic studies on the health effects of atomic bomb radiation commenced with investigations on germ cell damage (starting in the initial post-bombing period i.e. the second half of the 1940s). Studies have since been performed using various genetic indices[3], but no positive evidence of radiation-induced genetic effects has been forthcoming. However, the usually accepted hypothesis is that if such effects did occur, then there should at least be an increase in the diseases already identified as hereditary.

The recent 1990 BEIR-V[4] report describes risk calculations pertaining to the radiation-induced genetic effects in liveborn human infants. Based on this, let us consider a hypothetical population consisting of 100,000 first generation children whose parents are exposed to a dose of 0.4 Sv. Table 2 shows rough estimates of the numbers of both spontaneous and radiation-induced genetic disorders among this hypothetical population. The spontaneously induced genetic disorders refer to those

Table 2   Estimated genetic effects (number of cases) per 100,000 population in offspring born to parents exposed to a 0.4 Sv mean gonadal dose

Genetic disorder	Spontaneous	Radiation-induced
Autosomal dominant	1,000	24~140
X-linked	40	< 4
Recessive	250	< 4
Chromosomal		
Unbalanced translocations	60	< 20
Trisomies	380	< 4
Congenital abnormalities	2,000~3,000	40
Multifactorial inheritance*		
Heart disease	60,000	Not estimated
Cancer	30,000	Not estimated
Others	30,000	Not estimated

Estimated values quoted from BEIR V (1990) without consideration of differences between the effects of acute and chronic irradiation.
* Number of lifetime cases exceeds 100,000.

cases of unknown cause which are unrelated to radiation. Chronic exposure to radiation is also assumed here, while the risk coefficient for the acute atomic bomb irradiation is taken to be 2 to 3 times that value.

The cancer cases in Table 2 were classified according to multifactorial inheritance traits, but quantitative risk estimates were not performed due to uncertainties regarding the mode of inheritance. The maximum number of radiation-induced genetic diseases in this hypothetical population of 100,000 was less than 250. This rough estimate can be applied directly to the ≥ 0.01 Sv population in Table 1, since the number of births in the hypothetical population is approximately 3 times that in the ≥ 0.01 Sv population and offsets differences in risk coefficient due to chronic and acute irradiation.

Untoward pregnancy outcomes (stillbirths, congenital malformations, and neonatal deaths) have been considered an index of pre-birth genetic effects. In passing, a large systematic study which commenced in 1948 reported in 1956 on approximately 77,000 untoward pregnancy outcomes in atomic bomb survivors after the 140th day of pregnancy. Data have since been reanalyzed but no statistically significant increase in the frequency of untoward pregnancy outcomes has been observed with an increase in parental gonadal dose[5].

3. CANCER INCIDENCE STUDY

An increase in childhood leukemia has often been suggested for children for whom one parent had received medical X-ray irradiation[6]. At Sellafield in the United Kingdom an increased incidence of childhood leukemia and non-Hodgkin's lymphoma has been reported in children whose fathers worked at a nuclear fuel reprocessing facility[7]. Compared with these cases, however, the offspring of atomic bomb survivors exposed to a high single dose of acute radiation have not yet demonstrated a significant increase in leukemia risk with greater parental dose[6]. Leukemia is typical of radiogenic damage in somatic cells, but it is difficult to conceive that the damage caused to germ cells by radiation (the genetic effect) is manifested only as an increased incidence of leukemia.

Many cancers appearing in adults develop as a result of damage to somatic cells induced by radiation, chemical carcinogens, and viruses etc. However, certain childhood tumors (which frequently appear before age 15), such as retinoblastoma, Wilms' tumor, and neuroblastoma etc., are known to be occasionally transmitted by genetic means, and are regarded as suitable indices of radiation-induced damage in germ cells.

Based on this, a study was performed for the period 1946–82 on the cancer risk at all sites for subjects aged under 20[2]. As shown in Table 3, among the approximately 72,000 subjects there were 92 confirmed cancer cases, but no statistically significant increase in cancer risk was associated with parental gonadal dose. The cancers which epidemiological studies have thus far strongly indicated as being "heritable" (cancers regarded as having a genetic mode of transmission) accounted for approximately 20% (19 cases) of the cancers appearing before the age of 20. Also, since many of the "heritable" cancer cases resulted from pre- or post-natal damage to somatic cells, it was concluded that the number of cancers due to parental germ cell damage accounted for no more than 10–20%. In the case of other tumors with a lower genetic transmissibility (many of which were brain tumors) the figure was below 5%. In conclusion, since the cancer risk demonstrated no significant increase due to parental exposure, it is estimated that 3–5% of all cancer cases occurring under age 20 were due to spontaneous germ cell damage in the parents.

Table 3   Number of cancer cases among liveborn offspring of atomic bomb survivors (age < 20, 1946–82)

No. of children	Gonadal dose (Sv)		
	0	≥ 0.01	Total
	41,066	31,150	72,216
All cancers	49	43	92 (100%)
"Heritable" cancers	10	9	19 (21%)
Retinoblastoma	4	1	5
Wilms' tumor	1	4	5
Neuroblastoma	3	1	4
Osteosarcoma	1	1	2
Embryomal carcinoma, testis	1	1	2
Sarcoma, kidney	0	1	1
Leukemia	17	16	33 (36%)
Other cancers	22	18	40 (43%)

Including 15 brain tumors

4. MORTALITY STUDY

As previously mentioned, the untoward pregnancy outcome study covering the period from the 140th day of pregnancy to immediately after birth was extended to the postnatal mortality study. The primary objective of this study was to assess the hypothesis that one of the radiation-caused genetic effects is a life span reduction due to "dominant" deleterious mutations.

First, the offspring of atomic bomb survivors born in the period 1959–84 were added to the cohort, and for the approximately 72,000 subjects in Table 1 the results of the mortality follow-up study were summarized in 1990[1]. The analysis focused on the approximately 68,000 persons for whom it was possible to estimate the DS86 dose. The results are shown in Table 4.

Prior to discussing Table 4, let us consider the mortality rate by year of birth, which is an index of changes in the human living environment that constitutes an impossible-to-overlook confounding factor in the evaluation of the genetic effect on humans. Figure 1 shows the mortality rates from all causes for males throughout Japan up to 1985 according to birth cohort and age. For the first group of children born in 1946 the mortality rate reached a maximum at under 1 year of age, and decreased to a minimum at ages 10–14. The mortality rate rose slightly at ages 15–19, but remained virtually the same until the early 30s. At the cut-off time for

Table 4   Mortality rate among offspring of atomic bomb survivors, 1946–85

	Gonadal dose (Sv)						
	0	0.01–0.09	0.10–0.49	0.50–0.99	1.00–2.49	≥ 2.50	Total
No. of subjects	40,692	10,648	9,863	3,494	2,295	594	67,586
Non-malignant diseases							
No. of deaths	1,852	349	335	120	81	29	2,766
Mortality rate[a]	147.6	145.8	146.3	135.0	134.4	211.1	146.7
Fatal cancer							
No. of deaths	75 (27)[b]	17 (7)	14 (5)	5 (4)	4 (1)	0 (0)	115 (44)
Mortality rate	6.0	6.9	6.3	5.6	6.7	0.0	6.1

Analysis using Poisson regression model

		No. of deaths	Excess relative risk per Sv	Statistical significance
Non-malignant diseases	All diseases	2,766	0.03	None
	Respiratory disease (9th ICD 460–519)	515	0.15	None
	Digestive tract diseases (9th ICD 520–579)	359	0.15	None
Fatal cancers	All cancers	115	< 0.27[c]	None
	Leukemia	44	< 0.93[c]	None

a: Adjusted rate per 100,000 person-years
b: Parentheses indicate number of leukemia cases
c: 95% upper bounds
9th ICD = 9th International Classification of Diseases

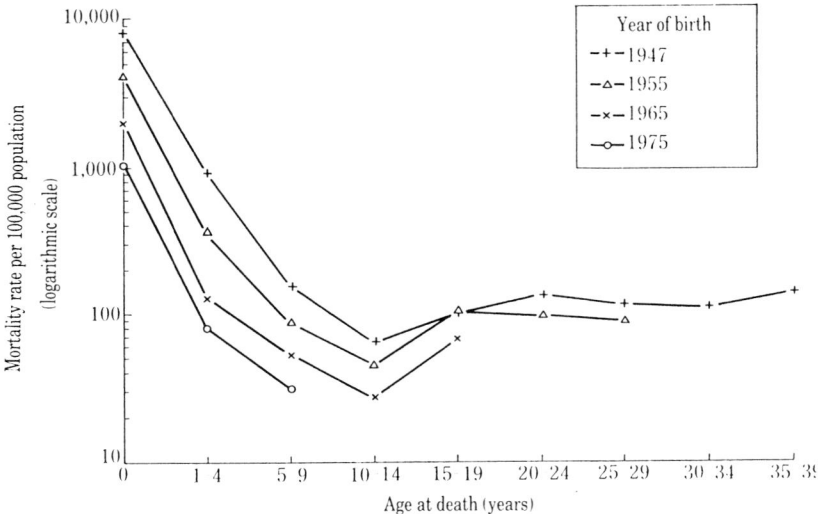

Figure 1   Motality rates for all causes of death by year of birth, 1946–85 (All Japan, males)

observation (1985), when subjects were aged 39, the mortality rate had again started to increase.

In particular, the mortality rate among male infants in 1947 (subjects aged < 1) was 8.1%, but due to improvements in the standard of medical care it had decreased by 1955, 1965, and 1975 to 4.2%, 2.2% and 1.1% respectively. Females displayed a similar age-related mortality pattern, although the levels were in general less than those observed in males. The figures in Table 4 have been adjusted to allow for this difference in mortality rate due to year of birth.

Let us now return to Table 4. Out of the above population of approximately 68,000, the total number of deaths was 3,852. Of these, 2,909 died from disease, 584 from extrinsic causes (i.e. causes unrelated to disease), and 359 from unknown causes. Of the disease-related deaths, non-neoplastic diseases accounted for 2,766 deaths and malignant neoplasms for 115. Excepting the 28 deaths from neoplasms of unspecified nature, approximately 70% were reported to have had brain tumors, with confirmed cases included in the afore-mentioned cancer incidence study. No significant increases with parental gonadal dose were observed in the mortality rates for either non-neoplastic disease or fatal cancer. However, the non-neoplastic disease mortality rate in the ≥ 2.5 Sv population was found to be approximately 1.4 times that in the 0 Sv population, which deserves some consideration.

This is believed to be due not to a radiation-induced genetic effect but to socioeconomic impoverishment of the parents as a result of the atomic bombing or else to socioeconomic characteristics of the proximally exposed population which had existed since before the bombing. Although it had been predicted that the mortality rate might increase with parental dose, until the previous study no increase in mortality rate had been observed. In the present study[1], an apparent increase in mortality rate was observed in the ≥ 2.5 Sv population due to the inclusion of subjects born between 1959 and 1984 and the relatively detailed dose categories. The 29 disease deaths in the ≥ 2.5 Sv population were children aged under 10. The apparent increase actually disappeared when birth weight and birth order of the infants was considered in addition to parental dose. Also, the non-neoplastic disease mortality rate among the population exposed to less than 2.5 Sv tended to be lower than in the 0 Sv population.

The lower part of Table 4 shows the excess relative risk (i.e. the relative increase after subtracting one from the relative risk) per 1 Sv of conjoint parental gonadal dose based on the Poisson regression model. The risk is strictly a calculated value based on data that includes the ≥ 2.5 Sv population, and thus does not demonstrate a statistically significant increase with dose. The excess relative risk at 1 Sv of non-neoplastic disease was 0.03 (an increased incidence of 1.03 times at 1 Sv); of these, diseases of the respiratory and digestive tracts showed an apparent increase of 0.15. For fatal cancers, the 95% upper bounds of the excess relative risk are shown, although the estimated risk coefficients were negative. That is, the excess relative risk at 1 Sv is ≤ 0.27 for all fatal cancers and ≤ 0.93 for leukemia.

Of the 3,852 deaths listed in Table 4 for the period 1946–85, 76% occurred before the age of 4. If the children born between 1959 and 1984 are discounted, this mortality data overlaps to a large extent with previous reported findings. A problem exists concerning the accuracy of causes of death listed in death certificates, but it is possible to ascertain fatal cancer data for both the entire period and for the whole of Japan. The present mortality study confirmed the results of the previously mentioned cancer incidence study.

5. GENETIC DOUBLING DOSE

The genetic doubling dose is employed as an index of the strength of the genetic effect of radiation. As shown in Fig. 2, the spontaneously induced germ cell damage load per gamete is assumed to be equal to □ for each of the parents. The genetic doubling dose (DD) is the radiation dose that newly causes damage to the germ cells amounting to ■, equal to □. Therefore as the genetic doubling dose (DD) decreases, the genetic effect of radiation increases.

As shown in Fig. 2, if only the father is assumed to have received a dose equal to 6 times the doubling dose (6DD), then the genetic load for the child is 4 times greater than for a child with an unexposed father. The increases in childhood leukemia and non-Hodgkin's lymphoma observed in children whose fathers worked in the Sellafield nuclear fuel reprocessing facility are in agreement with this. In particular, 4 cases of childhood leukemia were observed in children whose fathers worked in the nuclear reprocessing plant and were exposed to a cumulative pre-conception dose of ≥ 0.1 Sv; this figure is greater than the expected number of spontaneous leukemia cases (less than 1).

It is now hypothesized that all spontaneous childhood leukemia is related to spontaneous germ cell damage. The average paternal cumulative dose at the above facility was 0.2 Sv, and even assuming a low childhood leukemia incidence of 4 times the spontaneous rate, this leads to a doubling dose of $0.2/6 = 0.03$ Sv. This is

Frequency of parental germ cell mutation
(Frequency per gamete □ : Spontaneous ■ : Radiation-induced)

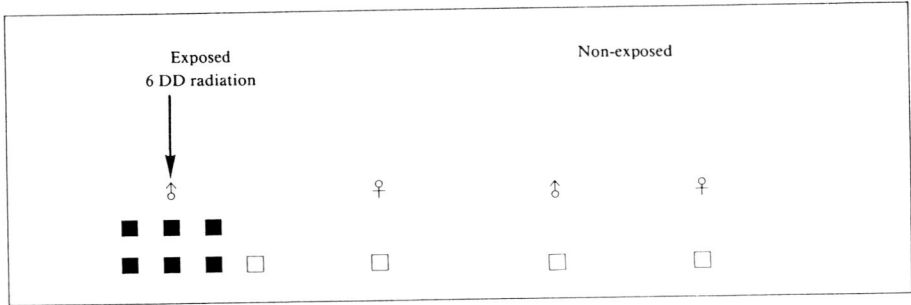

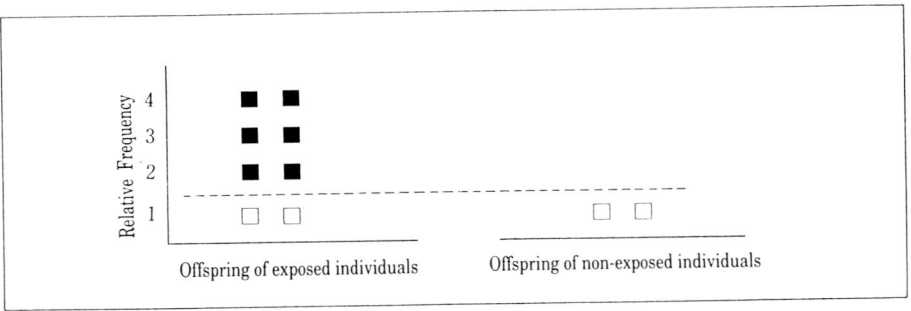

Relative incidence of genetic disorders in offspring (assuming the genetic component to be 100%)

Figure 2 Model for assessment of radiation-induced genetic effect based on the gamete genetic doubling dose (DD) method

an order of magnitude smaller than the doubling doses evident in animal experiments, leaving unresolved the problem of whether a causal relationship exists between parental radiation and childhood leukemia[8,9].

In the case of atomic bomb radiation, adoption of the maximum relative risk for leukemia yields a value of less than 2 times at 1 Sv of conjoint parental gonadal dose (i.e. not the exposure for one parent only). If it is hypothesized that the genetic load per unit dose of atomic bomb radiation is equal for both parents (in practice, the genetic load is not significant enough to necessitate discussion of differences between the parents), this leads to the conclusion that the genetic doubling dose is at least 1 Sv.

Furthermore, it is possible to broadly classify the causes of diseases suffered by humans during their lifetime into: 1) genetic damage transmitted from the parents via the germ cells; 2) embryological damage occurring during the prenatal period; and 3) postnatal somatic cell damage. Therefore, there are doubts about, for example, whether the afore-mentioned hypothesis, which states that all spontaneous childhood leukemias are a result of germ cell damage, can be directly applied to the model in Fig. 2 (the genetic component would be less than 10%). In the calculation of doubling dose, consideration was given to the extent to which germ cell damage contributes to the frequency of spontaneous disease.

For the genetic effect in the children of atomic bomb survivors, Neel and Schull *et al*[10] used various genetic endpoints and assumed the component due to germ cell damage at each endpoint, and subsequently estimated the genetic doubling dose for humans at 1.7–2.2 Sv. The figure is double this value for chronic irradiation. The doubling dose based on the observed genetic effect of exposure on one parent only is termed the gametic doubling dose, whereas that based on the data for the atomic bomb survivors is sometimes referred to as the zygotic doubling dose. The discussion concerning Table 2 is based on the assumption that the genetic doubling dose of chronic irradiation of humans is 1.0 Sv.

CONCLUSION

Fortunately, no positive evidence has been forthcoming regarding a genetic effect of atomic bomb radiation on the health of the children of atomic bomb survivors. However, it is difficult to prove that a genetic effect does not occur, and it is necessary to continue follow-up studies on the offspring of atomic bomb survivors.

(Yasuhiko Yoshimoto)

REFERENCES

1. Yoshimoto Y, Schull WJ, Kato H, *et al.* Mortality among the offspring (F₁) of atomic bomb survivors, 1946–85. *J Radiat Res* 1991; **32**: 327–51. (RERF TR 1–91, 1991).
2. Yoshimoto Y, Neel JV, Schull WJ, *et al.* The frequency of malignant tumors during the first two decades of life in the offspring of atomic bomb survivors. *Am J Hum Genet* 1990; **46**: 1041–52. (RERF TR 4–90, 1990).
3. Neel JV, Schull WJ. The effect of exposure to the atomic bombs on pregnancy termination in Hiroshima and Nagasaki. Washington, DC: National Academy of Sciences-National Research Council, Pub. No. 461, 1956.
4. National Academy of Sciences-National Research Council. Health effects of exposure to low levels of ionizing radiation. BEIR V. Washington. DC: National Academy Press, 1990: 70.
5. Otake M, Schull WJ, Neel JV. Congenital malformations, stillbirths and early mortality among the children of atomic bomb survivors: a reanalysis. *Radiat Res* 1990; **122**: 1–11.
6. Ishimaru T, Ichimaru M, Mikami M. Leukemia incidence among individuals exposed *in utero*, children of atomic bomb survivors, and their controls, Hiroshima and Nagasaki, 1945–79. RERF TR 11–81, 1981.
7. Gardner MJ, Snee MP, Hall AJ, *et al.* Results of case-control study of leukaemia and lymphoma among young people near Sellafield nuclear plant in West Cumbria. *Br Med J* 1990; **300**: 423–9.
8. Abrahamson S. Childhood leukemia at Sellafield. A genetically transmitted mutational disease? *Radiat Res* 1990; **123**: 237–8.
9. Nomura T. Of mice and men? *Nature* 1990; **345**: 671.
10. Neel JV, Schull WJ, Awa AA, *et al.* The children of parents exposed to atomic bombs: estimates of the genetic doubling dose of radiation for humans. *Am J Hum Genet* 1990; **46**: 1053–72.

19.4 BIOCHEMICAL STUDIES ON THE OFFSPRING OF ATOMIC BOMB SURVIVORS

INTRODUCTION

In order to comprehend the genetic effects of atomic bomb radiation, the Atomic Bomb Casualty Commission (the predecessor of the Radiation Effects Research Foundation, RERF) first performed epidemiological[1,2] and chromosomal studies[3], and then conducted biochemical genetics studies on the children of atomic bomb survivors. The objective of these studies was to clarify whether or not the gene mutation rate in germ cells was increased by exposure to radiation. If a mutation occurs at a gene locus in a germ cell of either the mother or the father, then a child born as a result of fertilization of that germ cell will, in all somatic cells, be heterozygous for normal and mutant alleles at that gene locus. If techniques capable of detecting these heterozygous mutant alleles were employed, the objective would be realized by testing the children of the atomic bomb survivors (the F_1 generation), negating the need for testing the F_2 generation (the grandchildren of atomic bomb survivors).

In protein level studies completed by 1985[4–6], mutant proteins in blood were employed as markers to identify mutations. The children were screened for variant proteins using starch gel electrophoresis and enzyme activity measurement, and investigations performed in order to determine whether or not the variant proteins resulted from mutations in the parental germ cells. The genetic effects of atomic bomb radiation can be estimated by comparing mutation rates between the exposed and control populations. At present, various techniques are available for the direct detection of mutations in DNA and RNA, and feasibility studies are being conducted to determine which would be the most effective for screening purposes. This section describes the protein level studies and also considers future studies at the molecular level (the DNA and RNA levels).

1. INDICATORS FOR MUTATION

Two types of indicators have been used for the detection of mutations in studies at the protein level. The first is a group of blood protein variants with altered electrophoretic mobilities from those of the normal types, and are "rare variants" with phenotype frequencies in the population of less than 1% (and allele frequencies of < 0.005). These variants indicate the existence of base substitutions, and of small base deletions and insertions in exons. The second indicators are erythrocytic enzyme deficiency variants with activities of less than 66% of normal. Individual differences were observed in human erythrocytic enzyme activity due to genetic heterogeneity and health condition (many enzymes displaying different activities in young and mature erythrocytes). However, for enzymes with a coefficient of variation (CV, the standard deviation expressed as a percentage of the mean value) of the enzyme activity of less than 11%, logically it is possible to detect heterozygotes with normal enzymes and mutant enzymes with no activity[7]. In this case, heterozygotes have a mean activity of less than 66%. This indicator reflects the partial or total deletion of genes. Furthermore, as is well known from the example of thalassemia genes, it also reflects point mutations that result in abnormal transcription and production of no enzymes with normal functions.

2. SUBJECTS AND PARENTAL EXPOSURE

First, two populations of children were selected from the subjects of the Life Span Study on the offspring of atomic bomb survivors living in Hiroshima or Nagasaki[8-10]. The first consisted of 16,702 children for whom either one or both parents were exposed within 2,000 meters of the hypocenters and who were born between June 1st 1946 and April 1st 1971. The second cohort consisted of 13,993 children born in the same period for whom either one or both parents were exposed in Hiroshima or Nagasaki at a distance greater than 2,500 m and who matched the first (proximally exposed) population in sex and age. Cooperation was forthcoming and tests conducted on 13,052 (78%) and 10,609 (76%) subjects in the two respective populations. These children are presently reclassified into two categories based on the DS86 doses[11]: an exposed population consisting of 11,364 children whose parents received a conjoint gonadal dose of $\geqslant 0.01$ sieverts (Sv), and a control population consisting of 12,297 children with a conjoint parental gonadal dose of < 0.01 Sv (Table 1). The maternal ovarian doses and the paternal testicular doses were calculated for the children in the study. In the case of parents for whom DS86 doses were not available, the DS86 gonadal dose equivalent was computed in sieverts according to the method of Otake et al[2], taking the relative biological effectiveness (RBE) of neutrons to be 20. The mean conjoint gonadal dose equivalent for parents of children in the exposed population was 0.491 Sv[12].

3. DETECTION OF MUTATIONS

Using acid citrate-dextrose (ACD) as an anticoagulant, 7 ml of blood was obtained from the subjects, separated into the plasma and erythrocyte layers by centrifugation, and preserved in liquid nitrogen. Using these materials, starch gel electrophoresis was performed to test for 30 different blood proteins, and rare variants were detected[13-16].

After leukocytes and platelets were removed by a cellulose column following the method of Beutler[17], a part of the erythrocyte layer was preserved in liquid nitrogen; this was then used for determination of enzyme activity. The activities of 9 enzymes in hemolysate were determined according to the method of Beutler et al[18], with detection of enzyme deficiency variants with less than 66% of average activities[7].

When rare variants or enzyme deficiency variants were observed in children, starch gel electrophoresis and enzyme activity measurements were also conducted on the parents, and investigations performed to determine whether or not the variants had been inherited from the parents. In cases where the variant was detected in the child but not the parents, tests were performed to confirm whether there was a biological parentage. The tests conducted were for 4 blood types (ABO, Rh, MNSs, Duffy), α-1-antitrypsin (P1) phenotype, human lymphocyte antigen (HLA) types (A, B, C loci), 9 protein phenotypes with polymorphism from among 30 proteins determined by starch gel electrophoresis, and chromosomes. When the variants were present in the child but not the parents and the tests demonstrated biological parentage, the presence of the variant was attributed to a mutation in the parental germ cells.

4. RESULTS OF PROTEIN STUDIES

Electrophoresis revealed rare variants in a total of 1,233 cases in the two populations, out of which parental tests were also performed in 964 cases (78%). In the majority of these the same variant was detected in both the child and one parent, clarifying that it was a hereditary variant. However, in 11 cases a variant was detected in the child but in neither parent. In 5 of these cases, the biological parentage was disproved in two or more test categories. "Fresh" mutations, i.e. mutations believed to have resulted from parental germ cells, were detected in 2 cases in the exposed population (1 case of glutamate-pyruvate transaminase-1, GPT1; and 1 case of phosphoglucomutase-2, PGM2) and in 4 cases in the control population (1 case each of haptoglobin, 6-phosphogluconate dehydrogenase, adenosine deaminase, and nucleoside phosphorylase). In each case a phenotype composed of the variant polypeptide and normal polypeptide was detected, showing that they were heterozygous for the mutant and normal alleles. With regard to the parents of the two children in the exposed population, in case 1 (GPT1) the mother had been exposed to a gamma ray dose of 0.03 Gy in Hiroshima whereas the father had not been exposed, and in case 2 (PGM2) both parents had been exposed in Nagasaki, the mother receiving a gamma ray dose of 0.73 Gy and a neutron dose of 0.002 Gy, and the father receiving a gamma ray dose of 0.03 Gy (a total of 0.8 Sv).

For both populations, the equivalent locus tests were totaled following calculations for each individual peptide constituting a protein[4–6]. As shown in Table 1-1, in the exposed population 544,779 equivalent locus tests were performed with the detection of 2 mutations, thus giving a mutation rate of 0.37×10^{-5} per locus per generation (0.04×10^{-5} to 1.33×10^{-5} per locus per generation at a 95% confidence limit); in the control population 589,506 equivalent locus tests were conducted with the detection of 4 mutations, giving a mutation rate of 0.68×10^{-5} per locus per generation (0.19×10^{-5} to 1.74×10^{-5} per locus per generation at a 95% confidence limit). Thus no significant difference in mutation rate was observed between the two populations.

Of the children examined by electrophoresis, the activities of a maximum of 9 erythrocyte enzymes were determined per person for 4,989 in the exposed population and 5,026 in the control population (Table 1-2). Enzyme deficiency variants were detected in 26 cases in the exposed population and in 21 cases in the controls; parental tests were performed in 42 of the cases, clarifying that in 41 of them the variant was transmitted from the parent to the child.

Table 1   Mutations in children of atomic bomb survivors

1.   Mutations altering electrophoretic mobility

	Exposed population	Control population
Conjoint parental gonadal dose	$\geqslant 0.01$ Sv	< 0.01 Sv
No. of children examined	11,364	12,297
Equivalent locus tests	544,779	589,506
Mutations	2	4
Mutation rate/locus/generation	0.37×10^{-5}	0.68×10^{-5}

2.   Mutations resulting in loss of enzyme activity

	Exposed population	Control population
No. of children examined	4,989	5,026
Equivalent locus tests	60,529	61,741
Mutations	1	0
Mutation rate/locus/generation	1.65×10^{-5}	0

An enzyme deficiency variant of triosephosphate isomerase (TPI) was observed in one child. Even though the TPI activity for this propositus born in 1960 was 65% of the mean value, the parents displayed normal activity (mother 92%, father 100%) and the younger brother had an activity of 104%. For each person the TPI electrophoretic mobility was normal, as was thermostability. Since there was no contradiction in tests for the biological parentage, the variant detected in the child was attributed to a mutation. The father had been exposed in Nagasaki to 0.03 Gy of gamma ray radiation, but the mother had not been exposed.

Out of 60,529 equivalent locus tests performed in the exposed population, 1 mutation was detected, giving a mutation rate of 1.7×10^{-5} per locus per generation. No mutations were detected in the 61,741 genetic loci examined in the control population.

In protein level studies using two types of indicators, no significant difference in mutation rate was observed between the exposed and control populations, and it was not possible to detect a genetic effect of atomic bomb radiation. Considering the parental doses, the possibility of such a result had been foreseen from the outset. However, the data obtained from the study, which has formed an important part of the RERF genetic program over a 40-year period, has been utilized in computation of the doubling dose of ionizing radiation[12].

The vast majority of the data yielded by the study was obtained by electrophoresis, with the data obtained using a second indicator capable of detecting gene deletions and insertions amounting to only approximately 1/10 of the total. Due to the late introduction of the automatic measurement equipment vital for screening erythrocyte enzyme activity, for approximately half of the subjects it was necessary to use blood specimens which had been preserved in liquid nitrogen, although this resulted in the decreased activity of some enzymes, necessitating a reduction in the number of tests performed. Also, a considerable individual difference exists in the genetically non-homogeneous human population, and only a limited number of enzymes meet the requirement that the coefficient of variation is 11% or less. These restraints made it impossible to increase the number of tests.

Electrophoretic data from the control population can be used for estimation of the human spontaneous mutation rate. Although the number of gene loci tested in this group (589,506) was the largest of any population, other studies also attempted to determine the spontaneous mutation rate using electrophoresis[19–21]. These studies involved testing a total of 716,126 loci and detected 1 mutation. Totaling all the results, 5 mutations were detected out of an aggregate of 1,305,632 loci tested, giving a mutation rate of 0.38×10^{-5} per locus per generation. If it is assumed that electrophoresis detects approximately 1/3 of single nucleotide substitutions, then the spontaneous mutation rate in humans is 3 times the above value, i.e. approximately 1.0×10^{-5} per locus per generation. Also, if the average number of nucleotides coding a polypeptide chain is taken to be 1,000, then a value of 1.0×10^{-8} per nucleotide per generation is obtained. However, in addition to the large errors incorporated in these estimates, the value gives no consideration to mutations other than single nucleotide substitutions such as gene duplications, deletions and rearrangements.

Radiation is thought to induce chromosomal damage in mammalian germ cells and produce gene deletions. Initial genetic studies certainly should have detected this effect, but no significant difference was observed. In the biochemical studies the second indicator was also the indicator for deletion mutations. At the present time, mutations in cells in culture which have been treated with radiation or chemical mutagens should be detected at the molecular level, and several reports have appeared regarding analyses by the Southern blotting method. Of the spontaneous mutations produced in the genes in germ cells and somatic cells which code hypoxanthine phosphoribosyl transferase, adenine phosphoribosyl transferase, and thymidine kinase, 20–40% are DNA deletions, insertions and inversions; however, it has been reported that these types of mutation account for 16–80% of the X-ray induced mutations in these genes in somatic cells. Factors affecting the mutation frequency, which varies greatly among types of cells and genes, are whether genes are heterozygous or hemizygous, and whether or not the gene is necessary for life. Also, in order to permit easy detection of mutations, selection systems were employed for the purpose of detecting mutant genes whose products have virtually no activity; consequently, the frequency is unknown for mutations such as the base substitutions or small deletions that have no effect on the activity of gene products. Out of the total of all mutations induced by ionizing radiation, the percentage that is detectable by means of protein electrophoresis still remains unknown.

5. MOLECULAR LEVEL GENETIC STUDIES

Genetic evaluation of the children of atomic bomb survivors is of great importance and should be clarified as far as possible. In preparation for future studies at the DNA and RNA levels, permanent cell lines are being established by using Epstein-Barr virus transformation from peripheral B-lymphocytes obtained from 1,000 families (the atomic bomb survivors, their spouses, and as many children as possible), with the lines preserved in liquid nitrogen. Intact lymphocytes and polymorpho-nuclear leukocytes are also being preserved so that untreated samples of DNAs and RNAs are readily available. In half of the families concerned, one or both parents was exposed to ≥ 0.01 Sv, and in the other half either both parents were unexposed or else received less than 0.01 Sv.

Furthermore, various techniques have been examined for their practicality in the screening for mutations at the DNA or RNA level. It has been concluded[22,23] that the most effective method for the detection of small mutations in DNA molecules (such as base substitutions, and small deletions and insertions) is the PCR-DGGE method[24], which is a combination of the polymerase chain reaction (PCR)[25] and denaturing gradient gel electrophoresis (DGGE)[26]. In the authors' laboratory, a fragment of 2,000–3,000 base pairs (bp) from the chromosomal DNA is amplified by PCR and examined by DGGE following cleavage into fragments of approximately 500 bp with restriction enzyme. Since the DNA fragments are then detected by staining the gel with ethidium bromide, it is not necessary to produce radioisotope-labeled probes, thus permitting rapid testing of many samples. As three DNA fragments (2,500 bp × 3 = 7,500 bp) can be examined on a single gel lane, 15 kilo-base pairs from the autosomal genes of one child can be examined at one time. Variations in mRNA can also be detected by the PCR-DGGE method, in which case the analysis is performed following conversion of the mRNA into complementary DNA by means of reverse transcriptases[27].

Since the radiation-induced mutations are predominantly deletions, techniques for detecting deletions need to be introduced. Adoption of the DGGE method permits detection of not just single base substitutions but deletions and insertions of up to 50 base pairs. Since attempts to apply the conventional Southern blotting to the detection of mutations such as deletions, insertions, and rearrangements have been successfully carried out[28], this method can also be applied to the authors' study at the molecular level. In addition, the authors established a method for determining the copy number of specific sequences in chromosomal DNA[29] in which the target sequences are quantitatively amplified by PCR and the amount of products are quantified. Adoption of this method permits detection of heterozygous gene deletions and insertions in various genes.

Selection of target sequences will determine the characteristics, value and effectiveness of molecular level research. Mutations occurring in functional genes will change gene products both quantitatively and qualitatively, with a high likelihood that they affect morbidity and mortality in the children.

Assuming that the mutation rate in functional genes is 2×10^{-8} per base pair per generation, and that the parents in the family from which cell lines are being produced were exposed to an average of 1/4 of the doubling dose (recently estimated at 1.7–2.2 Sv)[12], then in order to observe a significant difference in mutation rate between the exposed and control populations it is necessary to analyze 1.2 $\times 10^{10}$ base pairs per population[26]. In view of such a huge number it is possible that, as happened in the protein studies, molecular level research may fail to yield statistically significant differences. However, with the rapid advances in DNA analytical techniques, this prediction could easily change.

(Chiyoko Satoh)

REFERENCES

1. Neel JV, Schull WJ. The effect of exposure to the atomic bombs on pregnancy termination in Hiroshima and Nagasaki. Publ. No. 461, Washington, DC: National Academy of Sciences-National Research Council, 1956.
2. Otake M, Schull WJ, Neel JV. Congenital malformations, stillbirths, and early mortality among the children of atomic bomb survivors: a reanalysis. *Radiat Res* 1990; **122**: 1–11.
3. Awa AA, Honda T, Neriishi S, *et al.* Cytogenetic studies of the offspring of atomic bomb survivors. In: Obe B, Basler A, editors. Cytogenetics: basic and applied aspects. Berlin: Springer-Verlag, 1987: 166–83.
4. Neel JV, Satoh C, Goriki K, *et al.* The rate with which spontaneous mutation alters the electrophoretic mobility of proteins. *Proc Natl Acad Sci USA* 1986; **83**: 389–93.
5. Neel JV, Satoh C, Goriki K, *et al.* Search for mutations altering protein charge and/or function in children of atomic bomb survivors: final report. *Am J Hum Genet* 1988; **42**: 663–76.
6. Satoh C, Neel JV. Biochemical mutations in the children of atomic bomb survivors. *GANN Monograph on Cancer Res* 1988; **35**: 191–208.
7. Satoh C, Neel JV, Yamashita A, *et al.* The frequency among Japanese of heterozygotes for deficiency variants of 11 enzymes. *Am J Hum Genet* 1983; **35**: 656–74.
8. Kato H, Schull WJ, Neel JV. A cohort-type study of survival in the children of parents exposed to atomic bombings. *Am J Hum Genet* 1966; **16**: 214–30.
9. Neel JV, Kato H, Schull WJ. Mortality in the children of atomic bomb survivors and controls. *Genetics* 1974; **76**: 311–26.
10. Yoshimoto Y, Schull WJ, Kato H, *et al.* Mortality among the offspring (F_1) of atomic bomb survivors, 1946–1985. *J Rad Res* 1991; **32**: 327–51.
11. Roesch WC, editor. Final report of US-Japan reassessment of atomic bomb radiation dosimetry in Hiroshima and Nagasaki. Hiroshima: Radiation Effects Research Foundation, 1987.
12. Neel JV, Schull WJ, Awa AA, *et al.* The children of parents exposed to atomic bombs: estimates of the genetic doubling dose of radiation for humans. *Am J Hum Genet* 1990; **46**: 1053–72.
13. Ferrell RE, Ueda N, Satoh C, *et al.* The frequency in Japanese of genetic variants of 22 proteins. 1. Albumin, ceruloplasmin, haptoglobin, and transferrin. *Ann Hum Genet* 1977; **40**: 407–18.
14. Ueda N, Satoh C, Tanis RJ, *et al.* The frequency in Japanese of genetic variants of 22 proteins. II. Carbonic anhydrase I and II, lactate dehydrogenase, malate dehydrogenase, nucleoside phosphorylase, triosephosphate isomerase, hemoglobin A and hemoglobin A2. *Ann Hum Genet* 1977; **41**: 43–52.
15. Satoh C, Ferrell RE, Tanis RJ, *et al.* The frequency in Japanese of genetic variants of 22 proteins. III. Phosphoglucomutase-1, phosphoglucomutase-2, 6-phosphogluconate dehydrogenase, adenylate kinase, and adenosine deaminase. *Ann Hum Genet* 1977; **41**: 169–83.
16. Tanis RJ, Ueda N, Satoh C, *et al.* The frequency in Japanese of genetic variants of 22 proteins. IV. Acid phosphatase, NADP-isocitrate dehydrogenase, peptidase A, peptidase B and phosphohexose isomerase. *Ann Hum Genet* 1978; **41**: 419–28.
17. Beutler E. Red cell metabolism, a manual of biochemical methods, 2nd ed. New York: Grune & Stratton, 1975.
18. Beutler E, Blume KG, Kaplan JC, *et al.* International Committee for Standardization in Haematology. Recommended methods for red-cell enzyme analysis. *Br J Haematol* 1977; **35** (Suppl): 331–40.
19. Altland K, Kaempfer M, Forssbohm M, *et al.* Monitoring for changing mutation rates using blood samples submitted for PKU screening. In: Bonné-Tamir B, editor. Human genetics, part A: The unfolding genome. New York: Alan R Liss, 1982: 277–87.
20. Harris H, Hopkinson DA, Robson EB. The incidence of rare alleles determining electrophoretic variants: data on 43 enzyme loci in man. *Ann Hum Genet* 1974; **37**: 237–53.

21. Neel JV, Mohrenweiser H, Hanash S, *et al.* Biochemical approaches to monitoring human populations for germinal mutation rates: I. Electrophoresis. In: de Serres F, Sheridan W, editors. Utilization of mammalian specific locus studies in hazard evaluation and estimates of genetic risk. New York: Prenum Publ., 1983: 71–93.

22. Satoh C, Hiyama K, Takahashi N, *et al.* Approaches to DNA methods for the detection of heritable mutations in humans. In: Mendelsohn ML, Albertini RJ, editors. Mutation and the environment, part C: somatic and heritable mutation, adduction and epidemiology. New York: Wiley-Liss, 1990: 197–206.

23. Satoh C, Takahashi N, Asakawa J, *et al.* Variations among Japanese of the factor IX gene (F9) detected by PCR-denaturing gradient gel electrophoresis. *Am J Hum Genet* 1993; **52**: 167–75.

24. Sheffield VC, Cox DR, Lerman LS, *et al.* Attachment of a 40-base-pair G + C-rich sequence (GC-clamp) to genomic DNA fragments by the polymerase chain reaction results in improved detection of single-base changes. *Proc Natl Acad Sci USA* 1989; **86**: 232–6.

25. Saiki RK, Gelfand DH, Stoffel S, *et al.* Primer-directed enzymatic amplification of DNA with a thermostable DNA polymerase. *Science* 1988; **239**: 487–91.

26. Lerman LS, Silverstein K, Grinfeld E. Searching for gene defects by denaturing gradient gel electrophoresis. *Cold Spring Harbor Symp Quant Biol* 1986; **51**: 285–97.

27. Satoh C, Takahashi N, Asakawa J, *et al.* Detection of variations in mRNA employing denaturing gradient gel electrophoresis (DGGE) combined with polymerase chain reaction (PCR). *Jpn J Hum Genet* 1991; **36**: 26.

28. Mohrenweiser HW, Larsen RD, Neel JV. Development of molecular approaches to estimating germinal mutation rates. 1. Detection of insertion/deletion/rearrangement variants in the human genome. *Mutat Res* 1989; **212**: 241–52.

29. Asakawa J, Satoh C, Yamasaki Y, *et al.* Accurate and rapid detection of heterozygous carriers of a deletion by combined polymerase chain reaction and high-performance liquid chomatography. *Proc Natl Acad Sci USA* 1992; **89**; 9126–30.

20

Estimations of Radiation Dose

20.1 DS86 DOSIMETRY

INTRODUCTION

The term DS86 stands for Dosimetry System 1986, a system in which a super-computer at the Radiation Effects Research Foundation (RERF) is used to estimate the individual radiation doses received by the registered atomic bomb survivors who were exposed in Hiroshima and Nagasaki[1,2]. The results have been employed together with the findings of RERF's epidemiological studies on the same atomic bomb survivors (e.g. on cancer incidence etc.) in order to investigate the effects of radiation on the human body. A comparison between dose received and the increase in cancer incidence yields the cancer risk due to radiation. This risk has been determined by the International Commission on Radiation Protection (ICRP) and used by various countries to establish legal standards for exposure limits for workers occupationally exposed to radiation. It has permitted the establishment of safety limits for not only specialists such as workers in nuclear reactors and researchers in universities and other institutions who face occupational exposure, but also for the field of medical treatment, such as in X-ray imaging. If the risk from everyday use of radiation is known, then safety limits for radiation exposure can be established and herein lies the ultimate significance of evaluating the doses received by the atomic bomb survivors.

Several methods for determining atomic bomb doses have been proposed since the war, one of which was the "Tentative 1965 Dose" (T65D) method adopted in 1965, which became widely used in risk evaluation. However, in the latter half of the 1970s, inherent problems became evident in the T65D system, and a reassessment program was initiated. In 1987 a US-Japan working group devised the DS86 system, which aimed to correct these problems. The results of epidemiological studies based on DS86 doses have already been recomputed and recognized by the ICRP, and guidelines based on the results are about to be incorporated into Japanese law.

1. METHOD AND REASSESSMENT BY CATEGORIES

The reassessment of atomic bomb radiation doses by the joint US-Japan study considered ten categories. The final classification dealt with problems concerning errors, but later systematic errors were also detected, and since these have not yet been resolved, the results have not been published. This chapter therefore summarizes the contents of, and methods involved in, the first nine categories.

A. Energy Released by the Hiroshima and Nagasaki Atomic Bombs

The power of the Hiroshima and Nagasaki atomic bombs is usually expressed in terms of the equivalent number of kilotons of conventional TNT explosive; this corresponds to the total amount of energy (and total radiation) released by each explosion, and hence to the amount of nuclear fission (the quantity of uranium and plutonium undergoing combustion). The energy released by 1 kiloton of TNT

368

is equivalent to 4.2×10^{12} Joules of energy, or 10^{12} calories of heat; this is also equivalent to the fission of 56 grams of fissionable material, or the fission of 1.45×10^{23} atomic nuclei. The power of the Hiroshima and Nagasaki atomic bombs were initially estimated at equivalent to 12.5 and 21 kilotons of TNT respectively.

The power of the atomic explosions was determined from measurements of the shock wave created when the atomic bombs exploded, and the condition of wood surfaces scorched by heat, etc., and by comparisons with data obtained during atmospheric atomic tests. Since the data from nuclear tests all relate to Nagasaki-type bombs, the data for the Nagasaki type were determined first, and then the data for the Hiroshima type determined by comparison. As shown in Table 1, the present reassessment covered all aspects. The figures for the Hiroshima explosion were revised upward by 20% from 12.5 kilotons to 15 kilotons, but the figures for the Nagasaki bomb were little changed at 22 kilotons, instead of 21 kilotons.

B. Energy Spectra at the Source

The initial stages in the production of radiation were included in a supercomputer model of the atomic explosion process, but the Japanese researchers were allowed access only to the results. The process referred to covers the period from the start of nuclear fission to the release of radiation and the production of a fireball. The calculations of radiation released were performed using the Monte Carlo Code for Neutron and Photon Transport (MCNP), which is publicly available. The results pertaining to the energy spectra of the Hiroshima and Nagasaki atomic bombs were reported in the form of tables giving the data for neutron and gamma rays[1,2]. Figure 1 compares the neutron spectra for Hiroshima and Nagasaki.

Table 1   The best yield estimates for the Hiroshima and Nagasaki bombs[1]

Method	Yield (kt)	Method	Yield (kt)
Absolute methods		Radiochemistry	
Thermoluminescence	18	Trinity test	20.3
Pressure vs time	16	Crossroads Able test	20.4
Cypress charring	15	Crossroads Baker test	21.7
Sulfur activation	13		
Blast damage	12	Fireball	
		Trinity test	20.8
Relative methods		Crossroads Able test	21.4
Thermal effects	14		
Blast effects	15	Theoretical calculations	22
Theoretical calculations		Recommended yield	21
Weighted average	15		

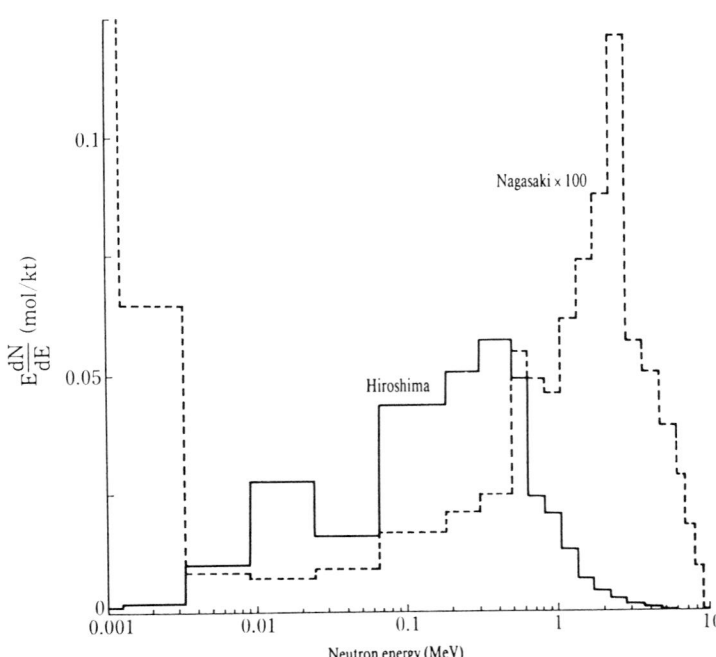

Figure 1   Distribution in the logarithm of the energy of neutrons emitted from the Hiroshima and Nagasaki bombs. The ordinates of the distribution for Nagasaki are multiplied by 100 to make the high-energy part of the spectrum visible (adapted from Ref. 1)

C. Calculations of Mid-Air Transmission of Radiation

The neutron and gamma rays produced in the atomic explosion collided with particles in the air, becoming scattered or absorbed. Subsequently both the unscattered radiation and the radiation with energy depleted by scattering reached the earth's surface. All these complex processes were incorporated into the transmission calculations, which were performed using the generally well-known ANISN and DOT-4 programs. The data input included such factors as the energy spectra (detailed in section B), air density, and nuclear data (basic data pertaining to scattering and absorption which indicates the changes occurring when radiation strikes atomic nuclei in the air). In order to ascertain air density, the temperature, atmospheric pressure and humidity at the time of explosion were investigated. For the nuclear data the ENDF/B-V files were employed. For each type of radiation arriving at the earth's surface, Table 2 shows the time between detonation and emission. The first radiation released consisted of prompt neutron and gamma rays formed as a result of nuclear fission. The results obtained from calculations describe the energy spectra of neutron and gamma rays close to the ground surface (for example, at a height of 1 meter). Every dose component was multiplied by the human soft tissue kerma coefficient for neutron and gamma rays and integrated to give the free-in-air (FIA) kerma (Fig. 2). The kerma coefficient has a generally

Table 2   Sources and emission times of ionizing radiation from a nuclear weapon

Source	Time emitted after detonation
Prompt neutrons from fission	< 1 μ sec
Delayed neutrons from fission products	< 1 min
Prompt gamma rays from fission process	< 1 μ sec
Gamma rays from inelastic scattering[a]	
From weapons[b]	< 1 μ sec
From air	< 10 μ sec
From ground	< 10 μ sec
Gamma rays from charged-particle reactions[a]	
From weapons[b]	< 1 μ sec
From air	< 10 μ sec
From ground	< 10 μ sec
Captured gamma rays[a]	
From weapon[b]	< 1 μ sec
From air	Few msec to 0.2 sec
From ground	Few msec to 0.2 sec
Activation gamma rays[a]	
Early time	0.2 sec to 1 min
Residual	1 min to years
Delayed gamma rays from fission products	
Early time	0.2 sec to 1 min
Residual	1 min to years

[a]These sources of gamma rays are of secondary origin and result from the interaction of neutrons with the air and ground and with the weapon itself.
[b]Included in source terms for the prompt neutrons and gamma rays which are emitted while the weapon is still intact and still able to sustain the fission process.

well-known value, and has been tabulated. The free-in-air kerma is close in value to the radiation dose (in Grays) received by the skin surface of those people exposed at ground level; this was previously termed the mid-air dose, but in the reassessment program was assigned its newer and more correct name. The FIA kerma for neutron and gamma rays in both Hiroshima and Nagasaki are shown in Table 3. The large changes are with respect to Hiroshima. Firstly, the neutron dose at a distance of 1 km from the hypocenter decreased to approximately 1/10 of the value, with the relationship between dose and distance no longer parallel to that observed with T65 doses, and ceasing to be linear. Secondly, although gamma rays showed almost no change at distances up to 1 km, the difference then gradually increased with distance, rising to more than twofold at 1.5 km. Also, as in the case of neutrons, the relationship was not linear. In Nagasaki the changes were not large in comparison, with the neutron dose declining by approximately 40% and the gamma ray dose exhibiting no great change.

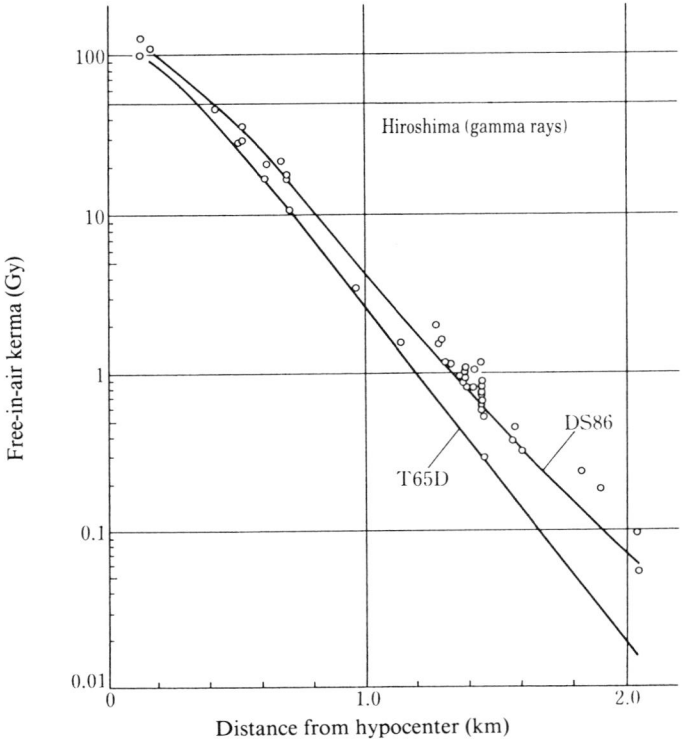

Figure 2   Comparison of theoretical free-in-air tissue kerma with thermoluminescence measurements (adapted from Ref. 1)

D. Thermoluminescence Observations of Gamma Ray Dose

Gamma ray dose observations were performed mainly in Japan, and had the important function of corroborating the American calculations. The method involves collection and pulverization of the exposed roof and wall tiles, and subsequent extraction of the minute quartz particles contained in the specimens. Following the application of heat, light is produced (thermoluminescence); the amount of light is measured since the quantity generated is proportional to the gamma ray dose received, thereby providing an estimate of the radiation dose from the atomic explosion. It is a method originally used in archaeology for dating pottery etc. by considering the fixed annual exposure to natural radiation. This system of measurement was available even at the time the T65D system was devised, but measured values were only obtained for the area within 1 km of the hypocenter; however, the observed, the T65D, and the DS86 values were all in agreement for the problematic case of Hiroshima. There were no observed values for distances greater than 1 km, and since these were undoubtedly different, the results for these locations were a problem. However, these areas were measured and agreement with the DS86 values confirmed (Fig. 4)[1,5,6]; values for

Table 3   Total kermas in tissue normalized to energy yields of 15 kilotons for the Hiroshima bomb and 21 kilotons for the Nagasaki bomb[1]

Distance from hypocenter (m)	FIA kerma in tissue (cGy) at one meter above ground			
	Hiroshima		Nagasaki	
	Gamma rays	Neutrons	Gamma rays	Neutrons
100	11,700	3,310	29,200	1,800
150	10,800	2,910	26,500	1,590
200	9,720	2,480	23,400	1,360
250	8,630	2,070	20,200	1,130
300	7,310	1,700	17,200	925
350	6,190	1,350	14,400	736
400	5,150	1,050	12,000	572
450	4,270	802	9,740	439
500	3,500	604	7,850	331
550	2,830	446	6,290	246
600	2,270	328	5,010	182
650	1,820	238	3,990	134
700	1,460	171	3,140	97.6
750	1,170	123	2,480	71.1
800	940	88.1	1,970	51.7
850	754	62.9	1,570	37.2
900	609	44.7	1,240	27.1
950	487	31.9	983	19.7
1,000	393	22.7	783	14.3
1,050	316	16.1	624	10.4
1,100	255	11.5	498	7.57
1,150	207	8.24	396	5.44
1,200	167	5.91	318	4.02
1,250	135	4.24	257	2.94
1,300	110	3.04	207	2.15
1,350	89.8	2.20	167	1.58
1,400	72.8	1.58	135	1.16
1,450	59.6	1.15	110	0.855
1,500	48.7	0.838	89.3	0.631
1,550	39.6	0.610	73.0	0.467
1,600	32.9	0.446	59.7	0.346
1,650	26.9	0.326	49.0	0.256
1,700	22.1	0.239	40.2	0.191
1,750	18.2	0.176	33.0	0.142
1,800	15.0	0.130	27.2	0.106
1,850	12.4	0.096	22.4	0.079
1,900	10.3	0.071	18.5	0.059
1,950	8.52	0.053	15.3	0.044
2,000	7.10	0.039	12.7	0.033
2,100	4.90	0.022	8.76	0.019
2,200	3.41	0.012	6.05	0.011
2,300	2.37	0.007	4.23	0.006
2,400	1.67	0.004	2.96	0.004
2,500	1.18	0.002	2.09	0.002

FIA kerma = free-in-air kerma

Nagasaki were similarly measured and again agreement with DS86 values confirmed (Fig. 3)[1,5,6].

E. Comparison of Measured and Calculated Neutron-Induced Radioactivity

The measured levels and experimentally determined values for neutrons were compared in the same manner as the thermoluminescence data for gamma-ray dose estimation. Neutron-induced radioactivity is classified into three categories in both the present and former systems of measurement:

(1)   the production of ^{32}P (phosphorus-32) due to the reaction of neutrons with the sulfur used to bond insulators to utility poles, in which ^{32}S absorbs a neutron (n) and emits a protein (p), thereby producing ^{32}P [this is expressed as ^{32}S (n, p) ^{32}P][1,2,7];

(2)   the production of ^{60}Co (cobalt-60) due to the reaction of neutrons with the cobalt used in steel for ferro-concrete bars etc. in concrete buildings, with the release of gamma rays [^{59}Co (n, γ) ^{60}Co][1,2]; and

(3)   the production of ^{152}Eu (europium-152) due to the reaction of neutrons with europium, a rare earth metal element present in minute quantities in rock, with the emission of gamma rays [^{151}Eu (n, γ) ^{152}Eu][8-11].

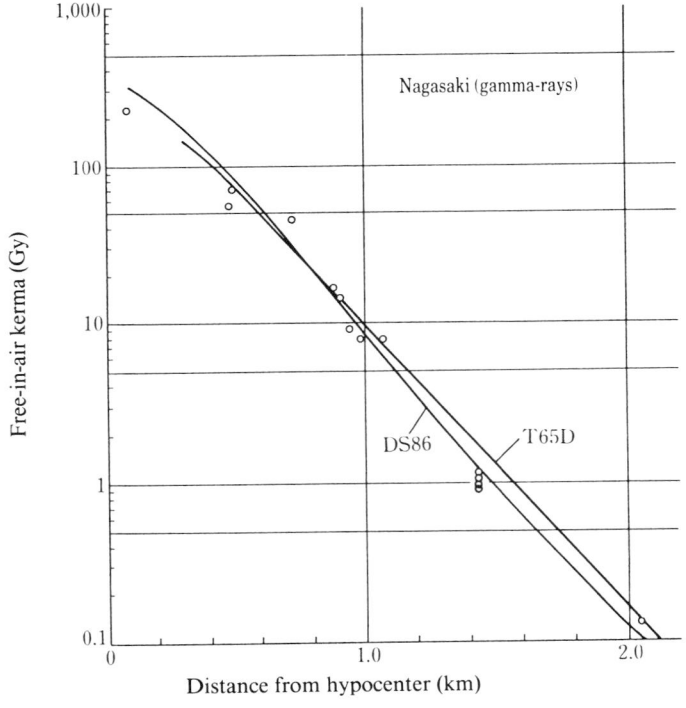

Figure 3   Comparison of theoretical free-in-air tissue kerma with thermoluminescence measurements (adapted from Ref. 1)

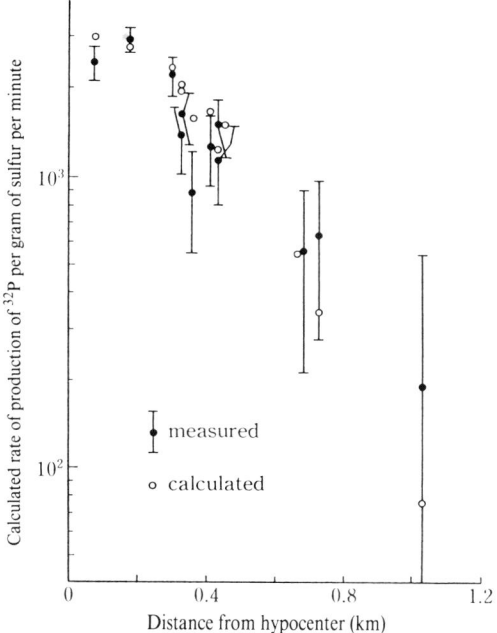

Figure 4   Comparison of theoretical and measured levels of ^{32}P produced by the reaction of neutrons with the sulfur used to bond insulators to utility poles (adapted from Ref. 1)

The half-lives for these forms of radioactivity are respectively 14.3 days, 5.3 years, and 13 years. Consequently, it is not possible today to measure the ^{32}P levels. The ^{60}Co levels were also determined when the T65D system was devised, and specimens again tested with the advent of the new system[1,2]. The third type (^{152}Eu) was determined for the first time; however, the data were not used since the values were too scattered. Moreover, the investigations at that time were inadequate, which later caused problems. Of the 3 types of radioactivity produced as a result of the atomic explosion, the first (^{32}P) was created due to fast neutrons (≥ 2 MeV), and the other two due to thermal neutrons (0.025 eV). The principal effect of exposure on the human body is due to neutrons of above approximately 0.5 MeV; lesser amounts of energy have little effect. Therefore, although the ^{32}P results indicate the doses themselves, the amounts of the other two types do not directly indicate the doses received by human bodies. For this reason the DS86 system was applied principally to the investigation of ^{32}P data[1,2,7]. Figure 4 shows a comparison between measured and calculated values; no difference is observed in the case of DS86 doses. For ^{60}Co, when a difference is found between experimental values and the values calculated on the basis of DS86 dosimetry, it is indicative of a system error. The discrepancy will be discussed later, but a similar difference was later detected in the case of another nuclide; the reasons for this are currently under investigation.

F. Exposure to Residual Radiation

There were two forms of residual radioactivity, depending on the means of production, i.e. radioactivity due to the absorption of neutrons and that due to nuclear fission products (typified by ^{137}Cs and ^{90}Sr) formed by the fission of uranium and plutonium. The differences in means of production resulted in differences in the locations where they are observed. The former was produced in surface soil close to the hypocenter, and the latter contained in the so-called "black rain." However, due to the difficulty of estimation, and since it is not clearly known where the black rain fell, the radioactivity resulting from nuclear fission products was not included in the DS86 dose assessments (this is discussed in detail in Chapter 20-3)[8,11].

G. Shielding due to Buildings and Topography

The majority of atomic bomb survivors were exposed inside buildings; individuals outdoors were also shielded if near to a building. The DS86 system allowed accurate computation of these effects due to the use of a supercomputer. The shielding effect for atomic bomb survivors was expressed using 9 parameters, with the method and data the same as that used with the T65D system. This topic is dealt with more fully in Chapter 20-2.

H. Organ Dose

Although the question of cancer risk requires consideration of the particular organ concerned, it is necessary to remember that before reaching an organ (e.g. the stomach) the radiation must first be transmitted from the skin surface. Thus when considering the development of gastric cancer, it is necessary to consider the dose actually received by the stomach itself, i.e. allowing for the absorption of some radiation during transmission from the skin to the stomach. This shielding effect by the human body itself is complex since there is also a dependence on bodily orientation relative to the hypocenter, but a detailed computation was performed on the supercomputer using a human model that incorporated organ data. Differences in the composition of bone and soft tissue were input, as were the configurations of the head, trunk, legs and hands.

Data were input into the supercomputer relating to fourteen target organs, and the human models classified in detail to allow for differences for different ages (adults aged 15 and above, children aged 5 and above, and infants aged 1), the posture at the time of exposure (lying, sitting, or standing), the orientation relative to the hypocenter, and the location within the building, etc. The actual values of the transmission factors are discussed in Chapter 20-2.

I. DS86 Dosimetry System

The dosimetry system employed by the Hiroshima Radiation Effects Research Foundation (RERF) for determining the individual doses received by each survivor is summarized in Fig. 5. As can be seen, first the mid-air dose (free-in-air kerma) was calculated, then the shielding effects due to housing and the body itself input, and the organ dose and error calculated. The whole process is referred to as the DS86 dosimetry system, and is that portion of Fig. 5 enclosed by a dotted line. Comparison of the DS86 doses with the data from RERF's epidemiological studies allowed assessment of the risk from radiation. Virtually all radiation risk standards used throughout the world are based on studies on the atomic bomb survivors.

2. UNRESOLVED PROBLEMS

The DS86 dosimetry system was devised as a result of a large-scale joint US-Japan reassessment project, but nevertheless two problems still remain unresolved. These are (1) the inconsistencies between the induced radioactivity data referred to in section (E) and the results of calculations based on the DS86 system, and (2) the non-agreement of thermoluminescence data at distances greater than approximately 1.5 km from the hypocenter (the data values being high).

With regard to point #1, as already discussed in section (E), the non-agreement with ^{60}Co data was already recognized by the DS86 system. Later several reports appeared concerning accurate data for ^{152}Eu in Hiroshima, which demonstrated the existence of the same system error[11]. Fears thus arose that the DS86 calculations themselves might contain essential flaws, and therefore studies are continuing. Figure 6, which shows a comparison between calculated and observed values, seems to reveal the same tendencies for ^{32}P data.

Due to the difference in gamma ray doses, point #2 poses a problem in the case of Hiroshima. As can be seen from Fig. 7, the values of the thermoluminescence data are even greater than the DS86-computed doses; this difference becomes apparent at

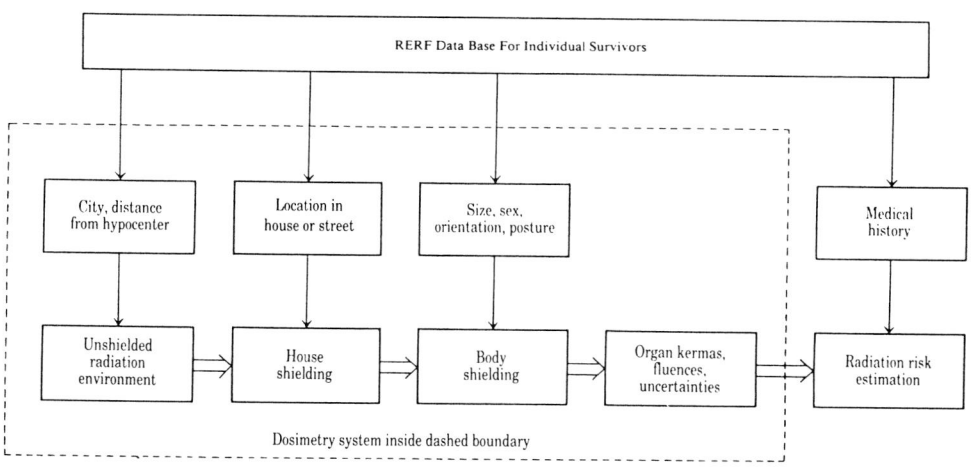

ATB = at the time of bombing

Figure 5   DS86 dosimetry system for RERF, Hiroshima and Nagasaki,[1,4].

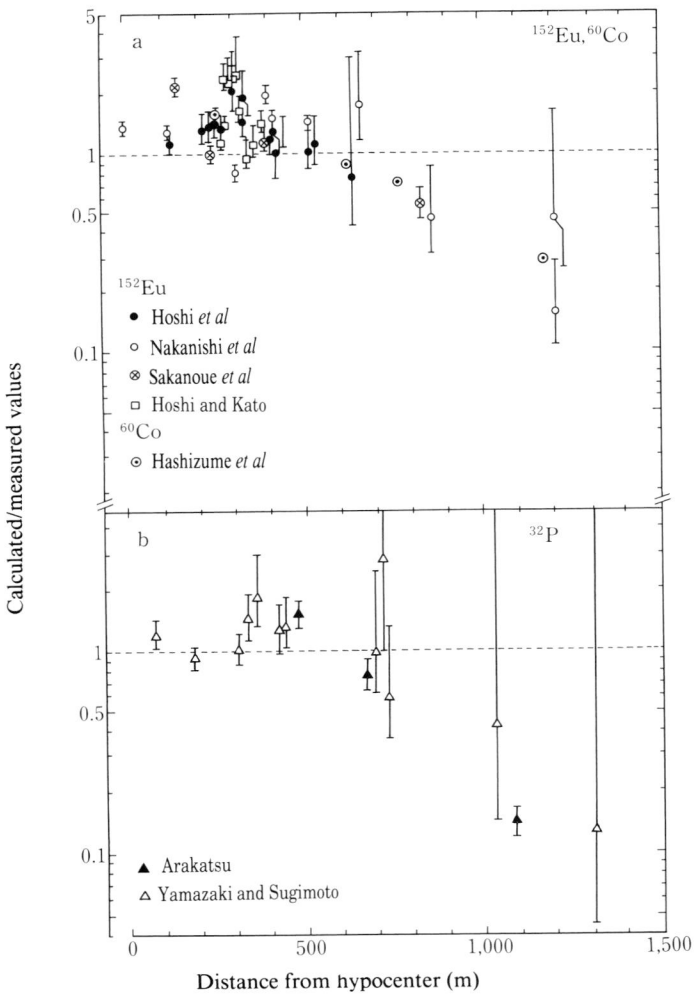

Figure 6   Ratio of calculated DS86 to measured ^{52}Eu and ^{32}P activities compared with ^{60}Co. The upper figure (a) shows comparisions for ^{152}Eu, and ^{60}Co data; the lower figure (b) shows the comparision for ^{32}P data[11]

approximately 1.4 km from the hypocenter, after which it increases with distance, becoming approximately 70% greater at around 2 km. This in itself results in an increased dose only for doses of approximately 0.1 Gy, and since higher doses produce little effect, it can be viewed as not causing a great problem in risk evaluation; however, as the cause of the discrepancy is probably due to neutrons, it is very likely that the problem involved with gamma rays is related to the problem of neutrons, and interest has focused on this point.

(Masaharu Hoshi)

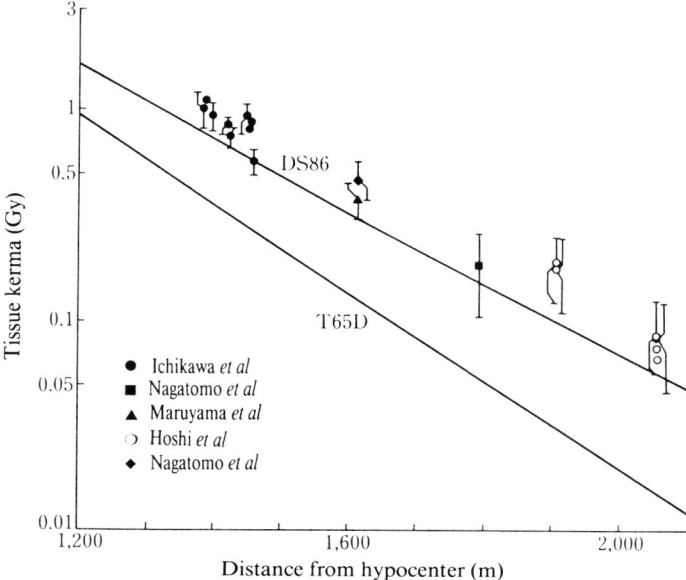

Figure 7   Comparison of experimental thermoluminescence measurements and the theoretical DS86 dose vs distance curve for doses from the Hiroshima atomic bomb[6]

REFERENCES

1. Roesch WC. US-Japan joint reassessment of atomic bomb radiation dosimetry in Hiroshima and Nagasaki, final report, Vol. 1. Hiroshima: Radiation Effects Research Foundation, 1987.
2. Roesch WC. US-Japan joint reassessment of atomic bomb radiation dosimetry in Hiroshima and Nagasaki, final report, Vol. 2. Hiroshima: Radiation Effects Research Foundation, 1987.
3. Milton RC, Shohoji T. Tentative 1965 radiation dose estimation for atomic bomb survivors of Hiroshima and Nagasaki. Hiroshima: Radiation Effects Research Foundation, ABCC TR 1-68, 1968.
4. Hoshi M, Sawada S. The dosimetry system 1986 (DS86) and its remaining problems. *Annual Report of Research Institute for Nuclear Medicine and Biology*, Hiroshima University 1986; **27**: 105-17. (*In Japanese*)
5. Maruyama T, Kumamoto Y, Noda Y. Reassessment of gamma-ray doses in Hiroshima and Nagasaki. *J Radiat Res* 1991; **32** (Suppl): 40-7.
6. Nagatomo T, Ichikawa Y, Hoshi M. Theromoluminescence dosimetry of gamma rays using ceramic samples from Hiroshima and Nagasaki: a comparison with DS86 estimates. *J Radiat Res* 1991; **32** (Suppl): 48-57.
7. Hamada T. Recalculation of data on ^{32}P activity induced in sulfur in Hiroshima. *J Radiat Res* 1991; **32** (Suppl): 103-7.
8. Sakanoue M, Komura K, Tan K. Residual radioactivity in neutron-exposed objects and residual alpha radioactivity in black rain areas. *J Radiat Res* 1991; **32** (Suppl): 58-68.
9. Nakanishi T, Ohtani H, Mizuochi R, *et al.* Residual neutron-induced radionuclides in samples exposed to the nuclear explosion over Hiroshima: comparison of the measured values with the calculated values. *J Radiat Res* 1991; **32** (Suppl): 69-82.
10. Tatsumi-Miyajima J, Okajima S. Physical dosimetry at Nagasaki: europium-152 of stone embank-

ment and electron spin resonance of teeth from atomic bomb survivors. *J Radiat Res* 1991; **32** (Suppl): 83–98.

11. Hoshi M, Hasai H, Yokoro K. Studies of radioactivity produced by the Hiroshima atomic bomb. 1. Neutron-induced radioactivity measurements for dose evaluation. *J Radiat Res* 1991; **32** (Suppl): 20–31.

12. Hasai H, Hoshi M, Yokoro K. Studies of radioactivity produced by the Hiroshima atomic bomb. 2. Measurements of fallout radioactivity. *J Radiat Res* 1991; **32** (Suppl): 32–9.

20.2 COMPARISON OF DS86 AND T65D DOSIMETRY

INTRODUCTION

The investigation of the health effects of atomic bomb radiation requires the most accurate estimate possible of the dose received by each individual. Until the development of a systematic method for doing this, the question of whether or not an atomic bomb radiation effect exists was investigated by considering a combination of factors such as the distance of the atomic bomb survivor from the hypocenter, the presence of acute symptoms, and the existence of heavy shielding etc. The T57D system of dose estimation was devised in 1957, but essentially it was not until after the development of the T65D dosimetry system[1] in 1965 that the health effects also became evaluated quantitatively. In 1976 at the Los Alamos National Laboratories in the United States, Preeg was the first to raise doubts concerning the T65D dose, and this led to a reassessment of atomic bomb radiation doses by a joint US-Japan working group[2-4]. In 1986 the new DS86 dosimetry system was devised[5-7], and the individual doses received by the atomic bomb survivors calculated; these are used in the evaluation of various health effects, including reassessments of cancer mortality rates, chromosomal aberrations, and epilation etc. This section considers estimates of the radiation doses received by atomic bomb survivors, focusing on a comparison of the DS86 and T65D systems.

The following briefly explains some terms frequently used to describe doses. Other than residual radiation, there were 3 forms of radiation in the initial period following detonation of the atomic bombs: 1) following the explosion, the gamma ray and neutron dose at any given distance from the hypocenter that reached the height above the ground at which a survivor's organs would have been exposed (correctly speaking, the free-in-air kerma in tissue) ["Kerma" (an abbreviation for "kinetic energy released in material") describes the energy released in a material as a result of irradiation, and the free-in-air kerma in tissue is taken to be the exposure dose received by the surface of the human body]; 2) the radiation dose that passes through the surrounding shielding material and reaches the point where the survivor was located (correctly speaking, this is also referred to as the free-in-air kerma in tissue); and 3) the doses absorbed by various organs. For the sake of convenience, radiation category #1 (free-in-air kerma) is distinguished from category #2 (shielded kerma, an abbreviation for free-in-air kerma in tissue adjusted for shielding). In the absence of shielding objects, the shielded kerma is the same as the free-in-air kerma. Radiation category #3 is termed the organ dose. When the term "dose" is used, it usually refers to the organ dose.

1. COMPARISON OF DOSE ESTIMATION METHODS

The T65D system of dose estimation is based on experimental data obtained in Nevada, USA using Nagasaki-type atomic bombs, and uses a formula calculating free-in-air kerma as a parameter of distance from the hypocenter together with a formula calculating the transmission factor (the ratio of shielded kerma to free-in-air kerma) of shielding materials such as Japanese-style housing etc. as a computer-coded parameter for atomic bomb survivors[1]. These formulae are different for Hiroshima and Nagasaki, and also for gamma rays and neutrons. The organ doses were not calculated, but later the transmission factor for radiation passing through body tissue to each organ (the ratio of organ dose to shielded kerma) was treated as a constant[8], with individual differences at the time of bombing such as posture and direction not considered.

On the other hand, the DS86 system of dosimetry involves processing of a computer data base constructed on the basis of elementary physical processes which considered the various processes involving the radiation from the moment of detonation to arrival at various human organs. During the US-Japan joint reassessment of atomic bomb dosimetry various experimental and measured data were used in verification of the code. For each atomic bomb survivor, each of the four types of radiation (i.e. prompt neutrons, prompt gamma rays, delayed neutrons and delayed gamma rays) was modeled in detail by supercomputer from the moment of detonation to arrival at various organs. For each 25-meter increment in distance from the hypocenter, calculations were performed for 1) the estimated free-in-air tissue kerma at the height above the ground at which a survivor's organs would have been exposed; 2) the free-in-air tissue kerma at the survivor's location adjusted for shielding materials; and 3) the energy and angular fluence distributions (the number of radiation particles incident on a unit sphere) at various organs. These fluence values allowed the free-in-air kerma, shielded kerma, and organ dose to be calculated as required. Health effect evaluations were performed using a combination of gamma ray and neutron doses.

At the Atomic Bomb Casualty Commission, ABCC (the forerunner of the Radiation Effects Research Foundation, RERF), detailed shielding data pertaining to individual atomic bomb survivors were recorded following interviews in Hiroshima and Nagasaki with a total of 28,000 survivors, which were conducted mainly in the 1950s[9]. All necessary data were coded and used in the T65D calculations. When exposure occurred inside a wooden house, the shielding data were expressed in the T65D calculations by 9 parameters; this applied to 18,000 cases. The nine parameters were the number of floors, slant penetration (the distance from the point of entry into the house to the survivor), the number of internal front walls, the number of internal lateral walls, the existence and size of front shielding structures (if any), the distance from any unshielded windows in the direction of the hypocenter, lateral shielding, and the height above the floor; also, for those outdoors but sheltered by a wooden structure, three-dimensional data (so-called global data) was coded (approximately 4,000 cases)[1].

The DS86 system of dosimetry was basically constructed on the basis of these coded data. In the above-mentioned detailed shielding records for individual atomic bomb survivors, besides the shielding data for housing etc., the posture of the survivor at the time of bombing and the orientation relative to the hypocenter were recorded, with this data being used in current calculations of organ dose. In the DS86 system these data were employed in the selection of the appropriate computer model for each atomic bomb survivor using approximately 1,000 different shielding conditions from two computer models [i.e. for house clusters (a collection of 6 independent houses) of typical wooden structures, and tenement clusters (a collection of tenements)], and a phantom computer model that considered age group (infants, children, adults) and posture (standing, sitting, lying) based on data such as the physical build of the Japanese in 1945.

2. SUBJECTS USED IN DOSE CALCULATIONS

The DS86 system can be used for direct calculation of received dose for survivors who were exposed within 2.5 km of the hypocenter and for whom detailed shielding records exist when the survivor was 1) in a wooden house, 2) outdoors with no shielding, 3) outdoors with shielding from a wooden house, 4) in a factory (Nagasaki only), and 5) shielded by terrain (Nagasaki only). Since the numbers of individuals fulfilling these requirements would be too small for the evaluation of the health effects on survivors, in the DS86 calculations performed at RERF: 6) the average transmission factor for wooden structures was applied to survivors who were exposed in wooden houses but for whom no detailed shielding records exist; 7) the average transmission factor was applied to distal survivors who were exposed outdoors; and 8) the received dose was defined as zero for survivors for whom the free-in-air kerma was zero or for whom it became zero on multiplication by the average transmission factor[10].

Now let us consider in detail the RERF Life Span Study sample, which consists of approximately 120,000 persons, to whom the DS86 system was applied (Table 1). Excluding non-exposed individuals, there were approximately 94,000 atomic bomb survivors, among whom T65D calculations had been performed on approximately 91,000. DS86 calculations have been conducted on approximately 87,000 individuals, i.e. 95% of the latter group (92% of the total exposed). This sub-population has been used in the reassessment of health effects. The individuals for whom T65D calculations were not performed were survivors who were inside trains, shielded by trees, or exposed under other complex shielding conditions; those for whom T65D calculations were conducted but for whom DS86 calculations were not performed included individuals in concrete structures and air raid shelters, and some of those in Nagasaki factories. For only the proximally exposed (i.e. those within 1.6 km of the hypocenter in Hiroshima, and within 2.0 km in Nagasaki), the DS86 calculations cover 95% of the cases evaluated by the T65D system in Hiroshima, but only 76% of those in Nagasaki. The shielding conditions which can be covered by the DS86

Table 1   Summary of dose estimation coverage for the RERF Life Span Study sample as of July 1, 1990

	Hiroshima	Nagasaki	Total
Total exposed	61,984	31,757	93,741
DS86 available	58,500	28,132	86,632
DS86 unknown	3,481	3,625	7,109
T65D unknown	(1,420)	(959)	(2,392)

system are mainly for Japanese-style housing; differences between Hiroshima and Nagasaki appear in the topography around the hypocenter and the time of day at which exposure occurred (i.e. 8:15 am in Hiroshima, and 11:02 am in Nagasaki).

3. COMPARISON OF ESTIMATED RECEIVED DOSES

Figure 1 shows a comparison between T65D and DS86 systems for free-in-air kerma[5]. For Hiroshima, there is a discrepancy in DS86 gamma ray kerma which increases with distance from the hypocenter, becoming 2–3 times the T65D value. The neutron kerma exhibits a substantial decrease, with the DS86 value becoming approximately 1/10 the T65D value. For Nagasaki, the DS86 gamma ray kerma is 10% to 30% less than the T65D value, and the DS86 neutron kerma 1/2 to 1/3 less, and thus the changes are quite small relative to those in Hiroshima.

In order to consider the effect of shielding due to buildings etc. in the vicinity of the survivors, it is best to examine the transmission factors of the radiation. Let us consider exposure in Japanese-style housing, which accounted for the majority of exposure conditions (69% of the proximally exposed in Hiroshima, and 44% in Nagasaki). Many people experienced other shielding conditions, e.g. those who were outdoors and shielded by Japanese-style housing, and those in Nagasaki who were exposed in more solidly built factories but for whom transmission factor consider-ations were omitted. In the case of DS86 dosimetry, the house transmission factors were not determined directly, but obtained from a calculation of the ratio of the shielded kerma of survivors inside wooden structures to free-in-air kerma. In the

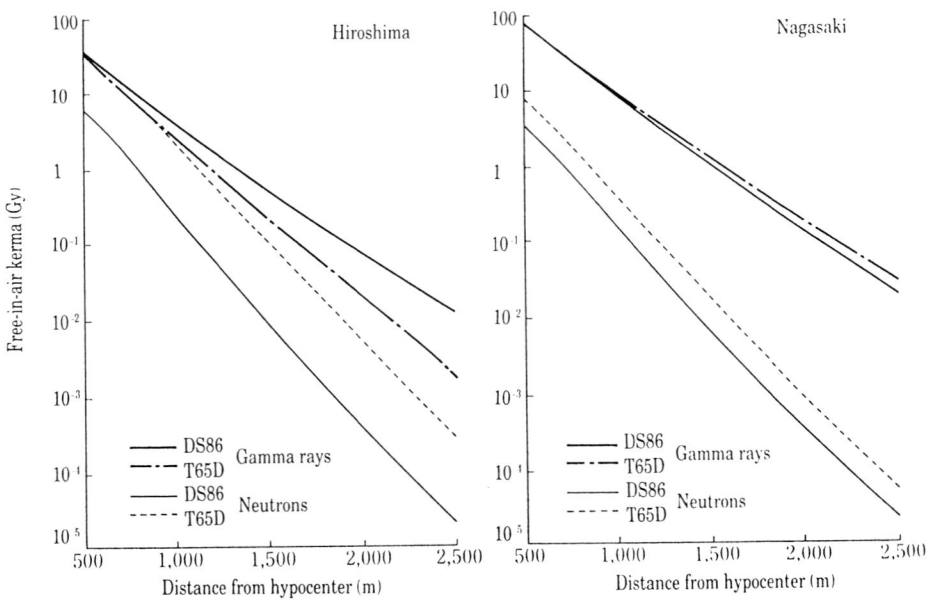

Figure 1   Comparison of DS86 and T65D values for the free-in-air kerma of gamma rays and neutrons

case of T65D dosimetry, experimentally-derived formulae were used to first calculate the housing transmission factor for each person, and the shielded kerma then computed by multiplication by the free-in-air kerma. Table 2 shows a comparison of the average house transmission factors[11], from which it can be seen that the DS86 gamma ray transmission factors are approximately half of the T65D values, whereas the neutron transmission factors are virtually unchanged.

With regard to the body tissue shielding of each organ, for the two examples of the bone marrow and large intestines the DS86 average transmission factors are compared with the T65D values reported by Kerr[8] and shown in Table 3[11]. The bone marrow dose was used in the studies on leukemia, and the intestinal dose for the assessment of non-leukemic cancers. The shielding effect of body tissue was greater in the case of the T65D system, i.e. the transmission factor was greater in DS86 dosimetry. The neutron transmission factor was 1.3 times greater for both organs, but the gamma ray transmission factor of bone marrow increased by 1.45 times, and for the intestines by 1.85 times; the ratio of transmission factors thus increased with increasing depth of the organ. Fifteen organs were selected in the DS86 calculations: the bone marrow, large intestine, stomach, lungs, breasts, bladder, ovaries, thyroid, liver, pancreas, testes, uterus, brain, eyes, and bone.

The doses received by individuals are an integration of the various above-mentioned factors, and a comparison follows of the DS86 and T65D results for doses received by subjects in the previously mentioned Life Span Study sample. With regard to shielded kerma, in Hiroshima the DS86 values are lower at high doses, but greater at low doses; overall the DS86 values are lower. In Nagasaki the DS86 values are clearly lower. Apart from female breast doses, the DS86 organ doses are slightly higher. These differences in DS86 and T65D exposure doses are mirrored in the differences in the DS86 and T65D health risk evaluations.

A reassessment of health effects such as cancer mortality etc. after introduction of the new system of dosimetry[11] revealed the following general tendencies. At the same level of dose, the T65D dose-response curve indicates a greater risk in Hiroshima than in Nagasaki; in the case of DS86 data, there is no statistically significant difference between them. When shielded kerma is considered, the DS86 cancer mortality risk is several tens of percentage points greater than in the case of T65D dosimetry, but when organ dose is used there is not much difference between the two. With the DS86 system, the neutron dose is extremely small (several per cent of the total), and it is not possible to reliably estimate the relative biological effectiveness (RBE). A large increase in the radiation-related cancer mortality risk has recently been reported[12,13]; however, this is certainly not due merely to switching

Table 2   Average house transmission factors

Radiation	Hiroshima		Nagasaki	
	DS86	T65D	DS86	T65D
Gamma rays	0.46	0.90	0.48	0.81
Neutrons	0.36	0.31	0.41	0.35

Table 3   Average body tranmisson factors for bone marrow and colon[11]

Radiation	Bone marrow		Colon	
	DS86	T65D	DS86	T65D
Gamma rays	0.81	0.56	0.74	0.40
Neutrons	0.37	0.28	0.19	0.14

from T65D to DS86 dosimetry, but rather to the realization that the radiation-related cancer risk is relative to the background level of radiation.

Finally, although the DS86 estimates of atomic bomb doses are regarded as far more accurate than those yielded by T65D dosimetry, they are not absolute values and do contain errors. These errors can be classified into the system errors related to factors such as the power of the explosion and in-air transport of radiation etc. which are common to all the survivors, and the random errors pertaining to factors such as the relative position of the survivor and the surrounding shielding etc.. Dose reassessment activities in Japan and the United States are continuing to attempt to reduce both types of error, and the former type in particular, with evaluations also being performed on the uncertainties in the dose computations. Also, with regard to the latter type of error, statistical treatment is being applied to risk evaluations.

(*Sho-ichiro Fujito*)

REFERENCES

1. Milton RC, Shohoji T. Tentative 1965 radiation dose estimation for atomic bomb survivors, Hiroshima and Nagasaki. ABCC TR 1–68, 1968.
2. Fujita S. Reassessment of atomic bomb radiation dosimetry in Hiroshima and Nagasaki — its background, present status, and future. *J Hiroshima Med Ass* 1986; **37**: 1256–62. (*In Japanese*)
3. Okajima S. Re-evaluation of atomic radiation. *Nagasaki Med J* 1986; **61**: 227–39. (*In Japanese*)
4. Preston DL, Pierce DA. The effects of changes in dosimetry on cancer mortality risk estimates in the atomic bomb survivors. *Radiat Res* 1988; **114**: 437–66.
5. Roesch WC, editor. US-Japan reassessment of atomic bomb radiation dosimetry in Hiroshima and Nagasaki: final report. Vol. 1. RERF Hiroshima, 1987.
6. Roesch WC, editor. US-Japan reassessment of atomic bomb radiation dosimetry in Hiroshima and Nagasaki: final report. Vol. 2. RERF Hiroshima, 1988.
7. Fujita S. Introduction of final report on US-Japan joint reassessment of atomic bomb radiation dosimetry. *J Hiroshima Med Ass* 1987; **40**: 78–93. (*In Japanese*)
8. Kerr GD. Organ dose estimates for Japanese atomic bomb survivors. *Health Physics* 1979; **37**: 487–508.
9. Noble K, editor. Shielding survey and radiation dosimetry study plan, Hiroshima and Nagasaki. ABCC TR 7–67, 1967.
10. Fujita S. Versions of DS86. RERF Update 1989; 1(2): 3.
11. Shimizu Y, Kato H, Schull WJ, *et al.* Life Span Study. Report 11. Part 1. Comparison of risk coefficients for site-specific cancer mortality based on the DS86 and T65DR shielded kerma and organ doses. *Radiation Research* 1989; **118**: 502–24.
12. Committee on the Biological Effects of Ionizing Radiation. Commission on Life Science. Health effects of exposure to low levels of ionizing radiation (BEIR-V). National Academy of Sciences-National Research Council. Washington, DC: National Academy Press, 1990.
13. United Nations Scientific Committee on the Effects of Atomic Radiation (UNSCEAR). Sources, effects, and risks of ionizing radiation. New York: United Nations, 1988.

20.3 RESIDUAL RADIATION

INTRODUCTION

In the Hiroshima explosion, the nuclear fission of uranium initiated a chain reaction. After the uranium reached a critical state, the bomb receptacle vaporized at high temperature, and in the approximately one microsecond (1 µs, i.e. one millionth of a second) that elapsed before completion of the chain reaction, neutrons and gamma rays were released. These were termed prompt radiation, and struck the ground ahead of the blast and the thermal radiation released by the explosion. Next, due to nuclear reactions caused by the action of these neutrons on materials in the air and ground, gamma rays were released within approximately 10 µs, and radioisotopes possessing a wide range of half-lives were produced. Isotopes with long half-lives can be detected even today. Radioactive fission products were also created as a result of nuclear fission of the uranium. Many of these ascended in the fireball and then were dispersed over a large area by air currents in the upper atmosphere, although some were transported to the ground in the rain that fell within several hours of the explosion. Such radioactive fallout caused high levels of radioactive contamination in specific limited areas.

In contrast to the prompt radiation, which was instantaneously released in the nuclear reaction as described above, radiation from the induced radioactivity and the fission products contained in the fallout was gradually released due to the decay of radioisotopes. Since their effects consequently continued over a period of time, they are termed residual radiation. This chapter discusses estimates of exposure due to residual radiation.

1. MEASUREMENTS OF RESIDUAL RADIATION

A. Early Studies

Soon after the detonation of the atomic bomb, numerous people began to measure radioactivity in various parts of the city, with the aim of acquiring conclusive evidence that it had been an atomic explosion. According to the Collection of Reports on Investigations of the Atomic Bomb Casualties[1], a study was begun on August 10th 1945 by a group from Osaka Imperial University, who found high levels of radioactivity in the vicinity of the hypocenter and near Koi station, where heavy rain fell. Following that, a survey was undertaken by Kyoto Imperial University and the Institute of Physical and Chemical Research. Radioactivity measurements were performed at Hiroshima and Nagasaki by an American team (the Manhattan Engineer District Investigating Group) in September and October of the same year, and by a joint Japanese-American group in October and November[2]. Fujiwara and Takeyama[3] of Hiroshima University of Literature and Science (Hiroshima Bunri Daigaku) conducted surveys in September 1945, and again in 1946 and 1948. These early studies revealed that besides the vicinity of the hypocenter, high levels of radioactivity were present in the Koi and Takasu areas of Hiroshima and the Nishiyama district of Nagasaki. Each of these areas was located approximately 3 km downwind from the hypocenter, and moreover was subjected to heavy rainfall within 30 minutes to 1 hour of the atomic explosion.

B. Fallout Studies Performed 30 years After the Atomic Bombing

In order to investigate the exposure effects on the residents in the areas that received rainfall and on the early entrants (i.e. those who entered the city soon after the bombing), in 1975 Takeshita[4] collected soil in the rainfall areas and measured ^{137}Cs levels. In 1976 the Committee for Residual Radioactivity Surveys in Hiroshima and Nagasaki was established by the Ministry of Health and Public Welfare, and studied ^{137}Cs and ^{90}Sr levels in soil samples collected within a radius of 30 km of the hypocenters in Hiroshima and Nagasaki[5]. Repeat studies were carried out in 1978, but by that time the effects of fallout from nuclear testing were already apparent, and no significant difference was observed due to the black rain that followed the Hiroshima explosion. Uranium was used in the Hiroshima bomb, and plutonium in the Nagaski explosion. Only a little of these atomic bomb materials underwent combustion, with the large majority being dispersed in the atmosphere. Therefore, using soil samples from Hiroshima, the proportion of naturally occurring uranium isotopes was investigated and tests conducted on the areas receiving fallout[6]. In Nagasaki plutonium levels were indeed found to be high in the fallout areas[7].

C. Recent Studies

Prior to the emergence of the atomic bomb dose reassessment problem that arose around 1981, Sakanoue and Komura of Kanazawa University[8] had in 1976 detected the existence of ^{152}Eu (europium-152)-induced radioactivity in exposed materials. Europium is a trace element contained in rocks etc. at a concentration of approximately 1 ppm (one part per million), but due to the high density of neutron absorption and the long half-life of the ^{152}Eu (13 years), it is relatively easy to detect by gamma-ray spectrometry using recently developed germanium (Ge) solid-state detectors. Consequently, measurements using this technique have been performed on ^{152}Eu levels in rock together with measurements by the previous method employing ^{60}Co, which has a half-life of 5 years[9,10]. In addition, since levels of neutron-induced ^{36}Cl and ^{41}Ca have been determined by mass spectrometry using recent accelerators[11,12], it is possible that convincing data will be forthcoming.

2. ESTIMATION OF DOSES DUE TO INDUCED RADIOACTIVITY

Induced radioactivity is an important consideration when estimating the doses received by atomic bomb survivors and early entrants. In 1958–67, Shohno[13] and Shohno and Iijima[14] performed calculations on induced radioactivty. Other computations were carried out by Arakawa[15], Hashizume et al[16,17] and Takeshita[18], with Gritzner and Woolson[19] performing DS86 calculations. This section describes the findings of Gritzner and Woolson. The method of calculating induced radioactivity was as follows:

First, the incident neutron spectrum was computed at each increment of distance from the hypocenter. From this, the energy, direction, and number of incident neutrons were determined. Next, the quantity of radioactivity produced was calculated based on the types and amounts of elements in the soil and their activation cross-sections. The transmission of gamma rays released by the induced radiation was then calculated until arrival at a point 1 meter above ground level, and from this the radiation rate was obtained in roentgens per hour. In order to permit consideration of the exposure effects on the human body, this was converted into a quantity known as the tissue kerma in air (in Grays), which is the amount of energy imparted to a unit mass of material when ionizing radiation in air strikes a piece of material which resembles human tissue.

The decrease with time in the dose rate (tissue kerma rate) at the hypocenter is shown in Fig. 1[19]. Changes in the dose rate are apparent in three bulges in the curve. The first bulge is due primarily to the contribution of ^{28}Al, which has a short life span (a half-life of 2.2 minutes); the second, occurring approximately 30 minutes later, is due to ^{56}Mn (a half-life of 2.6 hours) and ^{24}Na (15 hours); the third, occurring approximately one week later, is caused by ^{56}Fe (44 days) and ^{46}Sc (83 days). Approximately one year later the contributions of ^{54}Mn (312 days) and ^{134}Cs (2.05 years) become predominant. If the dose rates shown in Fig. 1 are integrated with respect to time, it is possible to obtain the cumulative dose for an individual who remained at the hypocenter for a fixed period of the time. Figure 2 shows the relationship between distance from the hypocenter and cumulative dose from immediately after the explosion[19]. Figure 3 shows the fraction of the cumulative dose received by an individual who entered the hypocenter area at a fixed interval after the explosion and continued to stay there[19]. The graph shows that the dose was high until approximately 100 hours (about 4 days) after detonation. For both Hiroshima and Nagasaki, dose estimations were performed for individuals for whom exact details were known regarding time of entry to the city, movements within the city, and length of stay. Results are shown in Table 1. In this calculation the DS86 cumulative doses at the hypocenter for the period from immediately after the explosion until infinity were assumed to be 0.8 Gy in Hiroshima and 0.4 Gy in Nagasaki. As can be seen from the table, approximately 80% of the cumulative dose was received on day 1, approximately 10% between days 2 and 5, and approximately 10% of the total dose on and after day 6.

3. ESTIMATION OF DOSES DUE TO RADIOACTIVE FALLOUT

The number of radioisotopes produced as a result of nuclear fission in the vicinity of mass numbers 90 and 140 exceeded approximately 200[21]. Since the majority of fission products were nuclides of short half-life, radioactivity levels rapidly decreased. Consequently individual exposure is related to whether or not fission products fell within several hours of the atomic explosion.

Two methods have been employed in the estimation of cumulative dose due to fallout:

1) Use of dose rate measurements from the early studies.
2) Use of ^{137}Cs activities recently determined by the germanium (Ge) solid-state detector The deposition of ^{137}Cs was estimated at 1 mCi/Km^2, suggesting that the cumulative gamma ray exposure from all the fission and activation products in the fallout was approximately 300 mR (milliroentgens)[20].

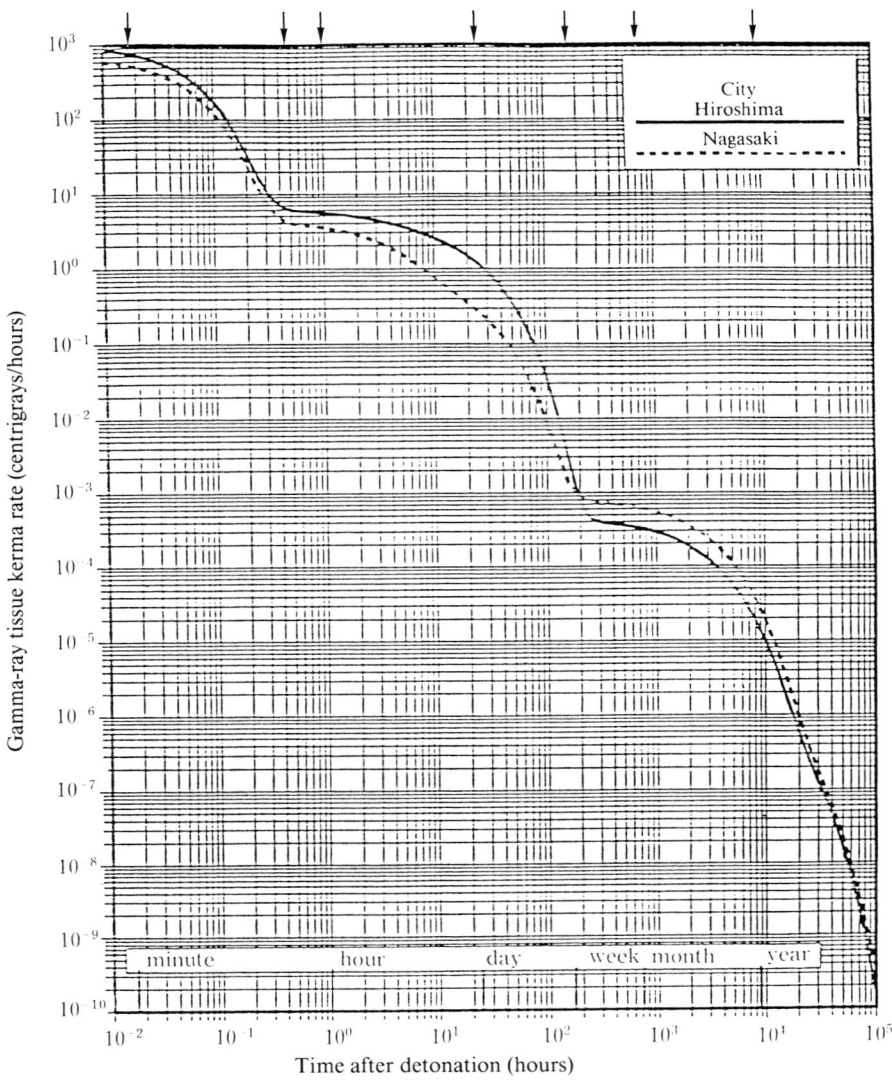

Figure 1   Exposure kerma rate obtained from soil activation versus time after detonation at hypocenter, Hiroshima and Nagasaki[19]

For Nagasaki it is possible to perform cumulative dose estimations by both of the above methods due to the existence of both dose rate measurement data from early studies and also ^{137}Cs spectrometric data obtained from soil samples collected before the effect from nuclear test fallout became significant. In the Nishiyama district of Nagasaki, early dose rate measurements led to an estimated cumulative dose of 20–40R (roentgens)[20]. The ^{137}Cs fallout values obtained by Miller using samples collected in the early post-detonation period (62 mCi/km^2 in the Nishiyama district,

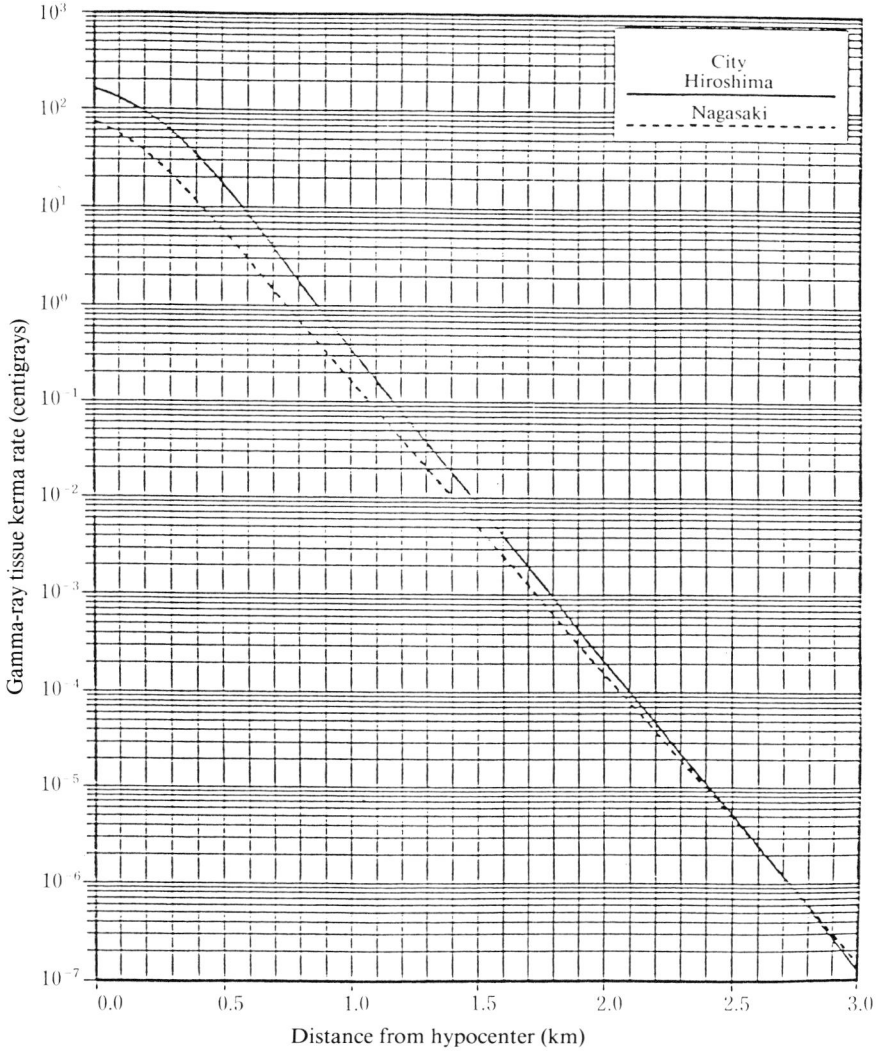

Figure 2   Infinite exposure kerma rate obtained from soil activation versus distance from hypocenter, Hiroshima and Nagasaki[19]

and 7 Ci/km[2] in Nagasaki) yielded a cumulative dose of 40R[20], with good agreement on estimated values thus obtained between the two methods.

For the Koi and Takasu districts of Hiroshima, only the early dose measurement data are available, with no ^{137}Cs spectrometric data for samples collected immediately after the atomic explosion. The dose rate measurement data yielded an estimated cumulative dose of 1–3R[20]. When a conversion factor is used to calculate back to the original dose, the estimated amount of ^{137}Cs depostion is 3–10 mCi/km[2]. Since this value is less than about 4% of the approximately 100 mCi/km[2] of ^{137}Cs

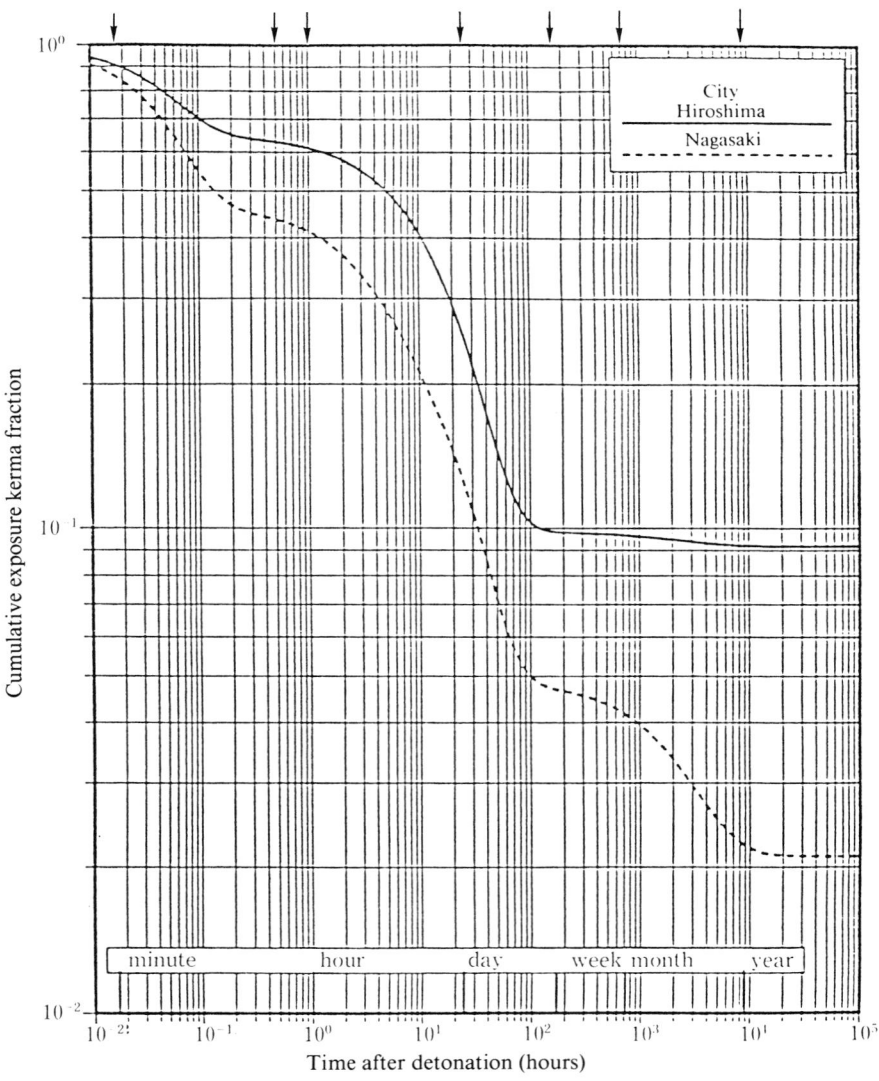

Figure 3   Cumulative exposure kerma fraction versus time after detonation, Hiroshima and Nagasaki[19]

due to deposition from later nuclear testing, it is difficult to detect in samples collected today.

Let us now consider the dose due to fallout in the vicinity of the hypocenter. The authors discovered exposed samples which had been collected soon after the atomic bombing[24] and kept in the Department of Geology at the Faculty of Science, Hiroshima University[24]. These samples yield an estimated ^{137}Cs fallout in the vicinity of the hypocenter of < 0.34 mCi/km^2. This was approximately 1/10 of the amount estimated to have fallen at Koi and Takasu, and is in agreement with the

Table 1   Estimated doses due to induced radioactivity

Distance from hypocenter (m)	City	aCumulative dose (cGy)	bDay 1	Day 2		Day 3		Day 4		Day 5		On and after day 6
				cDaytime	dNight	Daytime	Night	Daytime	Night	Daytime	Night	
0	Hiroshima	80	60	5.4	3.4	1.1	0.80	0.24	0.16	0.12	0.008	8.1 →
	Nagasaki	40	35	1.1	1.1	0.40	0.32	0.12	0.08	0.08	0.04	1.9 →
5 00	Hiroshima	9.1	6.8	0.62	0.39	0.13	0.09	0.03	0.02	1.0 →		
	Niroshima	3.4	2.9	0.095	0.095	0.034	0.027	0.010	0.007	0.17 →		
1,000	Hiroshima	0.17	0.13	0.012	0.007	0.024 →						
	Nagaski	0.096	0.083	0.003	0.003	0.007 →						
1,500	Hiroshima	0.0048	0.0036	0.0012 →								
	Nagasaki	0.0028	0.0024	0.0004 →								

a. Cumulative dose from immediately after explosion to present day.
b. From immediately after explosion to 8 a.m. the following morning.
c. From 8 a.m. the following morning to 6 p.m.
d. From 6 p.m. on the day after the explosion to 8 a.m. the following morning.
e. No mark indicates the cumulative dose from that day until the present.

estimate by Shohno based on early dose rate measurement data[13]. According to the previously mentioned data by Miller[10], even in Nagasaki it is believed that the fallout near the hypocenter was approximately 1/10 of that in the Nishiyama district.

Table 2 shows the cumulative doses due to induced radioactivity and fallout in Hiroshima and Nagasaki. It can be seen that the level of induced radioactivity in Hiroshima was approximately twice that in Nagasaki, but fallout in the Nishiyama area was about 10 times greater than in the Koi and Takasu districts of Hiroshima. Moreover, since the dose rate due to naturally occurring radioactivity is approximately 8 μR/h[18], the dose received over a period of 46 years is approximately 0.03 Gy, which is the amount corresponding to the cumulative dose in Koi and Takasu.

In the estimation of dose due to fallout, it is believed that besides the above, exposure occurs as a result of radioactive materials being introduced into the body via respiration, or ingestion of food and water. The amount of ^{137}Cs present in residents of the Nishiyama area of Nagasaki was meaured by Okajima et al[22,23,26], who found that the levels were almost twice as high as in other areas. It has been estimated that between 1945 and 1985 the cumulative dose due to internal exposure in this area was 1×10^{-4} Gy for men and 8×10^{-5} Gy for women[20]. No similar study has been performed in the Hiroshima fallout areas. Although there would be a wide variation in internal exposure according to individual lifestyle, it is believed that the amount of such exposure in the fallout areas in Hiroshima is less than 1/10 of that in Nagasaki.

CONCLUSION

Figure 4 shows the relationship between distance from the hypocenter and the atomic bomb radiation dose. Consult reference 27 for data concerning prompt radiation (neutrons and gamma rays), and reference 19 for data pertaining to induced radiation. Prompt radiation exposes humans to a large dose instanta-neously. Of the residual radiation, induced radioactivity leads to a small total exposure relative to that from prompt radiation, but it persists over a long period of time, and thus led to both atomic bomb survivors and early entrants being exposed.

Table 2   Cumulative external γ-radiaton exposure in the hypocenter and fallout areas. The value in the fallout area could be estimated in two ways: (a) from radiation rate measurement, and (b) from ^{137}Cs deposition data.

Source of radiation	Hiroshima		Nagasaki	
	Hypocenter	Koi-Takasu	Hypocenter	Nishiyama
Induced radioactivity	0.80	0	0.30–0.40	0
Fallout (a) Radiation rate (b) ^{137}Cs	— $\leqslant 0.001$	0.01–0.03 Not measured	— 0.05	0.20–0.40 0.40

(Units: Gy)

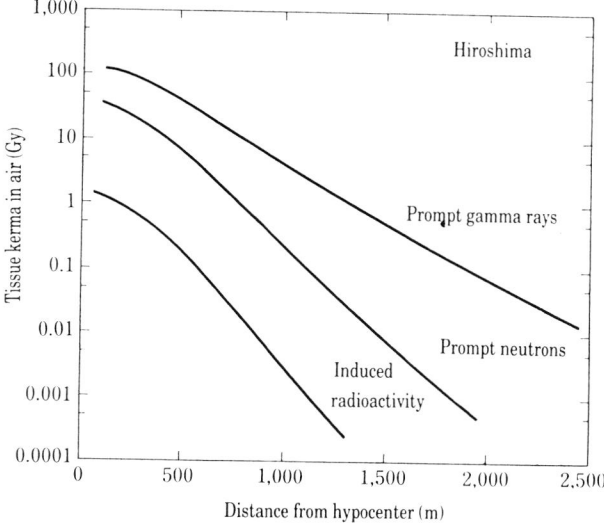

Figure 4   Tissue kerma in air versus distance from hypocenter

Also, although the effect due to fission products was localized, it was equivalent to short-term exposure to a dose of the same order of magnitude as long-term exposure to naturally occurring background radiation.

(Hiromi Hasai, Kiyoshi Shizuma)

REFERENCES

1. Japan Society for the Promotion of Science. In: *Genshibakudan saigai chousa* [Collection of the reports on the investigation of the atomic bomb casualties] Vol. 1. Tokyo: Japan Society for the Promotion of Science. 1953. (*In Japanese)*

2. Pace N, Smith RE. Measurement of the residual radiation intensity at the Hiroshima and Nagasaki bomb sites. Hiroshima: Atomic Bomb Casualty Commision. 1959. ABCC TR 26–59.

3. Fujiwara T, Takeyama H. Residual radioactivity around Hiroshima city. In: *Genshibakudan saigai chousa* [Collection of the repoprts on the investigation of the atomic bomb casualties] Vol. 1. Tokyo: Japan Society for the Promotion of Science. 1953: 75–83. (*In Japanese*)

4. Takeshita K. Doses to early entrants to the A-bomb areas and to residents of the fallout areas and ^{137}Cs in soil of the black rain area in Hiroshima. *J Hiroshima Med Ass* 1976; **29**: 298–306. (*In Japanese*)

5. Hashizume T, Okajima S, Kawamura S, *et al.* Estimation of residual radiation from the atomic bombs in Hiroshima and Nagasaki. *J Hiroshima Med Ass* 1978; **31**: 455–8. (*In Japanese*)

6. Takada J, Hoshi M, Sawada S, *et al.* Uranium isotopes in Hiroshima black rain soil. *J Radiat Res* 1983; **24**: 229–36.

7. Sakanoue M, Tsuji T. Plutonium content of soil at Nagasaki. *Nature* 1971; **234**: 92–3.

8. Sakanoue M, Maruo Y, Komura K. Distributions and characteristics of Pu and Am in soil. In: International Symposium of Methods for Low Level Counting and Spectrometry. Vienna: International Atomic Energy Agency, 1981: 105–24.

9. Nakanishi T, Moromoto T, Komura K, *et al.* Europium-152 in samples exposed to the nuclear explosions at Hiroshima and Nagasaki. *Nature* 1983; **302**: 132.

10. Hasai H, Iwatani K, Shizuma K, *et al.* Europium-152 depth profile of a atone bridge pillar exposed to the Hiroshima atomic bomb: ^{152}Eu activities for analysis of the neutron spectrum. *Health Phys* 1987; **53**: 552–6.

11. Ruhn W, Kato K, Korschinek G, *et al.* The neutron spectrum of the Hiroshima A-bomb and the dosimetry system 1986. *Nucl Instr Meth* 1990; **B52**: 557–62.

12. Straume T, Finkel RC, Eddy D, *et al.* Use of accelerator mass spectrometry in the dosimetry of Hiroshima neutrons. *Nucl Instr Meth* 1990; **B52**: 552–6.

13. Shohno N. On residual radiation. *J Hiroshima Med Ass* 1965; **20** (Suppl): 75–91. (*In Japanese*)

14. Shohno N, Iijima S. Nuclear radiation and atomic bomb disease. Tokyo: Nippon Hoso Shuppan Assn, 1975: 92.

15. Arakawa ET. Residual radiation in Hiroshima and Nagasaki. Hiroshima Atomic Bomb Casualty Commission. ABCC TR 2–62, 1962.

16. Hashizume T, Maruyama T, Kumamoto Y, *et al.* Estimation of gamma-ray dose from neutron induced radioactivity in Hiroshima and Nagasaki. *Health Phys* 1969; **17**: 761–71.

17. Hashizume T, Maruyama T. Dose estimation from residual and fallout radioactivity. 2. A simulated neutron activation experiment. *J Radiat Res* 1975; **16**: 32–4.

18. Takeshita K. Doses estimation from residual and fallout radioactivity. 1. Area surveys. *J Radiat Res* 1975; **16**: 24–31.

19. Gritzner ML, Woolson WA. Calculation of doses due to atomic bomb induced soil activation. In: Roecsh WC, editor. US-Japan joint reassessment of atomic bomb radiation dosimetry in Hiroshima and Nagasaki, final report. Hiroshima: Radiation Effects Research Foundation. 1987; **2**: 342–52.

20. Okajima S, Fujita S, Harley JH. Radiation doses from residual radioactivity. In: Roecsh WC, editor. US-Japan joint reassessment of atomic bomb radiation dosimetry in Hiroshima and Nagasaki, final report. Hiroshima: Radiation Effects Research Foundation. 1987; **1**: 205–26.

21. Eisenbud M. Environmental radioactivity. New York: Academic Press, 1973.

22. Okajima S. Fallout in the Nagasaki-Nishiyama district. *J Radiat Res* 1975; **16** (Suppl): 35–41.

23. Okajima S, Takeshita K, Antoku S, *et al.* Effects of the radioactive fallout of the Nagasaki atomic bomb. Hiroshima: Atomic Bomb Casualty Commission. ABCC TR 12–75, 1975.

24. Watanabe T, Yamasaki M, Kojima T, *et al.* Geological study of damages caused by atomic bombs in Hiroshima and Nagasaki. In: *Genshibakudan saigai chousa* [Collection of the reports on the investigation of the atomic bomb casualties] Vol. 1. Tokyo: Japan Society for the Promotion of Science. 1953: 143. (*In Japanese*)

25. Shizuma K, Iwatani K, Hasai H, *et al.* Fallout in the hypocenter area of the Hiroshima atomic bomb. *Health Phys* 1989; **57**: 1013–16.

26. Okajima S, Miyajima J, Morimoto I, *et al.* Effects of the radioactive fallout of the Nagasaki bomb. *J Hiroshima Med Ass* 1982; **35**: 334–6. (*In Japanese*)

27. Kerr GD, Dyer FF, Energy JF, *et al.* Activation of cobalt by neutrons from the Hiroshima bomb. Oak Ridge National Laboratory, ORNL-6590, 1990.

20.4 DOSE ESTIMATIONS USING EXTRACTED TEETH

INTRODUCTION

When investigating the late effects of radiation on the human body, it is necessary to determine each individually received dose as accurately as possible. The individual tissue absorbed doses are calculated on the basis of free-in-air tissue kerma, although these are in many cases extremely difficult to reproduce in a calculation due to complex shielding conditions. That is, shielding factor errors become important in the estimation of individual dose. There is thus a dire need for a more direct method of dose estimation, which can be met by the adoption of electron spin resonance (ESR) spectroscopy for the measurement of radiation--produced scars in teeth obtained from atomic bomb survivors. Even though these are classed as radiation damage, they are neither bodily effects nor remnants of radioactivity. When teeth are irradiated, electrons are ejected from their constituent atoms and captured by the minute traces of CO_3^{2-} ions present in teeth (approximately 2.5–3.5 weight percent), forming CO_3^{3-} radicals. These radicals are strongly bonded within the crystal lattice and thus exhibit long-term stability[1]. Since each radical has an unpaired electron, when the irradiated tooth is examined with an ESR spectrometer the signal intensity of the absorption spectrum of electromagnetic energy is proportional to the number of CO_3^{3-} radicals, and from this the radiation dose can be estimated[2-7].

After the teeth are washed with water and dried, only the enamel part is used for measurements. The samples used are obtained by crushing this into equal-sized grains with a diameter of ≤ 1 mm; enamel grains weighing 100–400 mg are obtained from one tooth. Figure 1 shows an example of an ESR signal from the enamel portion of a tooth from an atomic bomb survivor. The increase in signal intensity per unit dose is normalized using ^{60}Co gamma rays and converted into the radiation dose.

Electron spin resonance spectroscopy (ESR)

Electrons possess a spin, which creates a magnetic field around them. Since the magnetic poles in a material mutually oppose each other, the electron spin within a material does not generally exhibit a magnetic quality even if free electrons are present. Upon irradiation, an electron within the material is ejected (a process termed "ionization"), and the ionized electron captured within the material and stabilized. This captured electron and the hole from which it came are unpaired, and therefore the spin of the unpaired electron exhibits the qualities of a magnet. When an external magnetic field is applied, the electron spin is split into two energy levels. When a fixed quantity of electromagnetic wave energy is applied to the electron under the influence of this magnetic field such that the electromagnetic wave energy is equal to the difference in energy between the two levels, then the electromagnetic energy is absorbed with the electron raised to a high energy state. This phenomenon is termed electron spin resonance; when maintained under thermal equilibrium and a constant external magnetic field, the total energy of absorption accompanying the transition between the two energy states (the absorbed energy of the electromagnetic wave) is proportional to the total number of unpaired electrons, and therefore from the measurement of the amount of electromagnetic energy absorbed, the number of unpaired electrons (the number of radicals) can be determined[16].

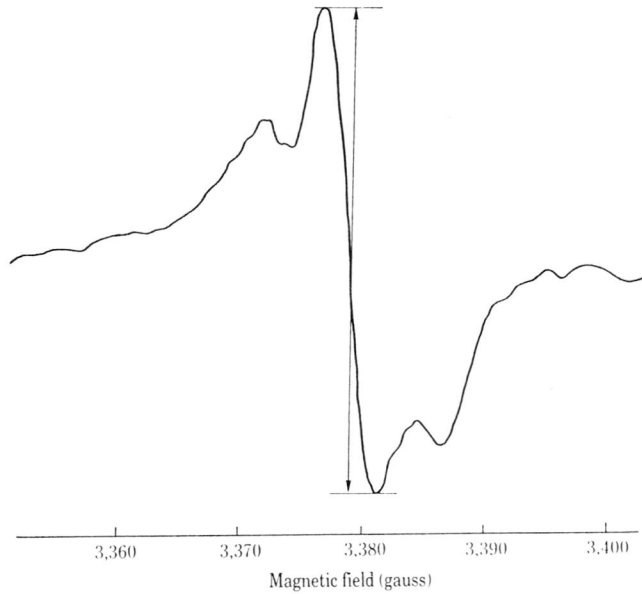

Figure 1   Typical ESR spectrum for tooth enamel from an atomic bomb survivor

1. SPECIMENS

By 1985 ESR measurements had been conducted on over 50 teeth from atomic bomb survivors and radiologic technologists, with confirmation that this method of dose estimation is accurate enough for practical adoption[2-8]. Accordingly, in order to clarify the dose received by many more survivors, the Scientific Data Center for the Atomic Bomb Disaster, Nagasaki University School of Medicine, has since 1985 systematically collected teeth from atomic bomb survivors. Appeals were made for teeth (following extractions etc.) from the proximally exposed population (i.e. those exposed within 1.5 km of the hypocenter), established from a database of the list of holders of the Nagasaki atomic bomb survivors' health handbooks. First, in December 1985 a questionnaire asking individuals whether they would cooperate in donating teeth and undergoing dental examinations was sent to a total of 1,681 persons, consisting of all the 1,368 proximally exposed survivors, 148 exposed outdoors at a distance of 1.5–2.0 km, and 165 survivors in the Nishiyama district of Nagasaki. The questionnaire received a response rate of 64%, reflecting the high interest of the atomic bomb survivors. A population of those willing to donate teeth was established from the 806 survivors who replied that they would cooperate in this project[9-11]. Furthermore, in order to permit continuous monitoring of this population, the Faculty of Dentistry at Nagasaki University has since February 1986 performed a series of dental examinations on the subjects; however, the percentage receiving examinations has only been about 30%. When extraction was deemed necessary at the time of examination, the tooth was extracted in the Faculty of

Dentistry and the tooth used as a specimen. For reference purposes, the survivors were asked at the time of examination about exposure conditions, and blood specimens were taken. Tooth specimens are also accepted at any time by mail.

In the initial period, the request for tooth donations evoked a considerable response from atomic bomb survivors, and within 4 months 28 individuals had donated 64 teeth by mail. Following that (i.e. after June 1986) a large number of teeth were obtained following extractions performed at the time of dental examinations. It is believed that the systematic collection of good specimens will permit determinations of radiation dose for many survivors.

2. RESULTS OF ESR DOSE MEASUREMENTS USING THE TEETH OF ATOMIC BOMB SURVIVORS

The results of dose evaluations for 40 survivors who provided teeth in good condition and for whom ESR measurements were possible are shown in Fig. 2. The

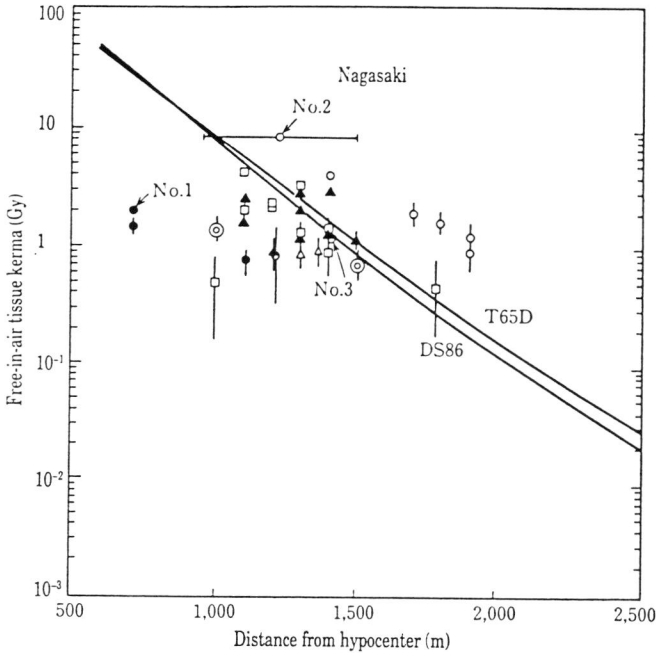

Figure 2 Comparison of ESR-determined doses for Nagasaki atomic bomb survivors with calculated T65D and DS86 free-in-air tissue kermas

The solid lines represent calculated values; other symbols indicate shielding conditions: ○ = no shielding, ◎ = shielding by trees or brick wall, □ = inside wooden structure, △ = inside munitions factory with roofs of slates supported by iron frames etc., ● = inside reinforced concrete structure. The specimen for which there was a large margin of error in the distance (specimen No. 2) was obtained from an individual who died within a week of the explosion from acute radiation illness, thus rendering ascertainment of the precise point of exposure impossible.

solid lines in the diagram indicate the calculated doses (the free-in-air tissue kerma determined by the T65D[12] and DS86[13] systems of dosimetry). Also, the number of subjects concerned and the doses determined by ESR are shown for no shielding (8 cases, indicated by single circles), shielding by trees or brick walls (3 cases, indicated by double circles), exposure inside a wooden Japanese-style house (10 cases, squares), inside munitions factories with galvanized sheet iron roofing or roofs with slates supported by iron frames (13 cases, triangles), and inside reinforced concrete structures (3 cases, solid dots). Three cases for whom individual conditions at exposure are well known have been assigned a number in the diagram.

Individual #1 was exposed in the former Nagasaki Medical University Hospital. The acute effects suffered by this individual were slight diarrhea and leukopenia, but the subject is now in good health. As shown in Fig. 3, when exposure occurs in a reinforced concrete structure, the walls and roof etc. act as a shield. However, it is believed difficult to estimate the thickness of the concrete through which the radiation passed, and furthermore, besides the direct gamma rays there was also

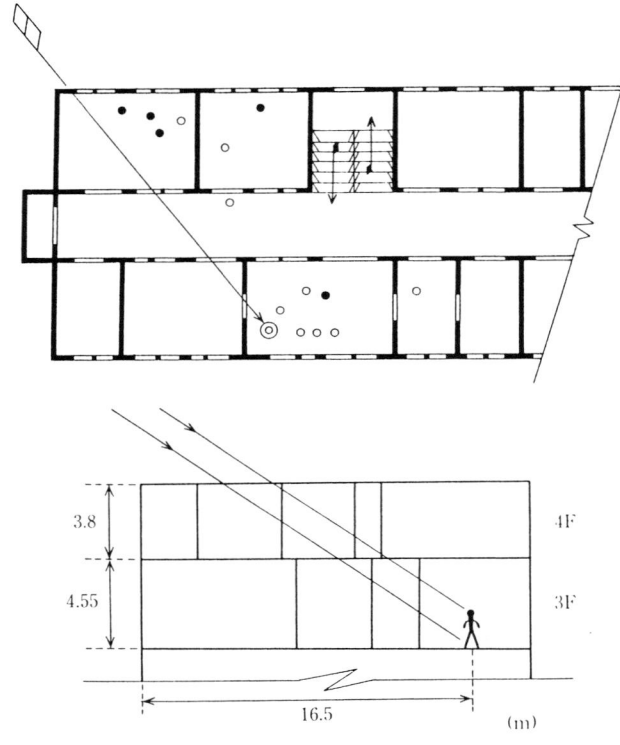

Dimensions in meters

Figure 3 Exposure status of the individual from whom teeth and shell buttons were collected
Individual No. 1 (indicated by ⊚) was exposed on the 3rd floor of the former Nagasaki Medical University Hospital, a reinforced concrete structure located 691 meters from the hypocenter, at which the DS86 free-in-air gamma ray dose was 32·8 Gy. The solid dots indicate individuals who died immediately after exposure[3,4].

scattered radiation; these factors rendered dose estimation difficult. The estimated DS86 free-in-air tissue dose of gamma radiation at a point 691 meters from the hypocenter was 32·80 Gy. The individual donated shell buttons from the clothing he was wearing at the time of the bombing and a tooth extracted 37 years after the explosion; the ESR-determined dose was 1·80 Gy.

Individual #2 was exposed in the former Mitsubishi Ohashi munitions factory and died 8 days later from acute effects. The distance from the hypocenter and shielding conditions are unknown. Since the site of the factory extended over a large area 950–1,500 m from the hypocenter, the estimated DS86 free-in-air tissue dose of gamma radiation covers the wide range from 9·83 Gy (at 950 m) to 0·89 Gy (at 1,500 m). After dying from the effects of the bombing, the individual was buried, making it possible to obtain the teeth and part of the surface of the femur; the ESR-determined dose was 7·80 Gy.

Individual #3 was exposed outdoors at a distance of 1,400 m (a brick wall was close, and the individual may have been shielded by it). Gingival bleeding occurred after 3–4 days. A tooth was donated 38 years after exposure. At this distance the estimated DS86 free-in-air tissue dose of gamma radiation was 1·35 Gy; the ESR-determined dose was 1·20 Gy.

Although not shown in the diagram, there are 2 cases of teeth measurements on survivors exposed in Hiroshima, one of these being a survivor whose exposure conditions are well known. The individual was exposed in a wooden one-story house at the eastern end of Bandai Bridge in Otemachi, 930 m from the hypocenter. Acute symptoms included epilation, anemia, gingival bleeding, and a reduced leukocyte count of under 400. A tooth extracted 39 years after exposure was received. At the point of exposure the DS86 estimated free-in-air tissue dose of gamma radiation was 5·33 Gy; the ESR-determined dose was 5·00 Gy.

As indicated in these examples, there is little discrepancy between the acute effects and doses estimated from teeth. Also, of the atomic bomb survivors who donated teeth, 4 in Nagasaki and 2 in Hiroshima were simultaneously tested for the frequency of chromosomal aberrations in peripheral blood (Fig. 4)[14]. The frequency of chromosomal anomalies increased with the ESR-estimated doses, with the latter in agreement with biological data.

A comparison of ESR-determined values according to shielding conditions reveals that the doses were inversely proportional to distance from the hypocenter. In particular, the curves for cases of no shielding and shielding by wood show a similar pattern of decrease, i.e. for each shielding material the rate of decrease with respect to distance was equal. Also, the ESR-determined doses decreased with increasing shielding effects e.g. a minimum for individuals exposed in reinforced concrete structures (which were believed to provide the most effective shielding). It is surmised that the wide variation in ESR-determined doses for individuals exposed in factories with galvanized sheet iron roofing or roofs with slate supported by iron frames is due to the fact that even at equal distances from the hypocenter there were cases where substantial shielding was afforded by machinery and manufacturing materials etc., thereby leading to different individual shielding conditions. The ESR-estimated doses for persons exposed while shielded by trees or brick walls was

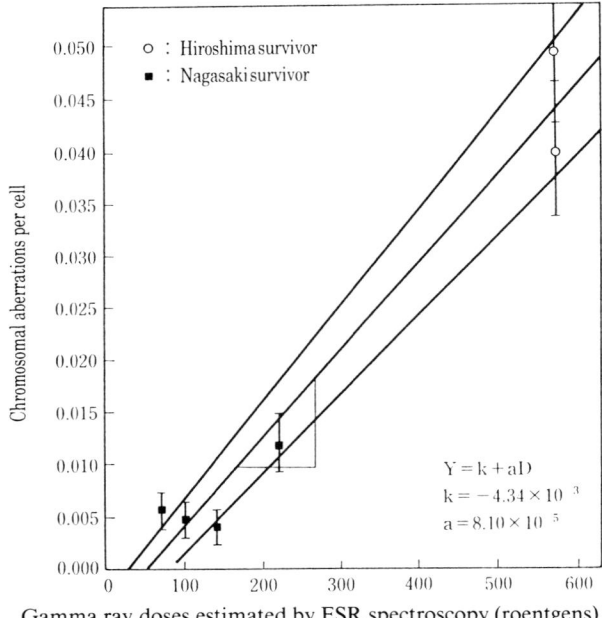

Gamma ray doses estimated by ESR spectroscopy (roentgens)

Figure 4   Chromosomal aberration frequency with respect to ESR-determined doses (for equivalent ^{60}Co gamma ray exposure). Analyses were performed on peripheral blood lymphocytes of 4 Nagasaki and 2 Hiroshima atomic bomb survivors. The solid lines were constructed using the least squares method[14].

10–28% of the value for the no-shielding condition. However, with one exception, all the ESR measurements for unshielded exposed persons were higher than the calculated values by a factor of 2 (for the proximally exposed) to 5 (for the distally exposed), the results thus being more striking with increased distance. One reason is that since the ESR sensitivity of tooth enamel is dependent on gamma and X-ray energy[6-9], it is necessary to correct for exposure to these forms of energy; however, at the present time changes in the atomic bomb gamma ray spectra due to distance and shielding have not yet been incorporated into the evaluations, and evaluations using ^{60}Co-gamma ray equivalents may influence ESR results.

3. ADVANTAGES AND PROBLEMS OF ESR DOSIMETRY

Dosimetry based on ESR teeth measurements is a completely new technique of individual dose determination involving direct measurement of specimens from living persons. In particular, it is useful for estimating the dose in a nuclear reactor accident when no dosimeter is carried and for estimating the cumulative dose received as a result of long-term occupational exposure (e.g. by radiologic technologists). It also has the advantage of allowing direct dose measurement even when the dose received by an atomic bomb survivor cannot be calculated due to complex shielding conditions. Furthermore, ESR differs from thermoluminescence dosimetry

(TLD) in that captured electrons cannot be released as a result of the absorption of only a little electromagnetic energy, thus permitting repeated measurements without a change in conditions. Also, since only inorganic materials such as roof tiles and bricks etc. can be measured in TLD, that technique suffers from the disadvantage that the determination of tissue dose received by survivors is performed indirectly. A further important characteristic of ESR dosimetry is that a direct relationship exists between the dose and the number of CO_3^{3-} radicals produced.

However, in many cases a long period of time elapsed between exposure to the atomic bomb and the teeth being extracted, and therefore the problem arises of the cumulative dose due to background radiation and X-ray radiography performed during dental examinations. The annual dose of background radiation is of the order of 0·001 Gy and does not pose a problem with the atomic bomb survivors, but although the energy in dental X-rays is low the number of radicals produced is 4–5 times as great. The dose received during one X-ray has been estimated at almost 0·005 Gy[15]; however, for teeth receiving multiple X-rays the number of radicals produced is thought to be large, and it is feared that individual doses are over estimated. More detailed studies of this problem are therefore required. It is necessary to estimate the effect of neutrons on radical formation when estimating the doses received by Hiroshima atomic bomb survivors. In an experiment involving neutron irradiation (4 Gy, 14 MeV), the author observed no increase in the number of CO_3^{3-} radicals; however, since the neutrons from the atomic bomb varied in energy from the level of thermal neutrons to 2 MeV, it is necessary in future to conduct studies on the rate of radical production by neutrons in this domain.

(*Junko Tatsumi-Miyajima*)

REFERENCES

1. Ikeya M, Miki T. Electron spin resonance dating of animal and human bones. *Science* 1980; **207**: 977.
2. Ikeya M, Miyajima J, Okajima S. Dose evaluation for atomic bomb survivors by ESR measurement. *J Atomic Energy Soc of Jpn* 1984; **26** (10): 878–9. (*In Japanese*)
3. Ikeya M, Miyajima J, Okajima S. ESR dosimetry for atomic bomb survivors using shell buttons and tooth enamel. *Jpn J Appl Phys* 1984; **23** (9): 697–9.
4. Miyajima J, Okajima S, Ikeya M. Atomic bomb radiation dose estimation by ESR measurement. *Nagasaki J Med* 1984; **59** (Suppl): 309–15. (*In Japanese*)
5. Tatsumi-Miyajima J, Okajima S. ESR dosimetry using human tooth enamel. In: Ikeya M, editor. ESR dating and dosimetry. Tokyo: Ionics, 1985: 397–405.
6. Tatsumi-Miyajima J, Zheng J, Shimasaki T, *et al.* Detail examination of ESR dosimetry for atomic bomb survivors. *J Hiroshima Med Ass* 1986; **39** (3): 418–22. (*In Japanese*)
7. Tatsumi-Miyajima J. ESR dosimetry for atomic bomb survivors and radiologic technologists. *Nucl Instr & Meth in Phys Res* 1987; **A257**: 417–22.
8. Tatsumi-Miyajima J, Okumura Y, Okajima S, *et al.* Dose estimation by electron spin resonance (ESR) from tooth enamel for radiologic technologists. *Nippon Acta Radiol* 1987; **47** (3): 527–30. (*English abstract*)
9. Tatsumi-Miyajima J, Okumura Y, Mine M, *et al.* Direct dose measurement by ESR (electron spin resonance) method. *Nagasaki J Med* 1986; **61** (Suppl): 459–66. (*In Japanese*)
10. Tatsumi-Miyajima J, Shimasaki T, Okumura Y, *et al.* Dose estimation for atomic bomb survivors using extracted teeth. 2. ESR dosimetry. *J Hiroshima Med Ass* 1988; **41** (3): 44–7. (*In Japanese*)

11. Mine M, Mori H, Kondo H, *et al.* Dose estimation for atomic bomb survivors using extracted teeth. 1. Collection of extracted teeth from exposed population by Nagasaki atomic bomb. *J Hiroshima Med Ass* 1988; **41** (3): 222–3. (*In Japanese*)

12. Auxier JA, Cheka JS, *et al.* Free-field radiation-dose distributions for the Hiroshima and Nagasaki bombings. *Health Phys* 1966; **12**: 425–9.

13. Kerr GD, Pace JV, Mendelsohn E, *et al.* Transport of initial radiations in air over ground. US-Japan joint reassessment of atomic bomb radiation dosimetry in Hiroshima and Nagasaki, final report. Vol. 1. Hiroshima: The Radiation Effect Research Foundation, 1987: 66–142.

14. Honda T, Sasaki M, Sadamori N, *et al.* Comparison of chromosome aberration frequencies with radiation dose estimated by electron spin resonance spectroscopy in A-bomb survivors. International Workshop on Reevaluation of Hiroshima and Nagasaki Cases by Chromosome Aberration Analysis for Dose Assessment and Risk Evaluation, Kyoto, Japan, Nov 28-Dec 3, 1985.

15. United Nations Scientific Committee on the Effects of Atomic Radiation, UNSCEAR. Ionizing radiation. Source and biological effects. 1982 report. New York: United Nations, 1982.

16. Kuwata K, Ito K. *Denshi supin kyoumei nyuumon* (Introduction to electron spin resonance spectroscopy). Tokyo: Nankoudou, 1980: 98–99. (*In Japanese*)

INDEX

Figures are indicated by 'f' after a page reference and tables by 't'.